Left Main Coronary Revascularization

Bernardo Cortese

Editor

Left Main Coronary Revascularization

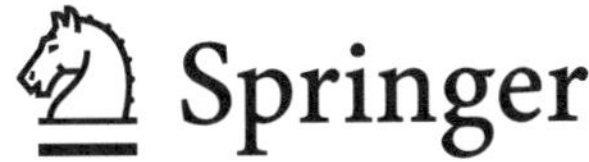 Springer

Editor
Bernardo Cortese
Fondazione Ricerca e Innovazione Cardiovascolare
MILANO, Milano, Italy

ISBN 978-3-031-05267-5   ISBN 978-3-031-05265-1   (eBook)
https://doi.org/10.1007/978-3-031-05265-1

This Springer imprint is published by the registered company Springer Nature Switzerland AG
The registered company address is: Gewerbestrasse 11, 6330 Cham, Switzerland

To Luigi and Guglielmo, my Sons
who inspire my life,
give me fuel,
give me heart,
and are the best gift God could give me.

Foreword

Although the first percutaneous treatment of unprotected left main coronary artery (ULMA) using balloon angioplasty dates back to the early Andreas Gruentzig days, this practice was promptly stopped due to initial disappointing results showing substantial procedural mortality, high restenosis rates, and poor long-term survival. The concomitant publication of randomized studies demonstrating higher survival rates in surgically treated patients with ULMA as compared to those treated medically proclaimed coronary artery surgery as the gold standard procedure for treatment of this insidious form of coronary artery disease. In the 1990s however percutaneous treatment of ULMA gained renewed momentum, fueled by the advent of coronary stents that reduced restenosis rates and by the use of dual antiplatelet therapy that decreased thrombotic complications. Since then, despite the publication of randomized trials comparing the two modalities of coronary revascularization and the thoughtful recommendations of international guidelines, this topic is still a subject of controversy and even of harsh confrontation between radical advocates of either interventional procedure. Two recent trials, NOBLE and EXCEL, rather than dissipate doubts, added fuel to the fire and sparked further discussion and opposing views. A recently published patient-level meta-analysis of four randomized trials with 5-year follow-up did not apparently cool off tempers.

Against this background the present book edited by Bernardo Cortese is an appropriate and timely initiative. It contains a series of chapters written by renowned experts in the field focusing on all aspects of the clinical decision making and analyzing technical details, also providing clues to operators to tackle practical difficulties. Although the Editor is a skillful interventional cardiologist, the book is well balanced, leaving equal room to PCI and surgical advocates in discussing respective advantages and limitations of the procedures. Both positions agree that Heart Team assessment taking into considerations clinical and anatomic findings has a crucial role in recommending the best treatment modality for patients with ULMA.

Five chapters in the book are devoted to intravascular imaging by both intravascular ultrasound and optical coherence tomography, in preoperative and postoperative assessment of patients treated with PCI. Intravascular ultrasound use has been shown to provide a clinical benefit particularly for distal left main treatment and is now endorsed by European Society of Cardiology guidelines. Recent data show that optical coherence tomography gives similar results and may even be superior to intravascular ultrasound thanks to a more detailed evaluation of stent apposition and final expansion. This is an area of current active research, whose recent achievements are presented and thoroughly discussed.

The book is a must-read for clinical and interventional cardiologists, but also for non-cardiologist members of the Heart Team who are facing in their practice the challenge of recommending or performing interventional procedures in these high-risk patients.

Department of Molecular Medicine   Stefano De Servi
University of Pavia
Pavia, Italy

Preface

hey guys, being a good interventional cardiologist
is not only a matter of how can I accommodate a stent there!
DEB School, since 2013

Since the birth of coronary revascularization techniques, left main stem has always been the most complex, risky, and intriguing lesion setting. I mean the Pattern of coronary revascularization.

Today, left main revascularization still represents the milestone of any technique, mainly for two reasons: (1) prognostically, its treatment is associated with the strongest, hardest outcome a patient with cardiovascular disease may incur, and (2) it is often complex to treat coronary lesions located there.

Moreover, left main treatment is a growing field of technical and scientific attention, given the high calcific burden, the frequent need for bifurcation lesion treatment, and the increased risk of further revascularizations. Recently, several studies have analyzed which technique (coronary artery bypass grafting or percutaneous coronary intervention) is associated with improved long-term outcome, the role of intravascular imaging (1) and the type of optimal technique for bifurcation management (2), in order to achieve a persistent result for years.

However, the main controversy here remains on who should be the gate keeper for left main revascularization: cardiac surgeon or interventional cardiologist? Long-term data of the Excel trial have generated so much controversies and a clear winner is not there yet (3).

In this book some among the most reliable experts on the matter will give their point of view according to the latest scientific developments.

Personally, I have several questions on the matter which will be hopefully answered:

- Why penetration of intravascular imaging is not 100% here?
- Is there a role for drug-coated balloons, to spare the total amount of metal in such a complex lesion setting?
- After left main revascularization with any technique, is short-to-mid-term invasive follow-up mandatory, to catch up eventual initial signs of restenosis, especially in case of percutaneous revascularization?
- Does a left internal mammary bypass to distal LAD make sense, if on top of left main disease the patient also has proximal or mid-LAD severe narrowings?
- In the setting of left main and 3-vessel coronary artery disease, does hybrid revascularization therapies, with mini-invasive CABG, small amount of

stents, and drug-coated balloons make sense, as an alternative to complex CABG or diffuse coronary paving?

Dear Reader, you may understand that the goal of this book is dual: to update you on the most recent developments in this field thanks to the inputs by some of the most eminent experts, and specifically, to understand that this setting is the most complex you will ever face.

So when you face a complex left main lesion, please stop, understand, think, plan, and go.

References

(1) Cortese B, de la Torre Hernandez JM, Lanocha M, Ielasi A, Giannini F, et al. Optical coherence tomography, intravascular ultrasound or angiography guidance for distal left main coronary stenting. The ROCK cohort II study. Catheter Cardiovasc Interv. 2021. doi: 10.1002/ccd.29959.

(2) Hildick-Smith D, Egred M, Banning A, Brunel P, Ferenc M, et al. The European bifurcation club Left Main Coronary Stent study: a randomized comparison of step-wise provisional vs. systematic dual stenting strategies (EBCMAIN). Eur Heart J. 2021;42(37):3829-3839.

(3) Stone GW, Kappetein AP, Sabik JF, Pocock SJ, Morice MC et al. Five-Year Outcomes after PCI or CABG for Left Main Coronary Disease. N Engl J Med. 2019;381(19):1820-1830.

Milano, Italy   Bernardo Cortese

Contents

History of Left Main Revascularization

Amr S. Gamal and Patrick S. Serruys

1.1 Introduction

Significant left main coronary artery (LMCA) stenosis is not uncommon, occurring in 5–10% of patients undergoing diagnostic coronary angiography [1]. LMCA is the main coronary artery supplying the left ventricle (LV); 84% of blood flow to the LV in a right dominant system and 100% of blood flow to the LV in a left dominant system [2, 3]. Due to the large area of jeopardized myocardium, patients with untreated severe stenosis of LMCA are at high risk of cardiovascular events.

1.2 The History of Left Main Stenosis

In 1921, James Herrick was the first to describe acute myocardial infarction in a 55-year-old male who died of cardiogenic shock. Autopsy revealed extensive necrosis of the left ventricle caused by LMCA occlusion by a thrombus overlying an area of atherosclerotic stenosis [4]. Since then, LMCA stenosis has been regarded as the most relevant prognostic disease of coronary arteries.

Medical management of obstructive LMCA stenosis has been reported to be associated with a three-year mortality rate of 50% which means that revascularization of significant LMCA stenosis is highly indicated [5, 6]. Historically, coronary artery bypass grafting (CABG) has been considered the gold standard treatment for LMCA disease. Multiple studies in the 1980s and 1990s of the past century have concluded a significant mortality benefit following treatment of LMCA disease with CABG compared to medical management [7–10]. At that stage, PCI was not advisable as a treatment option for such a high-risk patient cohort. However, recent advancements in percutaneous coronary interventions (PCI), stent technology, adjunctive pharmacotherapy, and use of intravascular imaging have all promoted many studies to evaluate the safety and efficacy of PCI in LMCA. This has resulted in a change in practice guidelines with recent studies showing comparable outcomes of PCI to CABG in LMCA [11–15].

Herewith, we will discuss the historical background and early experience of management of LMCA stenosis.

A. S. Gamal
Department of Cardiology, National University of Ireland, Galway (NUIG), Galway, Ireland

Consultant Interventional Cardiologist, Blackpool Victoria Hospital, England, UK

P. S. Serruys (✉)
Department of Cardiology, National University of Ireland, Galway (NUIG), Galway, Ireland

1.3 Overview of Early Trials in the Medical Management Era of LMCA Stenosis

Bruschke et al. evaluated the progress of 590 patients with documented coronary artery disease who were managed medically. Patients were followed up for 5–9 years post diagnostic coronary angiography. The 5-year mortality rates were 34.4% for the entire studied population and 56.8% for subgroup patients with ≥50% LMCA stenosis (37 patients) [16].

In 1975, Cohen et al. published the first follow-up data for 73 patients with narrowing of LMCA treated by either CABG (56 patients) or medical treatment (17 patients). Only 57% of medically treated patients were still alive at 18 months of follow-up [6].

In the same year, Talano et al. studied the prognosis of 145 patients medically treated with obstructive LMCA stenosis. Of these 145 patients, 32 patients were considered potential CABG candidates but they didn't have surgery. At 2 years, the survival rate for these 32 medically treated patients was 61% [17].

Another large series assessing the long-term prognosis of 141 medically treated patients with left main stenosis was reported by Lim et al. [18] The five-year mortality post diagnosis was 51%. The mortality rates were particularly high during the first 3 years post coronary angiography; 21.9%, 34.7%, and 43% at one, 2 and 3 years respectively.

In 1982, Takaro et al. described the 30 months follow-up for patients with significant LMCA stenosis who were recruited in the randomized Veterans Administration (VA) study; 53 of 113 patients were treated medically. The survival for the medically treated patients was only 65% at 2.5 years [9].

From November 1969 to June 1977, 3498 patients underwent cardiac catheterization at Duke University Medical Center and the Durham Veterans Administration Hospital. A total of 345 patients (9%) were found to have ≥50% luminal stenosis of LMCA; 163 patients with LMCA stenosis received medical management and were further stratified into ≥70% and 50–70% stenosis subgroups. The one- and three-year survival rates for medically managed patients with more than 50% LMCA stenosis were 79% and 50%, respectively. The survival rates were significantly higher for patients with 50 to 70% stenosis (one and three-year survivals of 91% and 66%) than for those with ≥70% stenosis (one and three-year survivals of 72% and 41%) [P < 0.05]. Besides, in patients with LMCA and three-vessel disease, LMCA stenosis <70% was not associated with an increased risk of mortality [19].

1.4 Overview of Early Trials of Supporting CABG Superiority in LMCA Stenosis

Oberman et al. retrospectively reviewed the survival data for patients diagnosed with significant LMCA stenosis at the University of Alabama Medical Centre from 1966 to 1975. A total of 179 patients were identified; 141 patients received CABG, 24 patients were treated medically but they could have been considered for surgical bypass (potentially surgical candidates) and 14 patients were treated medically but were unsuitable for bypass operation (non-surgical candidates). At 12 months, the survival rates were 89% in the surgical group, 73% in the medically treated group who were potentially surgical candidates, and 70% in the medically treated group who were inoperable. At 24 months, 86%, 65%, and 54% of each of the surgical group, surgical candidates, and non-surgical candidates respectively were still alive [20].

In 1977, a long-term follow-up for patients from the VA study of coronary artery bypass surgery was published. VA study was a randomized trial that assessed the efficacy of CABG versus medical treatment in 1015 patients with angina who were recruited from 1970 till 1974. Patients were further subdivided into high- and low-risk subgroups, with and without significant stenosis of LMCA. Four-year cumulative mortality rates for all patients showed that the presence of significant LMCA disease is the strongest predictor of survival benefit after CABG. In the subgroup of patients with LMCA disease, the four-year mortality was 7% with CABG and 36% with medical management (P < 0.005). When LMCA was excluded, the four-year mortality rates were not different in surgically and medically treated patients (15% and 14% respectively) [21].

CAMPEAU et al. performed a retrospective follow-up study for 301 patients who were diagnosed with isolated LMCA stenosis from January 1968 to December 1976. Out of these patients, 114 were treated medically and 197 were treated by CABG. The survival rates of operated patients were significantly higher than the unoperated (77.5% in the operated versus 48.5% in the unoperated cohort after 7 years). Differences in survival between the operated and unoperated groups remained significant in patients with LMCA stenosis < 70% or 70%. Similarly, survival was significantly improved in operated patients with associated significant stenosis of < 2 or ≥2 other coronary arteries. However, operated patients did not show significant survival benefit when there was no associated significant right coronary artery stenosis (> 70%) [22].

In another series, all patients who had coronary angiogram at the Peter Bent Brigham Hospital from 1970 till 1977 were reviewed. A total of 135 patients had a significant LMCA obstruction, defined as ≥ 50% of the luminal diameter measured in 2 planes. Patients were followed for an average of 36 months (minimum 12 months, maximum 90 months). Overall operative mortality 6.4% (9/141 patients); 10% in unstable group and 4% in stable group. The total late mortality rate was 3.5% (5/141 patients); 2 late deaths in unstable patients and 3 late deaths in stable patients. Actuarial survival rates were better in stable than unstable patients, in patients who were completely rather than incompletely revascularized, and in patients with isolated LMCA stenosis [23].

The Prospective Randomized Study of Coronary Artery Bypass Surgery in stable angina recruited 768 men aged under 65 from 1973 to 1976. All patients had mild to moderate angina pectoris with at least two-vessel disease and good left ventricular function. A total of 373 patients were assigned to medical treatment and 395 patients to surgical bypass. In contrast to VA study, patients with left ventricular dysfunction, single-vessel disease, and higher age were excluded. All patients were followed up for 3 years, 60% for 4 years, and 25% for 5 years. At 60 months follow-up, survival rates were significantly better with CABG compared to medical treatment (93.5% Vs 84.1% respectively; $P < 0.001$). In particular, LMCA ($p = 0.037$) and three-vessel disease subgroups ($P < 0.001$) had significant survival benefit with CABG [24] om the V.A. The Collaborative Study of Coronary Artery Surgery (CASS) study was an observational study that evaluated the cumulative survival rate in 1492 patients with left main coronary artery disease, defined as ≥50% of luminal diameter who received either CABG or medical management. The prognosis of patients with ≥50 LMCA stenosis was significantly better with CABG ($p < 0.001$). The 3-year survival rate was 91% and 69% and the 4-year survival rate was 88% and 63% in the surgical and medical treatment groups respectively [8].

1.5 Historical Background and Early Experience of LMCA PCI

In 1964, Dotter and Judkins invented the novel technique of transluminal angioplasty to treat atherosclerotic obstruction of the femoral arteries [25]. The original technic of Dotter and Judkins was further modified by Andreas Gruntzig with the introduction of the double-lumen dilatation catheter which had been used for the percutaneous dilatation of stenosis of femoropopliteal and iliac arteries since 1974 and coronary arteries since 1976 [26]. The first left main PCI was performed by Andreas Gruntzig in 1978 using the novel balloon dilatation technique. In his initial experience, Gruntzig performed balloon dilatation in 50 patients including 2 patients with LMCA stenosis over a period of 18 months (September 1977 to January 1979). The balloon dilation technique, similar to plain old balloon angioplasty (POBA), was successful in 32 patients. The mean left main stenosis improved from 84% to 34% ($p < 0.001$) and coronary pressure gradient decreased from a mean of 58 mmHg to 19 mmHg ($p < 0.001$). Out of 2 LMCA stenosis patients treated, one patient, 45-year-old man, died unexpectedly 2 months after the procedure. This patient had extensive hypertrophy of the medial muscle layer of the left main stem which was underestimated at the time of angiogram leading to incomplete vessel dilatation. However, autopsy showed no occlusion or dissection of LMCA with no evidence of infarction. Although the cause of death was reported as being not clear, Gruntzig felt that failure to dilate LMCA stenosis could have contributed to the patient's death 2 months later [27].

Angioplasty using POBA alone was associated with a number of mechanical complications including acute and subacute vessel closure, elastic recoil, late vascular remodeling, and re-narrowing of coronary arteries. These complications were mitigated by the development of coronary stents and their progressive refinement from bare-metal stents (BMS) to drug-eluting stents (DES). These newer stents addressed the shortcomings of BMS, specifically in-stent restenosis. Furthermore, the development of novel anti-platelet medications has led to significant reductions in the incidence of major adverse cardiac events (MACE). The possible occurrence of abrupt vessel closure or restenosis put patients with LMCA stenosis undergoing PCI with POBA at risk of severe perioperative complications including sudden death. The use of BMS in LMCA PCI remarkably lowered the incidence of abrupt vessel closure and the advent of DES decreased the risk of LMCA in-stent restenosis [28–31].

For more than 2 decades after the emergence of coronary angioplasty, patients with LMCA stenosis were excluded from all randomized trials comparing CABG Vs PCI as CABG continued to be the standard treatment option for these groups of patients at that time [32–35]. A number of observational studies and registries reported promising results with PCI for unprotected LMCA stenosis using BMS [36–41] and both BMS and DES [28–31, 42, 43].

1.6 Overview of Randomized Trials of LMCA PCI Using First Degeneration DES with/ without BMS

LE MANS (Left Main Coronary Artery Stenting) trial was the first prospective randomized trial comparing percutaneous vs surgical revascularization for LMCA. The trial randomized 105 patients with LMCA stenosis with or without multivessel coronary artery disease to either PCI ($n = 52$ patients) or CABG ($n = 53$ patients). PCI for LMCA disease was performed using DES if reference diameter was <3.8 mm or BMS if reference diameter was ≥3.8 mm. Left ventricular ejection fraction (LVEF) 12 months after the procedure significantly improved with PC compared with CABG (3.3 ± 6.7%; 95% CI 1.3 to 5.3 vs. 0.5 ± 0.8%; 95% CI 1.4 to 2.5; $p = 0.047$). Besides, PCI resulted in significantly lower rates of major adverse events (MAE) [8% vs. 28%; 95% CI 0.64 to 0.94; RR 0.78; $p = 0.006$] and MACCE [2% vs. 13%; 95% CI 0.79 to 0.99, RR 0.88; $p = 0.03$] and shorter hospitalizations (6.8 ± 3.7 days vs. 12.0 ± 9.6 days; $p = 0.0007$) compared to CABG [44].

In PRECOMBAT (Premier of Randomized Comparison of Bypass Surgery Versus Angioplasty Using Sirolimus-Eluting Stent in Patients With Left Main Coronary Artery Disease) trial, out of a total of 1454 patients with unprotected LMCA stenosis from 2004 to 2009, 600 patients were randomly assigned to either CABG (300 patients) or PCI with PCI with sirolimus-eluting stents (300 patients). PCI was noninferior to CABG in terms of major adverse cardiac or cerebrovascular events (MACCE) (death from any cause, myocardial infarction, stroke, or ischemia-driven target-vessel revascularization) at 1 and 2 years of follow-up. However, target vessel revascularization was significantly lower in the CABG group at 2 years. On 5 years follow-up, the same results were reproduced which again confirmed the non-inferiority of PCI in LMCA stenosis patients [45, 46].

SYNTAX (Synergy Between PCI With Taxus and Cardiac Surgery) trial randomly assigned 1800 patients with de-novo LMCA or three-vessel disease to undergo either CABG ($n = 897$ patients) or PCI with paclitaxel-eluting stents ($n = 903$ patients) after equivalent anatomical revascularization by either strategy was agreed by both interventional cardiologist and local cardiac surgeon. LMCA disease with or without diseased other vessels was present in 38.8% of the patients in the CABG group and 39.5% of the patients in the PCI group. In a sub-study of patients with LMCA disease, 12-month rates of MACCE didn't differ significantly between

CABG and PCI arms (13.7% and 15.8%, respectively; $P = 0.44$). However, repeat revascularization was significantly higher in LMCA patients treated with PCI (11.8%) versus CABG (6.5%), $P = 0.02$. On the other hand, rates of stroke were significantly higher in the CABG group (2.7%), compared to PCI (0.3%), $P = 0.01$ [13].

Five years follow-up of left main subgroup of SYNTAX trial has confirmed the findings of one-year follow-up. MACCE rates continued to be similar between the two treatment groups (31.0% in the CABG vs 36.9% in the PCI; $p = 0.12$). When patients with LMCA disease were sub-stratified by SYNTAX score, MACCE rates were significantly different between LMCA subgroups with high SYNTAX scores but not in subgroups with low or intermediate SYNTAX scores when compared to CABG. This proved that PCI could be an acceptable alternative to CABG for less complex LMCA patients [47].

References

1. Giannoglou GD, Antoniadis AP, Chatzizisis YS, et al. Prevalence of narrowing >or=50% of the left main coronary artery among 17,300 patients having coronary angiography. Am J Cardiol. 2006;98:1202–5.
2. Sianos G, Morel MA, Kappetein AP, Morice MC, et al. The SYNTAX score: an angiographic tool grading the complexity of coronary artery disease. EuroIntervention. 2005;1:219–27.
3. Leaman DM, Brower RW, Meester GT, et al. Coronary artery atherosclerosis: severity of the disease, severity of angina pectoris and compromised left ventricular function. Circulation. 1981;63:285–99.
4. Herrick J. Clinical features of sudden obstruction of the coronary arteries. JAMA. 1912;59:2015.
5. Taylor H, Deumite N, Chaitman B, et al. Asymptomatic left main coronary artery disease in the coronary artery surgery study (CASS) registry. Circulation. 1989;79:1171–9.
6. Cohen M, Gorlin R. Main left coronary artery disease: clinical experience from 1964–1974. Circulation. 1975;52:275–85.
7. Yusuf S, Zucker D, Peduzzi P, et al. Effect of coronary artery bypass graft surgery on survival: overview of 10-year results from randomised trials by the coronary artery bypass graft surgery Trialists collaboration. Lancet. 1994;344:563–70.
8. Chaitman BR, Fisher LD, Bourassa MG, et al. Effect of coronary bypass surgery on survival patterns in subsets of patients with left main coronary artery disease. Report of the collaborative study in coronary artery surgery (CASS). Am J Cardiol. 1981;48:765–77.
9. Takaro T, Peduzzi P, Detre KM, et al. Survival in subgroups of patients with left main coronary artery disease. Veterans administration cooperative study of surgery for coronary arterial occlusive disease. Circulation. 1982;66:14–22.
10. Caracciolo EA, Davis KB, Sopko G, et al. Comparison of surgical and medical group survival in patients with left main equivalent coronary artery disease. Long-term CASS experience Circulation. 1995;91: 2335–44.
11. Park DW, Kim YH, Yun SC, et al. Complexity of atherosclerotic coronary artery disease and long-term outcomes in patients with unprotected left main disease treated with drug-eluting stents or coronary artery bypass grafting. J Am Coll Cardiol. 2011;57:2152–9.
12. Morice MC, Serruys PW, Kappetein AP, et al. Outcomes in patients with de novo left main disease treated with either percutaneous coronary intervention using paclitaxel-eluting stents or coronary artery bypass graft treatment in the synergy between percutaneous coronary intervention with TAXUS and cardiac surgery (SYNTAX) trial. Circulation. 2010;121:2645–53.
13. Serruys PW, Morice MC, Kappetein AP, et al. Percutaneous coronary intervention versus coronary-artery bypass grafting for severe coronary artery disease. N Engl J Med. 2009;360:961–72.
14. Ferrante G, Presbitero P, Valgimigli M, et al. Percutaneous coronary intervention versus bypass surgery for left main coronary artery disease: a meta-analysis of randomised trials. EuroIntervention. 2011;7:738–46.
15. Park SJ, Kim YH, Park DW, et al. Randomised trial of stents versus bypass surgery for left main coronary artery disease. N Engl J Med. 2011;364:1718–27.
16. Bruschke A, Proudfit W, Sones F. Progress study of 590 consecutive nonsurgical cases of coronary disease followed 5-9 years. Circulation. 1973;47:1147–53.
17. Talano J, Scanlon P, Meadows W, et al. Influence of surgery on survival in 145 patients with left main coronary artery disease. Circulation 51 and. 1975;52(suppl I):1–105.
18. Lim J, Proudfit W, Sones F. Left main coronary arterial obstruction: long-term follow-up of I 4I nonsurgical cases. Am J Cardiol. 1975;36:131.
19. Conley M, Ely R, Kisslo J, et al. The prognostic spectrum of left main stenosis. Circulation. 1978 May;57(5):947–52.
20. Oberman A, Kouchoukos N, Harrell R, et al. Surgical versus medical treatment in disease of the left main coronary artery. Lancet. 1976;2:591–3.
21. Detre K, Murphy ML, Huitgren H. Effect of coronary bypass surgery on longevity in high and low risk patients. Lancet. 1977;2:1243–5.
22. Campeau L, Corbara F, Crochet D, Petitclerc R. Left main coronary artery stenosis: the influence of aortocoronary bypass surgery on survival. Circulation. 1978;57:1111–5.
23. Cohn LH, Kosier JK, Mee RB, Collins JJ Jr. Surgical management of stenosis of the left main coronary artery. World J Surg. 1978;2:701–7.

24. European Coronary Surgery Study Group. Prospective randomized study of coronary artery bypass surgery in stable angina pectoris. Lancet. 1980;2:491–5.
25. Dotters C, Judkins M. Transluminal treatment of arteriosclerotic obstruction. Description of a new technic and a preliminary report of its application. Circulation. 1964;30:654–70.
26. Grüntzig A. Idem: Die perkutane transluminale Rekanalisation chronischer Arterienverschluesse mit einer neuen Dilatationstechnik. Baden-Baden: G Witzsrock Verlag; 1977.
27. Grüntzig A, Senning A, Siegenthaler W. Nonoperative dilatation of coronary-artery stenosis — percutaneous transluminal coronary angioplasty. N Engl J Med. 1979;301:61–8.
28. Chieffo A, Colombo A. Treatment of unprotected left main coronary artery disease with drug-eluting stents: is it time for a randomized trial? Nat Clin Pract Cardiovasc Med. 2005;2:396–400.
29. Chieffo A, Stankovic G, Bonizzoni E, et al. Early and mid-term results of drug-eluting stent implantation in unprotected left main. Circulation. 2005;111:791–5.
30. Park SJ, Kim YH, Lee BK, et al. Sirolimus-eluting stent implantation for unprotected left main coronary artery stenosis: comparison with bare metal stent implantation. J Am Coll Cardiol. 2005;45:351–6.
31. Valgimigli M, van Mieghem CA, Ong AT, et al. Short- and long-term clinical outcome after drug-eluting stent implantation for the percutaneous treatment of left main coronary artery disease: insights from the rapamycin-eluting and Taxus stent evaluated at Rotterdam cardiology hospital registries (RESEARCH and T-SEARCH). Circulation. 2005;111:1383–9.
32. Hamm C, Reimers J, Ischinger T, et al. A randomized study of coronary angioplasty compared with bypass surgery in patients with symptomatic multivessel coronary disease. N Engl J Med. 1994;331:1037–43.
33. CABRI Trial Participants. First-year results of CABRI (coronary angioplasty versus bypass revascularisation investigation). Lancet. 1995;346:1179–84.
34. King S III, Lembo N, Weintraub W, et al. Comparison of coronary bypass surgery with angioplasty in patients with multivessel disease. N Engl J Med. 1996;335:217–25.
35. Bypass Angioplasty Revascularization Investigation (BARI) Investigators. Comparison of coronary bypass surgery with angioplasty in patients with multivessel disease. N Engl J Med. 1996;335(4):217–25.
36. Silvestri M, Barragan P, Sainsous J, et al. Unprotected left main coronary artery stenting: immediate and medium-term outcomes of 140 elective procedures. J Am Coll Cardiol. 2000;35:1543–50.
37. Park SJ, Lee CW, Kim YH, et al. Technical feasibility, safety, and clinical outcome of stenting of unprotected left main coronary artery bifurcation narrowing. Am J Cardiol. 2002;90:374–8.
38. Park SJ, Hong MK, Lee CW, et al. Elective stenting of unprotected left main coronary artery stenosis: effect of debulking before stenting and intravascular ultrasound guidance. J Am Coll Cardiol. 2001;38:1054–60.
39. Park SJ, Park SW, Hong MK, et al. Stenting of unprotected left main coronary artery stenoses: immediate and late outcomes. J Am Coll Cardiol. 1998;31:37–42.
40. Park SJ, Park SW, Hong MK, et al. Long-term (three-year) outcomes after stenting of unprotected left main coronary artery stenosis in patients with normal left ventricular function. Am J Cardiol. 2003;91:12–6.
41. Black A, Cortina R, Bossi I, et al. Unprotected left main coronary artery stenting: correlates of midterm survival and impact of patient selection. J Am Coll Cardiol. 2001;37:832–8.
42. Tan WA, Tamai H, Park SJ, et al. Long-term clinical outcomes after unprotected left main trunk percutaneous revascularization in 279 patients. Circulation. 2001;104:1609–14.
43. Takagi T, Stankovic G, Finci L, et al. Results and long-term predictors of adverse clinical events after elective percutaneous interventions on unprotected left main coronary artery. Circulation. 2002;106:698–702.
44. Buszman P, Kiesz S, Bochenek A. Acute and late outcomes of unprotected left main stenting in comparison with surgical revascularization. J Am Coll Cardiol. 2008;51(5):538–45.
45. Park SJ, Kim YH, Park DW, et al. Randomized trial of stents versus bypass surgery for left main coronary artery disease. N Engl J Med. 2011;364(18):1718–27.
46. Ahn JM, Roh JH, Kim YH, et al. Randomized trial of stents versus bypass surgery for left Main coronary artery disease: 5-year outcomes of the PRECOMBAT study. J Am Coll Cardiol. 2015;65(20):2198–206.
47. Mohr FW, Morice MC, Kappetein AP, et al. Coronary artery bypass graft surgery versus percutaneous coronary intervention in patients with three-vessel disease and left main coronary disease: 5-year follow-up of the randomised, clinical SYNTAX trial. Lancet. 2013;381(9867):629–38.

Historical Background of Left Main Stem Revascularization: A Step Further

Patrick W. Serruys, Masafumi Ono, Mattia Lunardi, Yoshinobu Onuma, and Scot Garg

2.1 Introduction of the Percutaneous Revascularization

In the early 1980s, there was really no debate as to the optimal treatment for patients with unprotected left main coronary disease (LMCAD). The CASS study reported clear prognostic benefits with CABG compared to medical therapy alone [2], and following a single case of sudden death (patient number 4, Fig. 2.1) 8 weeks after a successful percutaneous transluminal coronary angioplasty (PTCA) of an unprotected left main coronary artery lesion, this specific, but premature clinical application of the new-born technique was abandoned [1, 3]. In fact, the prognosis after PTCA of an unprotected LMCAD remained consistently very poor throughout the 1980s, with a case series in 1989 by O'Keefe et al. reporting 3-year survival rates after elective PTCA for unprotected and protected LMCAD, of 36% and 90%, respectively ($P < 0.0005$) [4]. The same authors also recommended surgeons remain on standby in case emergency CABG was required to salvage acute myocardial infarction induced by LMCAD. Therefore, entering into the twenty-first century CABG was appropriately the standard of care for the management of unprotected LMCAD, whereas percutaneous treatment was restricted and strongly discouraged (Class III in 2005 ACC/AHA/SCAI guidelines) until the advent of drug-eluting stents (DES) [5].

Fortunately, surgical therapy stagnated while all aspects of percutaneous coronary intervention (PCI) progressed exponentially. Balloon angioplasty was soon replaced by bare-metal stents and then drug-eluting stents (DES), the latter leading to marked improved outcomes through the reduction in restenosis [6]. The initial success of DES was however tempered by concerns about safety and stent thrombosis, which have been overcome with contemporary devices, the increased understanding about optimizing stent sizing and deployment with focus on plaque modification and the use of intra-coronary imaging and improvements in peri-procedural pharmacology [7]. All of these developments facilitated a more level playing

P. W. Serruys (✉)
Department of Cardiology, National University of Ireland, Galway (NUIG), Galway, Ireland

NHLI, Imperial College London, London, UK

M. Ono
Department of Cardiology, National University of Ireland, Galway (NUIG), Galway, Ireland

Department of Cardiology, Academic Medical Center, University of Amsterdam, Amsterdam, The Netherlands

M. Lunardi · Y. Onuma
Department of Cardiology, National University of Ireland, Galway (NUIG), Galway, Ireland

S. Garg
Department of Cardiology, Royal Blackburn Hospital, Blackburn, UK

© Springer Nature Switzerland AG 2022
B. Cortese (ed.), *Left Main Coronary Revascularization*,
https://doi.org/10.1007/978-3-031-05265-1_2

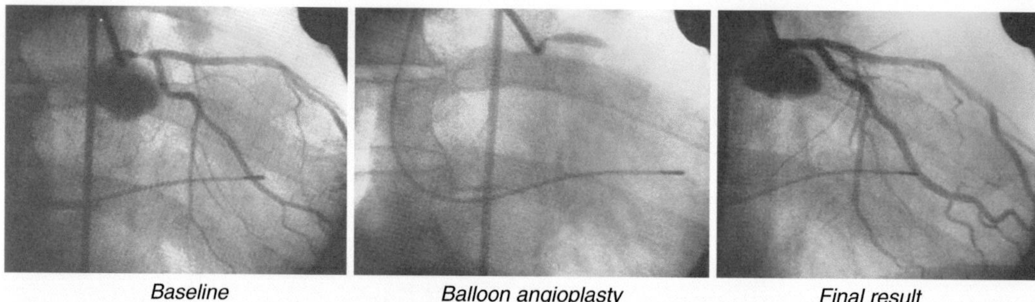

Fig. 2.1 Online Fig. 2.1. First percutaneous treatment of left main disease (patient number 4). Reprinted with the permission from Philippe Gaspard

field between percutaneous and surgical revascularization, enabling PCI to once again be considered in the management of unprotected LMCAD.

2.2 The First-Generation DES Versus CABG for Unprotected LMCAD: Were Interventional Cardiologists Overconfident?

In 2008, the LE MANS study [8] was the first to randomize patients with an unprotected LMCAD to CABG or PCI with stents (35% first-generation DES). The trial enrolled 105 patients (53 CABG and 52 PCI) and from the outset there were complaints from surgeons about the quality of surgery being performed, with less than three-quarters of the surgical cohort receiving a left internal mammary artery graft, despite its well-proven survival benefit [9]. The mechanistic primary endpoint was a change in ejection fraction (EF) and while this was unchanged between baseline and 12 months follow-up in the CABG cohort ($53.7 \pm 6.7\%$ versus $54.1 \pm 8.9\%$, $p = 0.85$), it increased significantly with PCI ($53.5 \pm 10.7\%$ to $58.0 \pm 6.8\%$, $p = 0.04$); the between-group difference at 12 months was also significant ($p = 0.01$) [10]. Very long-term follow-up at 10 years suggested a trend toward a higher EF with PCI ($54.9 \pm 8.3\%$ vs. $49.8 \pm 10.3\%$; $p = 0.07$); however, follow-up was incomplete ($N = 46$; 43.9%) [8]. Despite the criticism and the small sample size, it was interesting nevertheless to observe the absence of any significant between-group differ-

ence in rates of major adverse cardiac and cerebrovascular events (MACCE) at 3 and 10 years follow-up.

After the LE MANS study, large randomized trials including the SYNTAX, PRECOMBAT, NOBLE, and EXCEL trials were conducted to assess the efficacy of PCI with DES for unprotected LMCAD compared to CABG, which facilitated the change in position of PCI from "taboo" to a potential option, as reflected in current guidelines (Fig. 2.2).

The SYNTAX trial [11] was, and still is, a remarkable trial with a very long follow-up ($\geq$10 years in SYNTAXES: SYNTAX Extended Survival study) [12]. To try and reflect routine practice, and avoid the criticism directed at previous studies comparing PCI to CABG, which routinely excluded 88–98% of the screen population [13, 14], the study had minimal exclusion criteria. Moreover, to capture those patients not suitable for randomization, running parallel to the randomized group were two nested registries: a surgical one for patients where the extent and complexity of CAD was judged by the PCI operator to preclude a percutaneous approach, and a percutaneous one for patients whose comorbidities prohibited surgery [14].

In addition, the study mandated the use of the SYNTAX score, which was newly derived from an amalgam of existing angiographic scores, such as the Leaman score, with the aim that this would force the surgeons and interventional cardiologists to meticulously examine the extent and complexity of the patient's coronary disease, prior to their inclusion into the trial [15, 16].

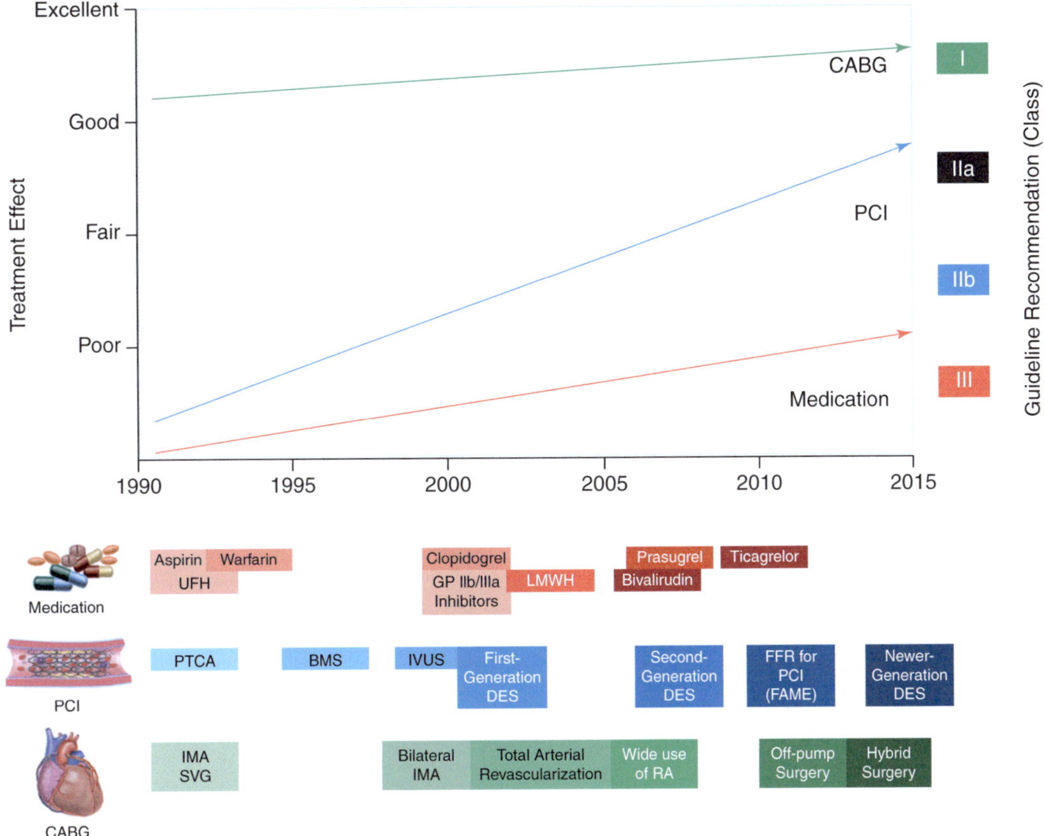

Fig. 2.2 Secular changes of treatment effect and guideline recommendations in relation to medical advances of each treatment stratum for left main coronary artery disease [5]

When the outcome of the trial was analyzed, the SYNTAX score transformed from a diagnostic tool to a prognostic one, helping identify those patients who had comparable safety when treated with PCI using first-generation TAXUS DES (Boston Scientific, Natick, MA) or CABG. In terms of patients with unprotected LMCAD this included all those with a SYNTAX score $\leq$ 32.

At a similar time, PRECOMBAT, which randomized 600 patients with unprotected LMCAD to either PCI with the first-generation Cypher (Cordis, J & J, Warren NJ) DES or CABG reported that PCI was non-inferior to CABG (PCI 8.7% vs. CABG 6.7%, $P_{non\text{-}inferiority}$ = 0.01) for the primary endpoint of MACCE, a composite of death, stroke, MI, and ischemia-driven target-vessel revascularization (TVR) [17]. Moreover, there were no between-group differences in MACCE at 5 years (PCI 17.5% vs.

CABG 14.3%; $P_{superiority}$ = 0.26) or at extended 10-year follow-up (29.8% vs. 24.7%; HR: 1.25; 95% CI: 0.93–1.69) [17].

The SYNTAX and PRECOMBAT trials opened a new avenue of revascularization options for unprotected LMCAD with favorable long-term results.

2.3 Tackling the Left Main Stem with the Second-Generation DES

The competitive role of PCI in unprotected LMCAD using first-generation DES drove the hunger for the EXCEL and NOBLE trials which were specifically designed to examine the outcomes in these patients randomized to CABG or PCI using second-generation DES [18, 19].

In the NOBLE trial, which randomized 1201 patients with unprotected LMCAD to CABG or PCI (11% first-generation DES, 89% biolimus-eluting stent), the primary endpoint, a composite of death, non-procedural MI (notably procedural MIs [PMIs] were not included), stroke, and repeat revascularization at 5 years occurred significantly more frequently with PCI than CABG (28% vs 19%; HR 1·58 [95% CI 1·24–2·01]) [19]. Moreover, while the similar rate of all-cause mortality at 5 years (PCI 9.4% vs. CABG 8.7%; HR: 1.08; 95% CI: 0.74–1.59) was re-assuring, the higher incidence of spontaneous MI was not (PCI 7.6% vs. CABG 2.7%; HR:2.99; 95% CI:1.66–5.39).

The EXCEL trial randomized 1900 patients with unprotected LMCAD and a SYNTAX score $\leq$ 32 [18], and demonstrated that PCI was non-inferior to CABG ($P_{\text{non-inferiority}}$ = 0.02 and $P_{\text{superiority}}$ = 0.98; HR:1.00; 95% CI:0.79–1.26) at 3 years for the composite primary endpoint of death, MI, and stroke. In the last 2 years of follow-up, the Kaplan-Meier curves for the composite endpoint crossed over and steadily diverged with a final hazard ratio at 5 years of 1.19 (95% CI: 0.95–1.50; $P_{\text{superiority}}$ = 0.13). While the rates of all-cause mortality favored surgery (13.0% vs. 9.9%; HR: 1.38; 95% CI: 1.03–1.85), the rate of cardiovascular death was similar.

The differing conclusions between the NOBEL and EXCEL trials are heavily dependent on the inclusion of PMI in the primary endpoint. Initially, the omission of PMI from their composite endpoint lead to heavy criticism of the NOBLE trialists; however, their decision has now been fully vindicated following the published debate and critical appraisal of PMIs and their definitions [20, 21]. Their clinical relevance, and impact on time-event curves and composite endpoints, is now more transparent than ever before [20, 21]. Contrast this with the EXCEL trial, where the higher initial in-hospital primary endpoint with CABG was driven by the EXCEL definition of PMI, which required an isolated enzyme release of CK-MB >10x upper limit of normal (ULN) without the necessity of other supporting evidence, whereas an elevation of CK-MB >5x ULN had to be accompanied by a new Q-wave.

References

1. Gruntzig A. Transluminal dilatation of coronary-artery stenosis. Lancet. 1978;1:263.
2. Chaitman BR, Fisher LD, Bourassa MG, et al. Effect of coronary bypass surgery on survival patterns in subsets of patients with left main coronary artery disease. Report of the collaborative study in coronary artery surgery (CASS). Am J Cardiol. 1981;48:765–77.
3. Grüntzig AR, Senning A, Siegenthaler WE. Nonoperative dilatation of coronary-artery stenosis: percutaneous transluminal coronary angioplasty. N Engl J Med. 1979;301:61–8.
4. O'Keefe JH Jr, Hartzler GO, Rutherford BD, et al. Left main coronary angioplasty: early and late results of 127 acute and elective procedures. Am J Cardiol. 1989;64:144–7.
5. Lee PH, Ahn JM, Chang M, et al. Left Main coronary artery disease: secular trends in patient characteristics, treatments, and outcomes. J Am Coll Cardiol. 2016;68:1233–46.
6. Morice MC, Serruys PW, Sousa JE, et al. A randomized comparison of a sirolimus-eluting stent with a standard stent for coronary revascularization. N Engl J Med. 2002;346:1773–80.
7. Serruys PW, Kogame N, Katagiri Y, et al. Clinical outcomes of state-of-the-art percutaneous coronary revascularisation in patients with three-vessel disease: two-year follow-up of the SYNTAX II study. EuroIntervention. 2019;15:e244–52.
8. Buszman PE, Buszman PP, Banasiewicz-Szkróbka I, et al. Left Main stenting in comparison with surgical revascularization: 10-year outcomes of the (left Main coronary artery stenting) LE MANS trial. JACC Cardiovasc Interv. 2016;9:318–27.
9. Meliga E, Valgimigli M, Buszman P, Serruys PW. Percutaneous coronary intervention or coronary artery bypass graft for unprotected left main coronary artery disease: the endless debate. J Am Coll Cardiol. 2008;52:582–4. author reply 584-6
10. Buszman PE, Buszman PP, Kiesz RS, et al. Early and long-term results of unprotected left main coronary artery stenting: the LE MANS (left Main coronary artery stenting) registry. J Am Coll Cardiol. 2009;54:1500–11.
11. Mohr FW, Morice MC, Kappetein AP, et al. Coronary artery bypass graft surgery versus percutaneous coronary intervention in patients with three-vessel disease and left main coronary disease: 5-year follow-up of the randomised, clinical SYNTAX trial. Lancet. 2013;381:629–38.
12. Thuijs D, Kappetein AP, Serruys PW, et al. Percutaneous coronary intervention versus coronary artery bypass grafting in patients with three-vessel or left main coronary artery disease: 10-year follow-up of the multicentre randomised controlled SYNTAX trial. Lancet. 2019;394:1325–34.
13. Hoffman SN, TenBrook JA, Wolf MP, Pauker SG, Salem DN, Wong JB. A meta-analysis of random-

ized controlled trials comparing coronary artery bypass graft with percutaneous transluminal coronary angioplasty: one- to eight-year outcomes. J Am Coll Cardiol. 2003;41:1293–304.

14. Serruys PW, Farooq V. Cherry-picking historical data to legitimize contemporary practice: should diabetic status influence decision-making in complex CAD? J Am Coll Cardiol. 2017;69:404–8.

15. Serruys PW, Onuma Y, Garg S, et al. Assessment of the SYNTAX score in the Syntax study. EuroIntervention. 2009;5:50–6.

16. Serruys PW, Chichareon P, Modolo R, et al. The SYNTAX score on its way out or … towards artificial intelligence: part I. EuroIntervention. 2020;16:44–59.

17. Park DW, Ahn JM, Park H, et al. Ten-year outcomes after drug-eluting stents versus coronary artery bypass grafting for left Main coronary disease: extended follow-up of the PRECOMBAT trial. Circulation. 2020;141:1437–46.

18. Stone GW, Kappetein AP, Sabik JF, et al. Five-year outcomes after PCI or CABG for left Main coronary disease. N Engl J Med. 2019;381:1820–30.

19. Holm NR, Mäkikallio T, Lindsay MM, et al. Percutaneous coronary angioplasty versus coronary artery bypass grafting in the treatment of unprotected left main stenosis: updated 5-year outcomes from the randomised, non-inferiority NOBLE trial. Lancet. 2020;395:191–9.

20. Hara H, Serruys PW, Takahashi K, et al. Impact of Peri-procedural myocardial infarction on outcomes after revascularization. J Am Coll Cardiol. 2020;76:1622–39.

21. Gregson J, Stone GW, Ben-Yehuda O, et al. Implications of alternative definitions of Peri-procedural myocardial infarction after coronary revascularization. J Am Coll Cardiol. 2020;76:1609–21.

Anatomical and Pathophysiological Considerations on the Left Main Coronary Artery

Luca Nai Fovino, Andrea Scotti, and Giuseppe Tarantini

3.1 Anatomy of the Left Main Coronary Artery

3.1.1 Normal Anatomy of the Left Main Coronary Artery

The definition "left main" refers to the initial segment of the left coronary artery. The left main is responsible for the blood supply of most of the left ventricle, but also of a considerable proportion of the right ventricle. Post-mortem angiographic studies showed that approximately 70% of the cardiac muscle (80–86% of the left ventricle) is irrigated by the left coronary artery in case of right dominant coronary circulation [1]. In left dominant systems, virtually the whole left ventricular muscular mass receives blood from the left main. Thus, its patency is necessary to grant sufficient perfusion of the heart, and severe left main coronary artery disease exposes patients to a high risk of mortality and major cardiovascular events.

The left main is conventionally divided into three segments: the ostium (i.e., its origin from the aorta), the trunk (also known as mid-shaft or mid-portion), and the distal portion. The latter usually bifurcates into the left anterior descending artery and the left circumflex artery [2]. However, in almost 30% of cases, a trifurcation exists. In the latter situation, a "ramus intermedius" arises between the left anterior descending artery and the circumflex artery, with a course similar to that of either a diagonal branch or a left marginal branch of the left circumflex. Notably, in 2% of subjects there are four branches.

Typically, the left main originates from the superior margin of the left aortic sinus of Valsalva, just below the sinotubular junction. It then runs anterior, superior, and leftward, within the left atrioventricular groove under the pulmonary artery, but its course can be altered by elongation or rotation of the aorta [3]. Understanding this course is of utmost importance for the interventional cardiologist, as it will help to obtain optimal angiographic views aiming to fully assess the presence of coronary artery disease.

3.1.2 Anatomical Variations of the Left Main Coronary Artery

Different congenital abnormalities of the left main take-off have been described. The angiographer should be aware of these variants in order to reduce procedural time and the amount of contrast agent. First, there may be no left main,

L. Nai Fovino · A. Scotti · G. Tarantini (✉)
Department of Cardiac, Thoracic, Vascular Sciences and Public Health, University of Padua Medical School, Padua, Italy
e-mail: giuseppe.tarantini.1@unipd.it

© Springer Nature Switzerland AG 2022
B. Cortese (ed.), *Left Main Coronary Revascularization*,
https://doi.org/10.1007/978-3-031-05265-1_3

when the left descending coronary artery and the left circumflex artery have separate origins. Second, anomalous origin of the left main can be found from the right sinus of Valsalva; in this case the vessel can have an inter-arterial course between the pulmonary trunk and the aorta, which is associated with increased risk of sudden death, particularly in children and young athletes [4]. Fortunately, this situation has a prevalence as low as 0.03%. Third, the left coronary artery can also arise from the non-coronary sinus of Valsalva without passing between the two major trunks, representing therefore a benign condition. Finally, in 0.013% of subjects, the left coronary artery originates above the left coronary sinus [4].

3.1.3 Histological Characteristics of the Left Main Coronary Artery

Histologically, the left main differs from the rest of the coronary tree in its elastic tissue content, which is greater at the ostium and diminishes distally [3]. Moreover, the ostium lacks adventitia and has aortic smooth muscle cells oriented perpendicularly. The extension toward the distal part of the left main of the aortic elastic fibers depends on left main length and thus might impact on stenosis distribution. The higher elastic tissue content at the ostium is likely responsible for the higher elastic recoil and high restenosis rates observed in the early days of percutaneous coronary angioplasty [5].

3.1.4 Normal Dimensions of the Left Main Coronary Artery

Left main length is highly variable. A pathology study evaluating 100 autopsy cases found an average length of 10.8 ± 5.2 mm (range 2–23 mm) [3], consistent with a more recent computed tomography angiography study retrospectively analyzing 300 consecutive patients without coro-

nary artery disease, where the mean left main length was 10.5 ± 5.3 mm [6].

The same two studies showed an average diameter of 4.9 mm and 3.7 mm, respectively. This discrepancy is likely related to post-mortem fixation of the pathology specimen. Notably, studies using quantitative coronary angiography analysis have found a mean diameter of 3.1–4.2 mm [7], and in a large intravascular ultrasound study the latter was 5 mm, ranging between 3.5 and 6.5 mm [8]. The left main caliper varies according to gender (i.e., it is smaller in women than in men), even after normalization for body surface area. This finding is consistent among autopsy and computed tomography reports. Moreover, the left main is larger in subjects with left ventricular hypertrophy or dilated cardiomyopathy [7] (Fig. 3.1).

It should be underlined that the left main is not a simple straight tube. Rather, its cross section has an elliptic shape, whose diameter varies between ostium, mid-shaft, and distal portion. Thus, four types of left main morphology have been identified: biconcave-shape appearance, tapering morphology, combined morphology, and funnel-shape appearance [9].

3.1.5 Anatomy of Distal Left Main Coronary Artery Bifurcation

The distal bifurcation angle is highly variable, with an average of $86.7 \pm 28.8°$ (range 40° to 165°). Interestingly, a positive correlation between left main length and this angle has been noted (i.e., the longer the left main, the larger the angle of division). Moreover, this angle is wider in males than in females (85 vs. 74°, $p < 0.001$) [3]. Notably, the bifurcation angulation is influenced by systolic motion of the heart, resulting in reduction of the distal angle. Furthermore, this angle varies with percutaneous coronary intervention, already after the insertion of an angioplasty guidewire [10]. Overall, angles get narrower with the implantation of one or more stents, but the narrowest pre-percutaneous intervention angles increase after the procedure. No

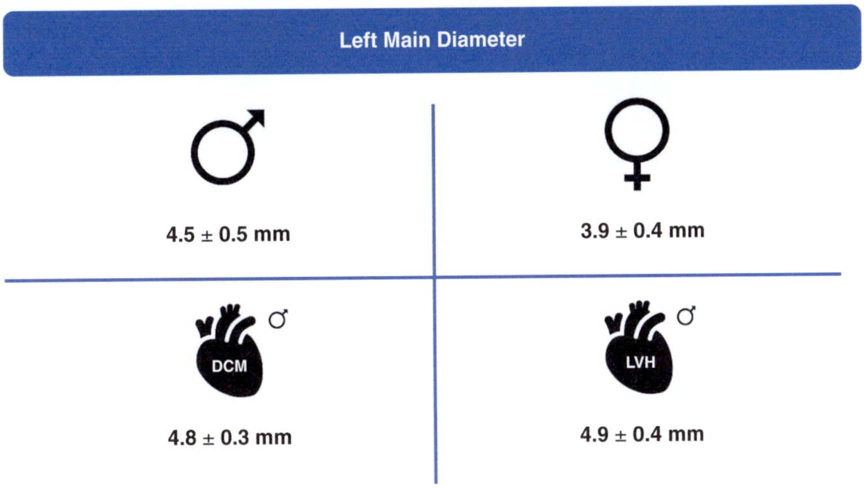

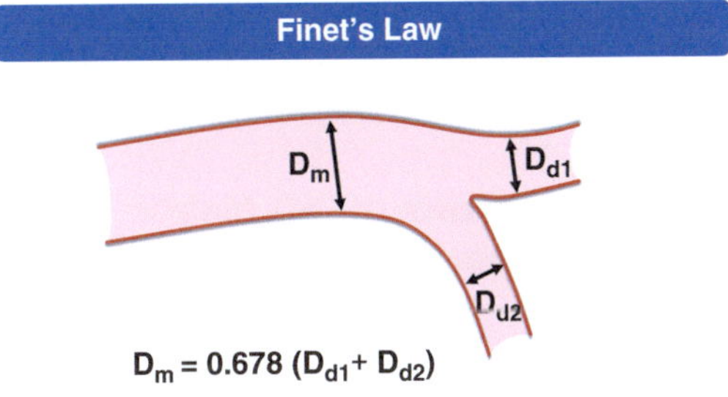

Fig. 3.1 Left main coronary artery diameter (mean ± standard deviation) in men (upper left corner), women (upper right corner), men with dilated cardiomyopathy (lower left corner), and men with left ventricular hypertrophy (lower right corner). *DCM = dilated cardiomyopathy; LVH = left ventricular hypertrophy*

clear difference in event rates across pre-percutaneous intervention angle values was found in a large intravascular ultrasound (IVUS) substudy of the synergy between PCI with Taxus and cardiac surgery (SYNTAX) trial, while patients with post-percutaneous intervention systolic diastolic range < 10° had a significantly higher rate of major cardiovascular events and repeat revascularizations [8].

The left main bifurcation, as any other coronary artery bifurcation, is characterized by peculiar hemodynamic features. The diameter reduction that occurs in each branch is governed by the law of conservation of energy and follows the principles of fractal geometry [11, 12]. In order to optimize stent size, it is of utmost importance for the interventional cardiologist to estimate the most truthful measure of each vessel diameter. Several efforts have been made in order to characterize the underlying pattern of these fractal objects. Murray was the first to propose a systematization of vascular bifurcations studying the interplay between workload and blood volumes in progressive diameter reduction. The most efficient relation found led to what is known today as Murray's law, which states that the cube of mother vessel radius coincides with the sum of the cubes of daughter vessels radii:

Fig. 3.2 Finet's formula on bifurcation vessels diameters. *Dd = diameter of daughter-vessel; Dm = diameter of mother-vessel*

$D_m^3 = D_{d1}^3 + D_{d2}^3$ [13]. The law of flow conservation derives from the application of conservation of energy to vascular bifurcations. It is a variant of Murray's law where squares are placed instead of the cubed values: $D_m^2 = D_{d1}^2 + D_{d2}^2$ [11].

In 2007, Finet and colleagues performed an angiographic study of coronary arteries where the true vessel diameters were calculated with the use of IVUS [14]. The aim of this work was to obtain these data in order to precisely quantify the bifurcation geometry and to derive it with a simple formulation. The results gave light to a new linear model which is known as Finet's law: $D_m = 0.678 (D_{d1} + D_{d2})$ (Fig. 3.2). This ratio (0.678) of mother-vessel diameter to the sum of the two daughter-vessel diameters was confirmed at every level of bifurcation, irrespectively of the mother vessel diameter. At a comparative analysis this linear model was the most precise if compared to Murray's law and the law of flow conservation, yielding differences between estimates and real values that were not statistically significant. Knowing two values, through this formula the diameter of the third one can be easily calculated. In case of vessels that are not angiographically normal, this calculation will result in underestimation at most without endangering the interventional procedures as would otherwise be the case. Moreover, the application of this law confirms the appropriateness of generalizing the final kissing balloon inflation which guarantees results closer to healthy vessels [15].

3.2 Pathophysiology of the Left Main Coronary Artery

3.2.1 Prevalence of Left Main Coronary Artery Disease

Significant (>50% of the luminal diameter) coronary artery disease involving the left main is observed at approximately 5% of coronary angiograms, more often in men than in women (5.1% vs 3.4%) [16]. Notably, men with left main stenosis are markedly younger than women, a finding consistent with the higher risk of men to develop atherosclerosis at a younger age and likely secondary to pre-menopausal estrogen protection. Isolated left main disease is found in less than 10% of cases, and predominantly involves the ostium. In the remaining cases, left main stenosis is associated with the presence of significant atherosclerosis in one or more coronary vessels, half of the times with three-vessel disease [16]. Notably, in the Coronary Artery Surgery Study (CASS) registry, only 3.6% of patients with left main involvement were asymptomatic [17].

3.2.2 Role of Endothelial Shear Stress in LM Bifurcation

Atherosclerosis is a chronic, fibroproliferative, inflammatory disease that mainly affects large- and medium-sized vessels. The dynamics of blood flow, together with other contributing factors, ensure different ways of atherosclerotic plaque distribution (Fig. 3.3). The regions of the arterial tree where these lesions arise are those where disturbed flow occurs as in the vicinity of branch points, the outer wall of bifurcations, or the inner wall of curvatures. Among the hemodynamic forces involved in this process, the flow-generated endothelial shear stress has a central role. The first evidence of such pathophysiological mechanism was provided by Caro et al. [18]. Endothelial shear stress is the tangential stress derived from the friction of the flowing blood on the endothelial surface of the arterial wall and is calculated as units of force/unit area (N/m^2 or Pascal [Pa] or dyne/cm2; $1 \; N/m^2 = 1 \; Pa = 10 \; dyne/cm^2$). Endothelial shear stress is proportional to the product of the blood viscosity and the spatial gradient of blood velocity at the wall (dv/dy). It is pulsatile with a magnitude that ranges from 15 to 70 $dyne/cm^2$ over the cardiac cycle and yields a positive time average. The most proatherogenic effect was found in areas with low endothelial shear stress (10–12 dynes/cm^2) which has a critical role in plaque development and progression to high-risk (vulnerable) plaques with a large necrotic core, increased inflammation, and thin fibrous cap [19]. Lateral walls of bifurcations are one of these areas dominated by low endothelial shear stress, whereas the carina exhibits the highest values of endothelial shear stress; this phenomenon can explain the carina sparing of atherosclerosis. The stimuli provided by low endothelial shear stress trigger numerous mechanoreceptors located on endothelial cell surfaces, which in turn activate a complex network of intracellular pathways, each of which cross-talk with the others (Fig. 3.4).

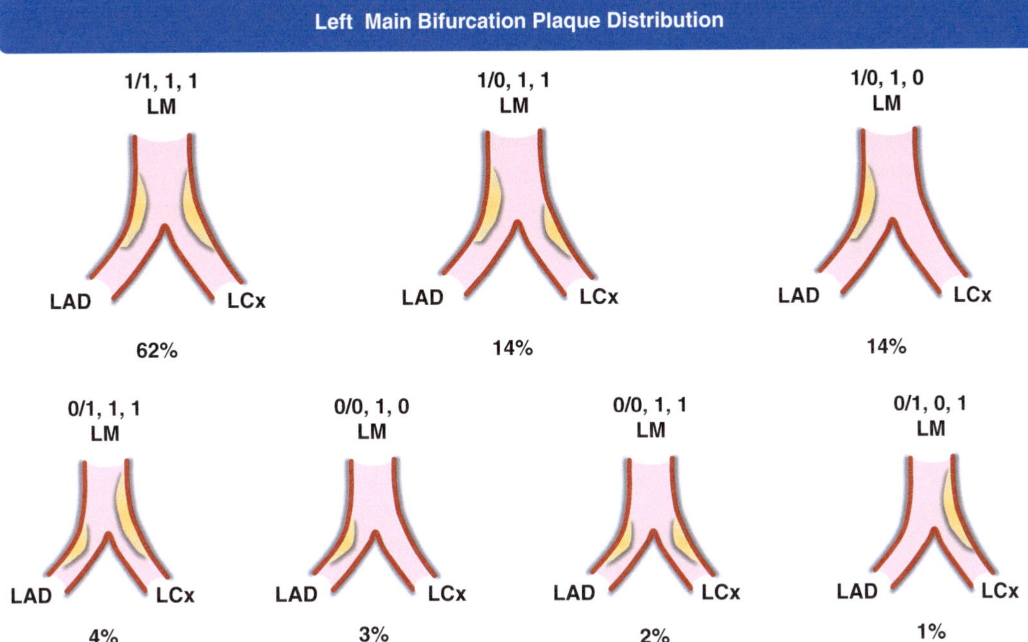

Fig. 3.3 Left main bifurcation plaque distribution (IVUS classification). Data from Oviedo et al. [22]. *IVUS = intravascular ultrasound; LAD = left anterior descending artery; LCx = left circumflex artery; LM = left main*

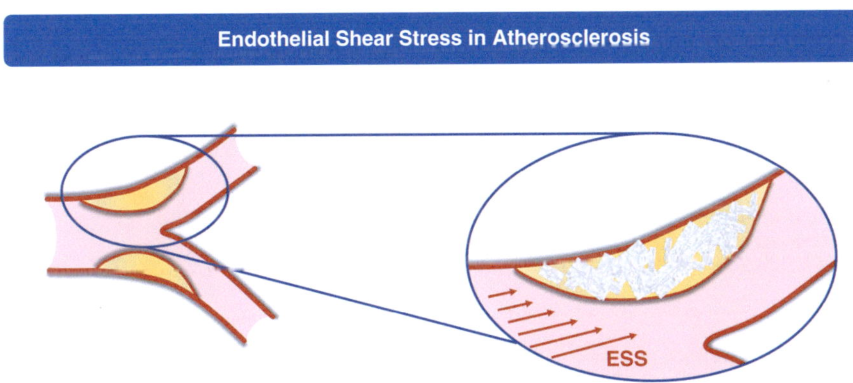

Fig. 3.4 Role of low endothelial shear stress in atherosclerosis. In arterial regions with disturbed laminar flow, low endothelial shear stress shifts the endothelial function and structure toward an atherosclerotic phenotype, thereby promoting atherogenesis, atherosclerotic plaque formation and progression, and vascular remodeling. *BMP = bone morphogenic protein; ET = endothelin; ICAM = intercellular adhesion molecule; IFN = interferon; IL = interleukin; LDL = low-density lipoprotein cholesterol; MCP = monocyte chemoattractant protein; MMP = matrix metalloproteinase; NO = nitric oxide; PDGF = platelet-derived growth factor; SREBP = sterol regulatory elements binding protein; TF = transcription factor; TGF = transforming growth factor; TNF = tumor necrosis factor; t-PA = tissue plasminogen activator; VCAM = vascular cell adhesion molecule; VEGF = vascular endothelial growth factor; VSMC = vascular smooth muscle cell*

The resulting effects are as follows:

- Attenuation of nitric oxide-dependent atheroprotection.
- Attenuation of extracellular matrix synthesis in vascular wall and plaque fibrous cap.
- Promotion of low-density lipoprotein cholesterol uptake, synthesis, and permeability.
- Promotion of oxidative stress.
- Promotion of inflammation.
- Promotion of vascular smooth muscle cell migration, differentiation, and proliferation.
- Promotion of plaque neovascularization.
- Promotion of plaque calcification.
- Promotion of atherosclerotic wall remodeling.
- Increase of plaque thrombogenicity.

3.2.3 Left Main Plaque Distribution

Atherosclerosis within the left main is usually diffuse and frequently affects the bifurcation as a result of low endothelial shear stress. Ostial lesions in turn are promoted by flow separation due to the rather sharp angulation of the lower leading edge of the left main artery as it originates from the aortic sinus. With the progression of atheroma within the vessel course, we can run into a phenomenon of positive remodeling (usually in the shaft) which tries to preserve lumen dimensions or, on the contrary, a localized negative remodeling (left main ostium, left anterior descending artery and left circumflex ostia) on its edges. Studies based on IVUS imaging demonstrated that when the disease is located on the lateral wall of bifurcation (where low endothelial shear stress is more pronounced) its extension into the divisional branches is very common (left stenosis tends to spread to the left anterior descending in up to 90% of the cases). Yet, plaques confined on the ostia of left anterior descending or left circumflex artery are very rare [20–22].

The distribution of plaques within the left main varies according to their length (Fig. 3.5). Short anatomic LM arteries (<10 mm) are mainly affected by stenosis near the ostium (ostium 55%, bifurcation 38%). On the contrary, the development of atherosclerosis in a long left main (≥10 mm) takes place more frequently near the bifurcation (ostium 18%, bifurcation 77%). Stenosis on the mid part of LM was rarely found (5–7%) [23]. The morphology of the stenosis differed by location. On IVUS imaging ostial lesions were found to be eccentric and associated with female sex, less plaque burden, less calcification, and more negative remodeling [23]. The applica-

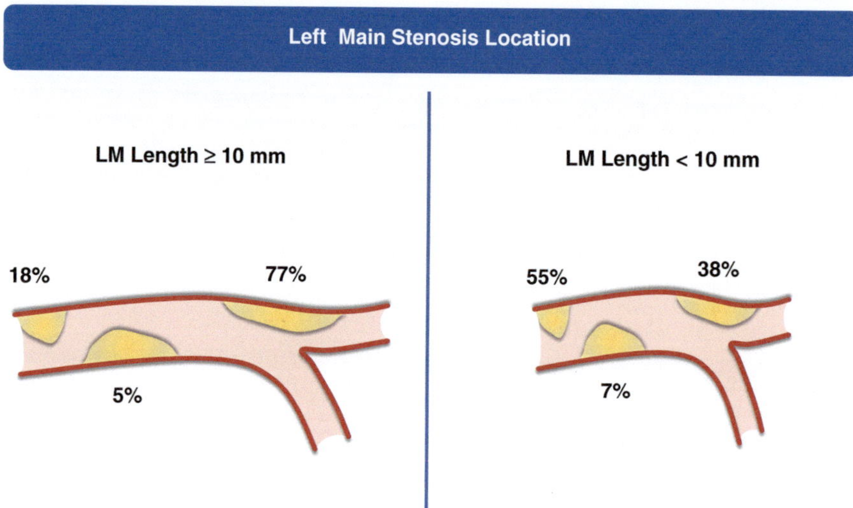

Fig. 3.5 Coronary stenosis distribution (ostial, shaft, distal/bifurcation) according to left main length (on the left ≥10 mm, on the right <10 mm). Data from Maehara et al. [23]. *LM = left main*

tion of Poiseuille's equation (left main length is directly related to pressure drop and inversely proportional to volume flow) can easily explain the presence of a small pressure drop and a large flow at the bifurcation in the short left main. Conversely, the long left main is characterized by a big pressure drop and low endothelial shear stress at bifurcation. This may explain the different atherosclerotic plaques distribution as a function of coronary length [24].

3.2.4 The Medina Classification for Left Main Bifurcation Disease

Among all the definitions and classifications of bifurcation lesions that have been proposed, the Medina classification stands out for its simplicity [25].

Its goal was to create a common language that could be widely adopted for clinical and research purposes. Each component of the bifurcation is assigned a value 0 or 1 in case of absence or presence of stenosis >50%, respectively. Since a bifurcation is made up of three parts, three different 0/1 values will result. The order in which they are assigned starts from the proximal segment, followed by the main distal segment and at the end the side branch; these values are separated by commas (e.g., 1,1,0 in case of stenosis of proximal and distal main segment with sparing of the side branch). Simple visual angiographic analysis allows to define the classification. However, in some circumstances, the side branch assessment could be difficult to carry out. For this reason, the use of dedicated quantitative coronary angiography software, IVUS, optical coherence tomography, or multi-slice computed tomography can be implemented for an optimal analysis.

3.2.5 Uncommon Causes of Left Main Coronary Artery Disease

Atherosclerotic disease is by far the primary cause of left main stenosis. However, since its 2 to 4 mm is within the aortic wall, the left main is subject to other conditions that affect the aorta. For instance, other etiologies include Takayasu disease, giant cell arteritis, syphilitic aortitis, mediastinal irradiation, trauma from coronary angiography, or aortic valve replacement. Moreover, the left main can suffer extrinsic compression by aneurysm, tumors, as a result of prior surgery, etc.

References

1. Leaman DM, Brower RW, Meester GT, Serruys P, van den Brand M. Coronary artery atherosclerosis: severity of the disease, severity of angina pectoris and compromised left ventricular function. Circulation. 1981;63(2):285–99.
2. DeMots H, Rösch J, McAnulty JH, Rahimtoola SH. Left main coronary artery disease. Cardiovasc Clin. 1977;8(2):201–11.
3. Reig J, Petit M. Main trunk of the left coronary artery: anatomic study of the parameters of clinical interest. Clin Anat. 2004;17(1):6–13.
4. Cheezum MK, Liberthson RR, Shah NR, Villines TC, O'Gara PT, Landzberg MJ, et al. Anomalous aortic origin of a coronary artery from the inappropriate sinus of Valsalva. J Am Coll Cardiol. 2017;69(12):1592–608.
5. Macaya C, Alfonso F, Iñiguez A, Goicolea J, Hernandez R, Zarco P. Stenting for elastic recoil during coronary angioplasty of the left main coronary artery. Am J Cardiol. 1992;70(1):105–7.
6. Medrano-Gracia P, Ormiston J, Webster M, Beier S, Young A, Ellis C, et al. A computational atlas of normal coronary artery anatomy. EuroIntervention. 2016;12(7):845–54.
7. Dodge JT, Brown BG, Bolson EL, Dodge HT. Lumen diameter of normal human coronary arteries. Influence of age, sex, anatomic variation, and left ventricular hypertrophy or dilation. Circulation. 1992;86(1):232–46.
8. Girasis C, Serruys PW, Onuma Y, Colombo A, Holmes DR, Feldman TE, et al. 3-dimensional bifurcation angle analysis in patients with left main disease: a substudy of the SYNTAX trial (SYNergy between percutaneous coronary intervention with TAXus and cardiac surgery). JACC Cardiovasc Interv. 2010;3(1):41–8.
9. Zeina AR, Rosenschein U, Barmeir E. Dimensions and anatomic variations of left main coronary artery in normal population: multidetector computed tomography assessment. Coron Artery Dis. 2007;18(6):477–82.
10. Louvard Y, Lefèvre T, Morice MC. Percutaneous coronary intervention for bifurcation coronary disease. Heart. 2004;90(6):713–22.

11. Kamiya A, Togawa T. Optimal branching structure of the vascular tree. Bull Math Biophys. 1972;34(4):431–8.

12. Zhou Y, Kassab GS, Molloi S. On the design of the coronary arterial tree: a generalization of Murray's law. Phys Med Biol. 1999;44(12):2929–45.

13. Murray CD. The physiological principle of minimum work: I. the vascular system and the cost of blood volume. Proc Natl Acad Sci U S A. 1926;12(3):207–14.

14. Finet G, Gilard M, Perrenot B, Rioufol G, Motreff P, Gavit L, et al. Fractal geometry of arterial coronary bifurcations: a quantitative coronary angiography and intravascular ultrasound analysis. EuroIntervention. 2008;3(4):490–8.

15. Takebayashi H, Kobayashi Y, Dangas G, Fujii K, Mintz GS, Stone GW, et al. Restenosis due to under-expansion of sirolimus-eluting stent in a bifurcation lesion. Catheter Cardiovasc Interv. 2003;60(4):496–9.

16. Giannoglou GD, Antoniadis AP, Chatzizisis YS, Damvopoulou E, Parcharidis GE, Louridas GE. Prevalence of narrowing >or=50% of the left main coronary artery among 17,300 patients having coronary angiography. Am J Cardiol. 2006;98(9):1202–5.

17. Taylor HA, Deumite NJ, Chaitman BR, Davis KB, Killip T, Rogers WJ. Asymptomatic left main coronary artery disease in the coronary artery surgery study (CASS) registry. Circulation. 1989;79(6):1171–9.

18. Caro CG, Fitz-Gerald JM, Schroter RC. Arterial wall shear and distribution of early atheroma in man. Nature. 1969;223(5211):1159–60.

19. Chatzizisis YS, Jonas M, Coskun AU, Beigel R, Stone BV, Maynard C, et al. Prediction of the localization of high-risk coronary atherosclerotic plaques on the basis of low endothelial shear stress: an intravascular ultrasound and histopathology natural history study. Circulation. 2008;117(8):993–1002.

20. Burzotta F, Lassen JF, Banning AP, Lefèvre T, Hildick-Smith D, Chieffo A, et al. Percutaneous coronary intervention in left main coronary artery disease: the 13th consensus document from the European bifurcation Club. EuroIntervention. 2018;14(1):112–20.

21. Scotti A, Nai Fovino L, Pavei A, Tarantini G. Left main bifurcation PCI with the culotte technique using two self-apposing stents. EuroIntervention. 2020;15(16):1458–9.

22. Oviedo C, Maehara A, Mintz GS, Araki H, Choi SY, Tsujita K, et al. Intravascular ultrasound classification of plaque distribution in left main coronary artery bifurcations: where is the plaque really located? Circ Cardiovasc Interv. 2010;3(2):105–12.

23. Maehara A, Mintz GS, Castagna MT, Pichard AD, Satler LF, Waksman R, et al. Intravascular ultrasound assessment of the stenoses location and morphology in the left main coronary artery in relation to anatomic left main length. Am J Cardiol. 2001;88(1):1–4.

24. Asakura T, Karino T. Flow patterns and spatial distribution of atherosclerotic lesions in human coronary arteries. Circ Res. 1990;66(4):1045–66.

25. Medina A, Suárez de Lezo J, Pan M. A new classification of coronary bifurcation lesions. Rev Esp Cardiol. 2006;59(2):183.

CABG Vs. PCI for Left Main Revascularization

4

Anastasios Roumeliotis, Rishi Chandiramani, George Dangas, and Roxana Mehran

4.1 Introduction

Coronary artery bypass grafting (CABG) has traditionally been the preferred mode of revascularization for patients with left main coronary artery disease (LMCAD). This was primarily due to the extensive myocardial territory supplied by the artery [1] and the technical difficulties with the percutaneous approach, especially in lesions affecting the distal segment of the vessel. However, owing to the shorter recovery time, less invasive nature, and lower procedural risk with percutaneous coronary intervention (PCI), it may be the favored mode of revascularization for both physicians and patients if the results were to be similar [2]. Recent advancements in stent technology [3–8], procedural techniques [9], imaging modalities [10–12], and antiplatelet pharmacotherapy [13–15] have helped PCI emerge as a viable alternative for the treatment of this high-risk population. Nonetheless, uncertainty regarding the durability of the intervention and its impact on subsequent long-term cardiovascular outcomes remains. This chapter discusses the most contemporary evidence available for the patients with LMCAD in particular and aims to identify the subgroups within this population that may derive the maximum benefit from each approach.

4.2 Current Evidence Comparing PCI to CABG for LMCAD

4.2.1 Real-World Evidence

Despite the fact that CABG constitutes the current gold standard for the treatment of unprotected LMCAD, performing such an invasive procedure is not feasible in multiple clinical scenarios, such as presence of a large number of comorbidities that may render the case inoperable or unwillingness of the patient to undergo a major surgical operation. As a result, evidence on the safety, efficacy, and technical challenges of PCI in these complex cases have gradually accumulated over time. Multiple observational registries have reported excellent short- and long-term outcomes in LMCAD patients treated with drug-eluting stents (DES) [16–18]. The Drug Eluting Stent for Left Main Coronary Artery (DELTA) 2 all-comer, international, multicenter registry included approximately 4000 patients and associated PCI with an acceptable rate of cardiovascular events after a median follow-up of 17 months; benefit for CABG was evident in target vessel

A. Roumeliotis · R. Chandiramani · G. Dangas ·
R. Mehran (✉)
Center for Interventional Cardiovascular Research and Clinical Trials, The Zena and Michael A. Wiener Cardiovascular Institute, Icahn School of Medicine at Mount Sinai, New York, NY, USA
e-mail: roxana.mehran@mountsinai.org

© Springer Nature Switzerland AG 2022
B. Cortese (ed.), *Left Main Coronary Revascularization*,
https://doi.org/10.1007/978-3-031-05265-1_4

revascularization (TVR) while PCI patients had lower risk for stroke [19]. Meanwhile, the Revascularization for Unprotected Left Main Coronary Artery Stenosis: Comparison of Percutaneous Coronary Angioplasty versus Surgical Revascularization (MAIN-COMPARE) registry evaluated 2240 patients with unprotected LMCAD treated either percutaneously or surgically. After a 5-year follow-up, PCI had similar rates of death, myocardial infarction (MI), or stroke but a higher incidence of TVR when compared to CABG [20].

4.2.2 Randomized Clinical Trials

Selection bias is always an issue in registry-driven data for LMCAD as either the simplest anatomic cases or the clinically terrible cases that are inoperable may be chosen for PCI. Therefore, randomized trials are of outmost importance in this subject (Table 4.1). Synergy between PCI with TAXUS and Cardiac Surgery (SYNTAX) remains one of the landmark trials on this topic [21]. As part of the trial, 1800 patients with three-vessel disease and/or LMCAD were randomly

assigned to percutaneous or surgical revascularization. At 5 years, major adverse cardiac and cerebrovascular events (MACCE), defined as a composite of all-cause mortality, stroke, MI, or repeat revascularization favored CABG (37.3% vs. 26.9%; $p < 0.0001$), primarily driven by the higher rates of repeat revascularization in the PCI arm. After stratifying for anatomical features, the majority of the benefit from CABG was derived from patients with three-vessel CAD while no statistically significant difference was demonstrated in patients with LMCAD [22]. Within the LM subgroup, only patients with a high SYNTAX score ($\geq$33) [23] benefited from CABG [22]. Longer-term follow-up confirmed that CABG provided mortality benefit in patients with multivessel disease but did not modify outcomes in those with LMCAD [24].

Other trials comparing PCI to CABG for unprotected LMCAD demonstrated very similar results. The Premier of Randomized Comparison of Bypass Surgery versus Angioplasty Using Sirolimus-Eluting Stent in Patients with Left Main Coronary Artery Disease (PRECOMBAT) trial randomized 600 patients to CABG or PCI and tested a non-inferiority hypothesis in terms

Table 4.1 Randomized clinical trials comparing PCI to CABG in LMCAD

Randomized clinical trial	Enrollment period	Follow-up duration	Number of patients with LMCAD	Type of stent	Primary clinical endpoint Definition	Primary outcome [PCI vs. CABG]
LE MANS [30]	2001–2005	10 years	105	TAXUS	Mortality, MI, stroke, or TVR	51.1% vs. 64.4%
Boudriot et al. [28]	2003–2009	1 year	201	SES	Death, MI, or repeat revasc	19% vs. 13.9%
PRECOMBAT [26]	2004–2009	5 years	600	SES	Death, MI, stroke, or TVR	17.5% vs. 14.3%
SYNTAX [22]	2005–2007	5 years	705	TAXUS	Death, MI, stroke, or repeat revasc	36.9% vs. 31%
NOBLE [33]	2008–2015	5 years	1201	Biomatrix	Death, non-periprocedural MI, or repeat revasc	28.4% vs. 19%
EXCEL [31]	2010–2014	5 years	1905	EES	Death, MI, or stroke	22% vs. 19.2%

CABG coronary artery bypass grafting, *EES* everolimus-eluting stent, *LMCAD* left main coronary artery disease *MI* myocardial infarction, *PCI* percutaneous coronary intervention, *revasc* revascularization, *SES* sirolimus-eluting stents, *TVR* target vessel revascularization

of MACCE. Although the cumulative event rate at 1 year was 8.7% in the PCI group vs. 6.7% in the CABG group ($p_{\text{non-inferiority}} = 0.01$), the clinical implications of the trial were limited due to the wide non-inferiority margin adopted [25]. The five-year follow-up results of the PRECOMBAT trial showed no significant difference in terms of MACCE, with the numerically higher event rate in the PCI group (17.5% vs. 14.3%; $p = 0.26$) being driven by the increased TVR [26]. A pooled analysis from the PRECOMBAT trial and LM arm of the SYNTAX trial showed that CABG was associated with a lower incidence of repeat revascularization (10.8% vs. 19.5%; $p < 0.001$) but similar rates of death, MI, or stroke (15.1% vs. 14%; $p = 0.45$) compared to PCI [27].

Around the same time, Boudriot and colleagues compared PCI with sirolimus-eluting stent and CABG for patients with unprotected LMCAD in a prospective randomized study. The study concluded that CABG was superior to PCI at 1-year follow-up with respect to the primary endpoint of major adverse cardiac events (MACE), defined as the composite of all-cause death, MI, or repeat revascularization (13.9% vs. 19%; $p_{\text{non inferiority}} = 0.19$) The results of this trial were also primarily affected by the difference in rates of repeat revascularization [28].

Left Main Stenting (LEMANS) was the first trial to thoroughly investigate the low to intermediate SYNTAX score population with LMCAD by comparing 52 patients undergoing PCI to 53 patients undergoing CABG. The PCI group demonstrated better results in terms of the primary endpoint of left ventricular ejection fraction (LVEF) modification 12 months post-revascularization [29]. From a clinical standpoint, after 10 years of follow-up, no difference was documented in the key secondary endpoint of MACCE (51.1% PCI vs. 64.4% CABG; $p = 0.28$) but the small number of patients enrolled limited the power of the study [30].

Based on the higher risk of repeat revascularization with PCI compared to CABG for LMCAD overall and the higher rates of mortality with PCI in the high SYNTAX score subgroups, newer studies focused specifically on patients with low to intermediate SYNTAX scores as these patients seemed to benefit the most from a percutaneous approach during previous trials. The Evaluation of XIENCE versus Coronary Artery Bypass Surgery for Effectiveness of Left Main Revascularization (EXCEL) trial enrolled 1905 patients with LMCAD of low or intermediate anatomical complexity and assigned them to either PCI with everolimus-eluting stents or CABG. After a 5-year follow-up period, the trial found no significant difference between the groups for the composite primary endpoint of death, MI, or stroke (PCI 22.0% vs. CABG 19.2%; $p = 0.13$). Similarly, a numerically higher, albeit statistically non-significant, mortality rate was demonstrated for the PCI arm at 5 years (PCI 13.0% vs. CABG 9.9%; 95% CI: 0.2 to 6.1). In more detail, as shown in Fig. 4.1, patients undergoing CABG had an incremental risk early after randomization primarily due to a higher incidence of periprocedural MI (PCI 3.9% vs. CABG 6.1%, Odds Ratio (OR) = 0.63 [95% CI: 0.41 to 0.96]) that attenuated between 2 and 3 years after and subsequently reversed due to lower spontaneous MI in the CABG group [31]. Interpretation and incorporation of this data in everyday clinical practice has been a subject of rigorous debate, particularly regarding the early and late MI definitions in PCI versus CABG settings. Myocardial injury and MI detection periprocedurally is quite complex in its pathogenesis and prognostic significance and this affects the disparity reflected in the fourth Universal MI definition [32].

Another notable trial comparing CABG with PCI for the treatment of LMCAD in the contemporary DES era was the Nordic–Baltic–British Left Main Revascularization (NOBLE) trial [33]. The study enrolled 1201 patients (598 PCI and 603 CABG) that were followed up for a median of 4.9 years with a primary endpoint of MACCE (all-cause mortality, non-procedural MI, repeat revascularization, or stroke) that excluded peri-procedural enzymatic MI events. The predefined threshold for non-inferiority with regard to MACCE was exceeded primarily due to the higher incidence of subsequent MI (8% vs. 3%, $p = 0.0002$) and repeat

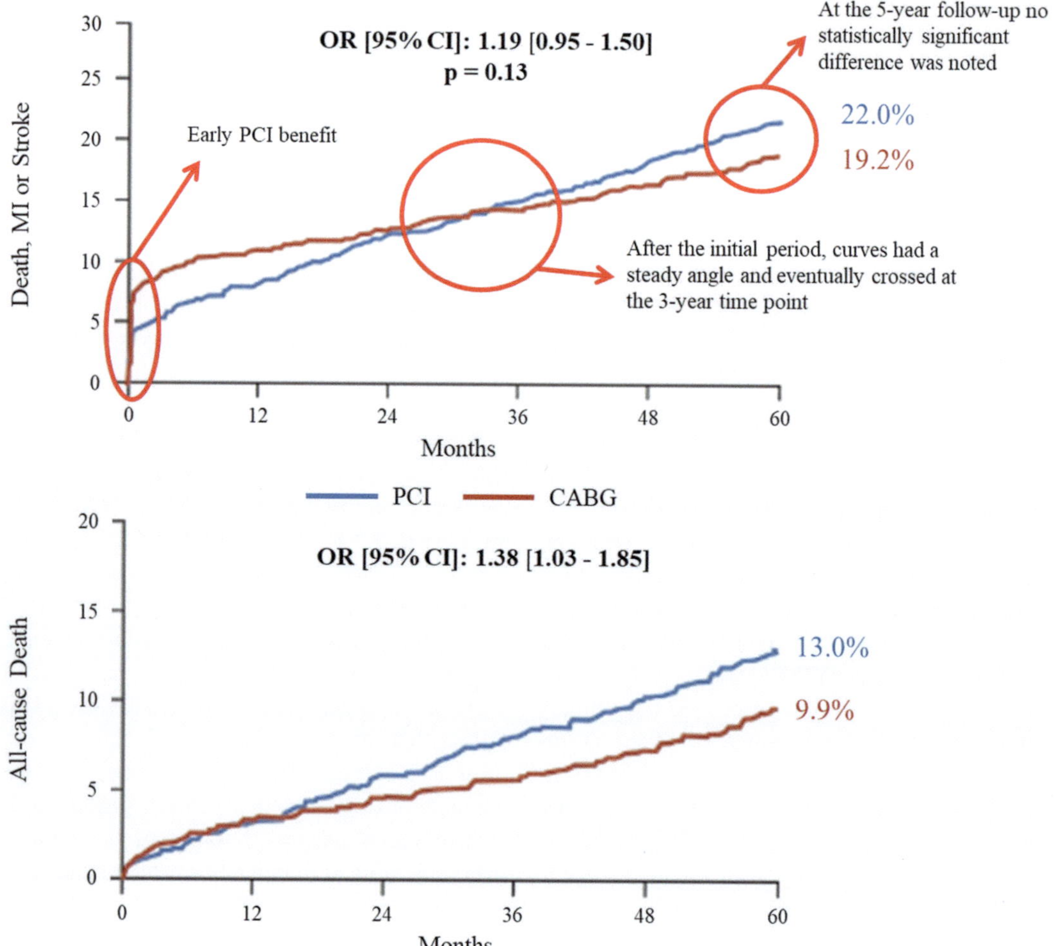

Fig. 4.1 Five-year results of the EXCEL trial

revascularization (17% vs. 10%; $p = 0.0009$) in the PCI group, although no difference was noted in mortality (9% vs. 9%; $p = 0.68$) [33]. While these results might appear contradictory to the results of the EXCEL trial, the similar number of events reported in the two studies [34] signal that the differences should probably be attributed to the differences in trial design and endpoints adopted (no periprocedural MI included in the primary endpoint of NOBLE and no repeat revascularization included in the primary endpoint of the EXCEL) (Fig. 4.2).

A contemporary meta-analysis combining the findings of the SYNTAX, PRECOMBAT, EXCEL, and NOBLE trials supports that PCI and CABG carry similar risk of death, MI, or stroke but CABG is superior with regard to repeat revascularization and that PCI represents a valid alternative to CABG especially in patients with a low or intermediate SYNTAX score [35]. Regardless, periprocedural MI continues to be difficult to evaluate particularly after CABG.

Clinically relevant findings that appear to be consistent across randomized trials are the early harm in terms of extended hospitalization as well as peri-procedural complications and the late steady benefit over time with the more invasive approach (CABG). As a result, follow-up length may impact the absolute risk/benefit ratio and the two time periods should be analyzed separately to allow for optimal patient-centered decision-making [36].

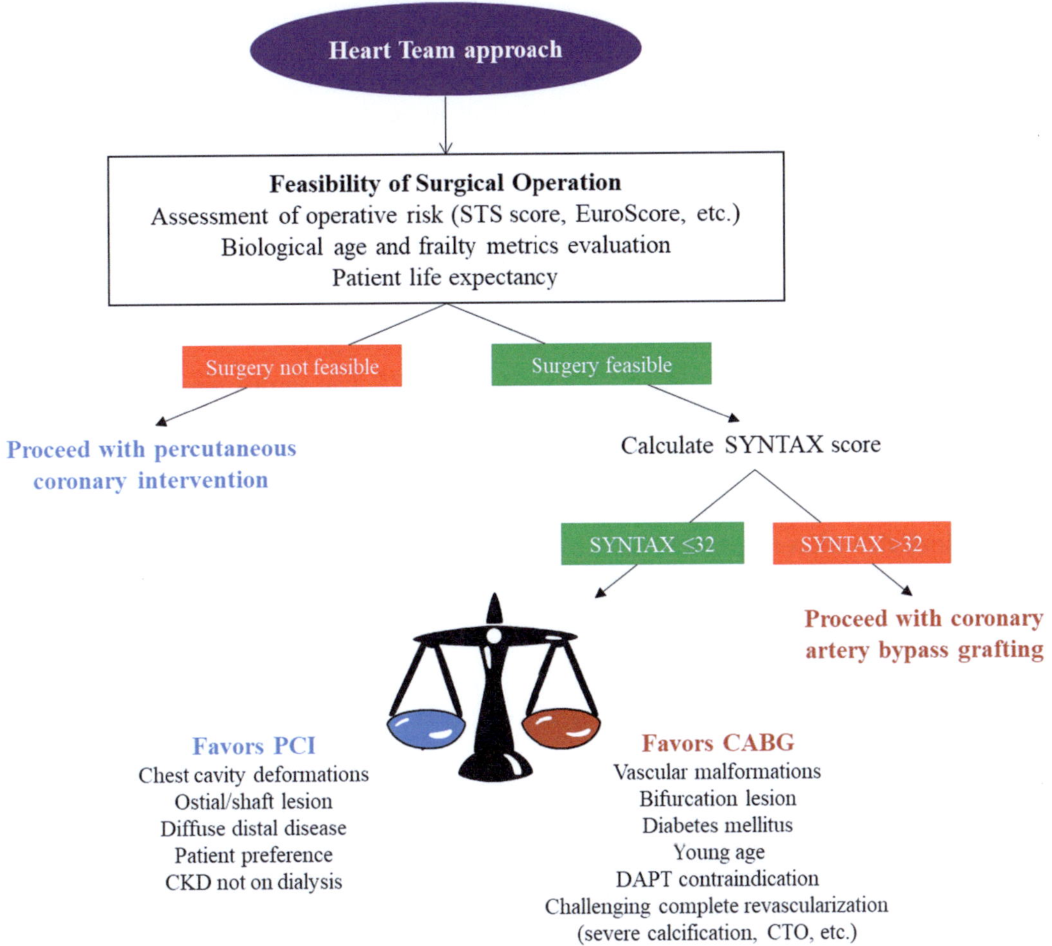

Fig. 4.2 PCI vs CABG decision making algorithm

4.3 Guideline Recommendations on LMCAD Revascularization

The most recent European Society of Cardiology guideline recommendations on the optimal treatment approach to LMCAD were published in 2018 and were primarily based on the explorative analyses of the SYNTAX trial as well as the early results of the EXCEL trial [22, 37]. CABG received an IA recommendation for all clinical scenarios while recommendations on PCI varied according to the SYNTAX score of the patient. In LMCAD patients with a low SYNTAX score, i.e., 0–22, PCI was indicated with a high level of evidence (IA) while in those with an intermediate SYNTAX score, i.e., 23–32, PCI should be considered as a treatment option (IIaA). PCI was not recommended (IIIB) in LMCAD patients with a high SYNTAX score, i.e., ≥33. Furthermore, it was advised that a Heart Team approach that takes individual clinical characteristics as well as patient preferences into account be adopted during the decision-making process. In general, parameters such as the presence of major (often rare) comorbidities, frailty, limited mobility, and challenging anatomical features of the chest cavity should favor a percutaneous approach while diabetes mellitus (DM), reduced LVEF (≤35%), contraindications to dual antiplatelet therapy, severe calcification, recurrent in-stent restenosis, and vascular malformations should favor surgery [38].

The most recent ACCF/AHA/SCAI guidelines for PCI were published in 2011 [39], when very little randomized evidence on LMCAD was available. Recommendations for this high-risk subgroup were that PCI should be considered in patients with low SYNTAX score (IIaB), may be considered in those with intermediate SYNTAX score (IIbB) and should be avoided in high SYNTAX score patients (IIIB) [39]. The upcoming ACCF/AHA/SCAI coronary artery revascularization guidelines are expected to provide better insight into the optimal approach for LMCAD patients after incorporating recent data from contemporary randomized trials.

4.4 Individualized Patient Approach

Multiple factors such as predicted surgical risk, complexity and location of CAD, procedural urgency, additional clinical characteristics, and feasibility of complete revascularization should be taken into consideration when deciding the optimal management strategy for patients with LMCAD. A plethora of available evidence highlights the complexity of this topic and underscores the need for a multidisciplinary Heart Team approach. All LMCAD cases should be subject to dedicated discussion between the primary care physician, clinical cardiologist, interventional cardiologist, and cardiothoracic surgeon and never be planned for ad-hoc PCI. Patients should be provided with all the pertinent information, receive the Heart Team recommendation, and given ample time to process the situation and make the optimal decision tailored to their individual preferences and requirements when possible [40].

4.4.1 Predicted Surgical Risk

Accurate periprocedural risk estimation is crucial for patients with LMCAD, as presence of high surgical risk shifts the decision toward a minimally invasive approach regardless of coronary anatomy. In everyday clinical practice, risk scores primarily used to assess prognosis after myocardial revascularization include the European System for Cardiac Operative Risk Evaluation (EuroSCORE II) and the Society of Thoracic Surgeons (STS) scores. EuroSCORE II is a cardiac risk model designed to assess in-hospital mortality based on the patient's clinical characteristics and may be calculated online (www. euroscore.org/calc.html). An update on the initial EuroSCORE risk model, EuroSCORE II was derived from an international database of 22,381 patients [41] and has been validated in external cohorts of CABG patients [42, 43].

The STS score is a widely used risk algorithm in the United States incorporating patient age, sex, variables reflecting comorbidities as well as acuity and severity of cardiac disease, and can also be calculated online (http://riskcalc.sts.org) to estimate the risk of perioperative mortality. The score is regularly calibrated to reflect contemporary clinical practice [44]. Since no standard cutoffs exist for either of these scores, their clinical use should only be considered complimentary to medical judgment. Notably, both the above surgical databases only include patients who did undergo CABG, so their results should not be generalized to patients who are poor candidates for surgery.

4.4.2 Anatomy of CAD

Currently, anatomical complexity constitutes the only parameter modifying the guideline recommendations for PCI in LMCAD. The SYNTAX score (http://www.syntaxscore.com) was originally created from the SYNTAX trial to help quantify the extent of CAD and has since become one of the most widely adopted scores in the field of interventional cardiology [23]. Individual trials presented earlier in this chapter as well as a patient-level meta-analysis of randomized clinical trials including 11,518 patients have repeatedly validated that a higher SYNTAX score is associated with better outcomes after CABG compared to PCI [45]. To summarize, surgical revascularization, if feasible, is clearly the optimal mode of revascularization in patients with a high SYNTAX score, while PCI may be a viable alternative in cases with low to intermediate SYNTAX score [38]. The Global Risk Classification (GRC) and the Clinical SYNTAX score constitute combined risk models that allow us to account for both clinical and angiographic parameters. The GRC was derived by combining the EuroSCORE with the SYNTAX score and has been associated with significant refinement in the assessment of cardiac mortality following myocardial revascularization [46]. The Clinical SYNTAX score was created by integrating important clinical variables (age, creatinine clearance, and LVEF) with the SYNTAX score and exhibited enhanced ability to predict MACCE and mortality when compared to the SYNTAX score alone [47]. In particular, for the subgroup of patients undergoing PCI for left main coronary artery stenosis, combined risk assessment may achieve enhanced risk discrimination capability [48].

In addition to the burden of disease, lesion location should also be taken into consideration. Distal lesions of the LM bifurcation treated with PCI have been associated with inferior cardiovascular outcomes compared to ostial and body disease [49–51]. This probably reflects the higher lesion complexity and unique technical difficulties encountered during interventions on the distal segment of the LM coronary artery [52]. A secondary analysis from the 3-year results of the EXCEL trial investigated the comparative efficacy of PCI and CABG according to the location of the LM lesion. While no difference was reported for lesions in the ostium or the shaft, patients in the PCI arm with a distal LM lesion experienced a higher incidence of ischemia-driven revascularization (13.0% vs. 7.2%; $p = 0.0001$) [53]. Final kissing balloon inflation did not appear to improve long-term outcomes of distal LM bifurcation stenting in both 1-stent and 2-stent techniques [54].

4.4.3 Completeness of Revascularization

Complete revascularization to minimize residual myocardial ischemia should be considered a universal goal [38]. Real-world evidence supports the prognostic value of complete revascularization in multivessel CAD by showing that incomplete revascularization with PCI had a higher incidence of MI when compared to CABG; however, these differences were attenuated in PCI patients with complete revascularization ($p = 0.02$ for interaction) [55]. Multiple randomized trials have also highlighted the value of an aggressive strategy aiming toward the treatment of all anatomically and functionally significant lesions in ST-segment elevation MI patients [56–60], with a large meta-analysis of randomized clinical trials involving 89,993 patients reporting that complete revascularization was associated with reduced mortality (Relative Risk (RR): 0.71; 95% CI: 0.65 to 0.77; $p < 0.001$) and repeat revascularization (RR: 0.74, 95% CI: 0.65 to 0.83; $p < 0.001$) [61].

In all randomized trials comparing PCI to CABG for the treatment of LMCAD, complete revascularization is highly recommended or even required by the study protocol (Table 4.2). Interestingly, the higher rates of complete revascularization with surgery may also explain the superior results of CABG in high SYNTAX score patients. Pooled data from the several trials reported that PCI had similar long-term survival rates to CABG only when complete revascularization was achieved [62]. In patients undergoing PCI, a residual SYNTAX score may be used as a measure of revascularization completeness and has shown the ability to identify individuals at increased risk for 5-year mortality [63]. Unfortunately, however, no such validation is available for patients undergoing CABG. Furthermore, diffuse as well as distal disease that cannot be surgically modified poses a unique problem that should be considered pre-operatively.

Table 4.2 Completeness of revascularization in randomized clinical trials comparing CABG to PCI

Randomized clinical trial	Complete revascularization (%) PCI arm	Complete revascularization (%) CABG arm	Definition of complete revascularization
LE MANS [30]	79%	89%	N/A
Boudriot et.al [28]	98%	97%	CABG or PCI of all lesions with >50% stenosis in vessels with a diameter of $\geq$2.0 mm required
PRECOMBAT [26]	68.3%	70.3%	Revascularization of vessels 2.5 mm and lesions >50% diameter stenosis
SYNTAX [22]	56.7%	63.2%	Revascularization of all vessels at least 1.5 mm in diameter with stenosis of 50% or more
NOBLE [33]	91.7%	N/A	Treatment of all anatomically of functionally significant lesions stenosis
EXCEL [31]	N/A	N/A	PCI: [1] $\geq$70% angiographic diameter stenosis (visually assessed) [2] <70% diameter Stenosis associated with noninvasive functional evidence of ischemia in the territory of the lesion or intra-procedure FFR $\leq$0.80 or IVUS minimal luminal area $\leq$ 4.0 mm^2 with plaque burden >60% CABG: Coronary arteries with $\geq$50% stenosis and $\geq$ 1.5 mm in diameter should be revascularized.

CABG coronary artery bypass grafting, *FFR* functional flow reserve, *IVUS* intravascular ultrasound, *N/A* not available

In summary, complete revascularization seems to play a crucial role in the outcomes of patients treated for CAD, and feasibility of thorough revascularization should be one of the major factors determining the mode of LMCAD management. In cases where complete revascularization is technically impossible to achieve, maximal revascularization should be aggressively pursued.

4.4.4 Procedural Urgency

In emergency cases of STEMI and cardiogenic shock secondary to LM coronary artery occlusion, immediate revascularization should be prioritized. Subsequently, these patients must be directed to primary PCI often with the adjunctive use of a left ventricular assist device such as Impella, extracorporeal membrane oxygenation, or intra-aortic balloon pump unless initial medical stabilization is required due to advanced patient age, extensive comorbid conditions, and dubious goals of care [64]. Such dire emergencies represent exclusion criteria for all randomized controlled trials since acute hemodynamic instability, altered mental status often encountered in the context of cardiac arrest or cardiogenic shock, along with potent anticoagulants and antiplatelets utilized as part of acute coronary syndrome protocols, preclude safe CABG procedure. After immediate culprit lesion revascularization, staged CABG may be considered in the presence of severe residual CAD with the Heart Team discussing the possibility for a hybrid revascularization technique [65].

4.4.5 Clinical Characteristics

In addition to the anatomical features and surgical risk, clinical parameters and patient comorbidities impact long-term outcomes and should be evaluated by the multidisciplinary Heart Team.

4.4.5.1 Diabetes Mellitus

DM not only constitutes one of the greatest risk factors for CAD but is also known to be associated with considerably worse outcomes [66]. CABG has always been the preferred mode of revascularization when compared to PCI in this population. However, as the majority of the available data comes from multivessel disease [67–70], whether this advantage extrapolates to LMCAD remains unclear. Interestingly, a pooled analysis from 3 randomized clinical trials showed that in patients with DM, multivessel disease, and a low SYNTAX score, PCI could be an acceptable option [71]. In contrast, an analysis from the EXCEL trial focusing on DM patients reported comparable MACCE between PCI and CABG but a higher mortality rate for the PCI arm [72]. Previously published data from the Future REvascularization Evaluation in patients with Diabetes mellitus (FREEDOM) trial associated CABG with a steady advantage over PCI in terms of MACCE regardless of SYNTAX score among diabetics presenting with multivessel CAD [73]. Therefore, despite the absence of concrete guideline recommendations on the preferred mode of revascularization for this population, existing evidence does support that LMCAD in diabetics should be indicated for CABG.

4.4.5.2 Heart Failure with Reduced Ejection Fraction

Systolic heart failure (HF) is commonly caused by ischemic heart disease and has been associated with increased morbidity and mortality post myocardial revascularization. Since the publication of the STICH trial, CABG has been the preferred treatment strategy for most patients with complex CAD and reduced ejection fraction (EF). During the study, despite experiencing a higher rate of peri-operative complications, patients assigned to the revascularization cohort exhibited a lower mortality rate after long-term follow-up [74]. However, no randomized evidence comparing PCI to CABG is currently available for patients with LMCAD and low EF, mainly because these patients are mostly excluded from trials. Interestingly, a large multicenter registry of 5795 patients with LMCAD identified prior HF as an independent predictor of MACCE after PCI but not after CABG [75]. Conversely, other data support that even though

heart failure is highly associated with adverse cardiovascular outcomes, different modes of revascularization have a uniform effect regardless of baseline LVEF owing to the high operative risk and smoother hospital course with PCI and its possible application with intraprocedural hemodynamic support [76]. Finally, when evaluating patients with reduced EF we need to differentiate between hibernating myocardium post-acute coronary syndrome that may gradually improve, non-viable myocardium, and concomitant non-ischemic cardiomyopathy especially in cases of intermediate severity LM lesions since management may differ on a case by case basis.

4.4.5.3 Chronic Kidney Disease

Chronic kidney disease (CKD) is known to complicate the course of patients undergoing surgical or percutaneous revascularization. Excess hemodynamic fluctuation during CABG [77] or the use of contrast media during PCI contributes to the development of acute kidney injury (AKI) [78], primarily in patients with an already compromised kidney function [79, 80]. It is also important to note that the risk for AKI has been higher after CABG [81].

4.4.5.4 Bleeding Risk

In addition to the ischemic risk, it is paramount that the bleeding risk of the patients is taken into consideration when deciding on a revascularization strategy. Previous trials have shown that severe bleeding may be equally, if not more strongly, associated with mortality when compared to an MI [82]. Criteria rendering patients at high bleeding risk have been recently described in detail in the consensus document from the Academic Research Consortium for High Bleeding Risk [83]. For patients with LMCAD, both revascularization techniques pose a significant bleeding hazard. A surgical approach increases early post-procedural events while an interventional approach comes with a long-term risk due to the duration of dual antiplatelet therapy (DAPT) required post-PCI. Short-term DAPT followed by P2Y12 monotherapy has recently emerged as an alternative regimen for

PCI patients. In the subgroup of patients undergoing complex PCI in the TWILIGHT trial, 3 months of ticagrelor and aspirin followed by ticagrelor monotherapy exhibited improved bleeding outcomes compared to long-term DAPT with aspirin and ticagrelor without compromising ischemic efficacy [84]. Nonetheless, data on this novel strategy that focuses exclusively in LMCAD patients remains scarce.

4.4.5.5 General Status of the Patient

When evaluating a patient with LMCAD, the Heart Team should adopt a more individualized and holistic approach toward the optimal revascularization strategy. We know that there is trade-off between early perioperative complications of the surgical approach and long-term durability concerns with the percutaneous approach and all trials demonstrating a benefit for CABG have done so around the 5-year follow-up. Keeping this in mind, biological age, frailty, general condition, and life expectancy of the patient play an integral part in Heart Team decision-making.

4.5   Conclusions

The choice of revascularization strategy for unprotected LMCAD constitutes one of the classic examples where one size does not fit all patients. The role of a multidisciplinary Heart Team in understanding the overall risk profile of the presenting case and optimizing treatment modalities after considering individual patient preferences and often discordant early and late outcomes after PCI vs. CABG becomes of paramount importance.

Disclosures Dr. Roumeliotis and Dr. Chandiramani report no conflicts of interest. Dr. Dangas reports receiving consulting fees from Biosensors, Abbott Vascular Laboratories, and Boston Scientific; grant support, paid to his institution, from AstraZeneca, Bayer, and Daiichi-Sankyo; owning common stock of Medtronic (entirely divested). Dr. Mehran reports receiving consulting fees from Abbott Vascular, Boston Scientific, Medscape/WebMD, Siemens Medical Solutions, Phillips/Volcano/Spectranetics, Roviant Sciences, Sanofi Italy, Bracco Group, Janssen, and AstraZeneca; grant support, paid to her institution, from Bayer, CSL Behring, DSI, Medtronic, Novartis Pharmaceuticals, OrbusNeich, Osprey Medical, PLC/RenalGuard, and Abbott Vascular; grant support and advisory board fees, paid to her institution, from BMS; fees for serving on a data and safety monitoring board from Watermark Research Funding; advisory fees and lecture fees from Medintelligence (Janssen); lecture fees from Bayer.

References

1. Collet C, Capodanno D, Onuma Y, Banning A, Stone GW, Taggart DP, et al. Left main coronary artery disease: pathophysiology, diagnosis, and treatment. Nat Rev Cardiol. 2018;15(6):321–31.
2. Ohlow MA, Farah A, Kuntze T, Lauer B. Patients' preferences for coronary bypass grafting or staged percutaneous coronary intervention in multivessel coronary artery disease. Int J Clin Pract. 2018;72(4):e13056.
3. Meliga E, Garcia-Garcia HM, Valgimigli M, Chieffo A, Biondi-Zoccai G, Maree AO, et al. Longest available clinical outcomes after drug-eluting stent implantation for unprotected left main coronary artery disease: the DELFT (drug eluting stent for LeFT main) registry. J Am Coll Cardiol. 2008;51(23):2212–9.
4. Kim YH, Dangas GD, Solinas E, Aoki J, Parise H, Kimura M, et al. Effectiveness of drug-eluting stent implantation for patients with unprotected left main coronary artery stenosis. Am J Cardiol. 2008;101(6):801–6.
5. Valgimigli M, van Mieghem CA, Ong AT, Aoki J, Granillo GA, McFadden EP, et al. Short- and long-term clinical outcome after drug-eluting stent implantation for the percutaneous treatment of left main coronary artery disease: insights from the rapamycin-eluting and Taxus stent evaluated at Rotterdam cardiology Hospital registries (RESEARCH and T-SEARCH). Circulation. 2005;111(11):1383–9.
6. Chieffo A, Park SJ, Valgimigli M, Kim YH, Daemen J, Sheiban I, et al. Favorable long-term outcome after drug-eluting stent implantation in nonbifurcation lesions that involve unprotected left main coronary artery: a multicenter registry. Circulation. 2007;116(2):158–62.
7. Kim YH, Park DW, Lee SW, Yun SC, Lee CW, Hong MK, et al. Long-term safety and effectiveness of unprotected left main coronary stenting with drug-eluting stents compared with bare-metal stents. Circulation. 2009;120(5):400–7.

8. Tamburino C, Di Salvo ME, Capodanno D, Marzocchi A, Sheiban I, Margheri M, et al. Are drug-eluting stents superior to bare-metal stents in patients with unprotected non-bifurcational left main disease? Insights from a multicentre registry. Eur Heart J. 2009;30(10):1171–9.

9. Chen SL, Zhang JJ, Han Y, Kan J, Chen L, Qiu C, et al. Double kissing crush versus provisional stenting for left Main distal bifurcation lesions: DKCRUSH-V randomized trial. J Am Coll Cardiol. 2017;70(21):2605–17.

10. de la Torre Hernandez JM, Baz Alonso JA, Gomez Hospital JA, Alfonso Manterola F, Garcia Camarero T, Gimeno de Carlos F, et al. Clinical impact of intravascular ultrasound guidance in drug-eluting stent implantation for unprotected left main coronary disease: pooled analysis at the patient-level of 4 registries. JACC Cardiovasc Interv. 2014;7(3):244–54.

11. Park SJ, Kim YH, Park DW, Lee SW, Kim WJ, Suh J, et al. Impact of intravascular ultrasound guidance on long-term mortality in stenting for unprotected left main coronary artery stenosis. Circ Cardiovasc Interv. 2009;2(3):167–77.

12. de la Torre Hernandez JM, Hernandez Hernandez F, Alfonso F, Rumoroso JR, Lopez-Palop R, Sadaba M, et al. Prospective application of pre-defined intravascular ultrasound criteria for assessment of intermediate left main coronary artery lesions results from the multicenter LITRO study. J Am Coll Cardiol. 2011;58(4):351–8.

13. Wiviott SD, Braunwald E, McCabe CH, Montalescot G, Ruzyllo W, Gottlieb S, et al. Prasugrel versus clopidogrel in patients with acute coronary syndromes. N Engl J Med. 2007;357(20):2001–15.

14. Wallentin L, Becker RC, Budaj A, Cannon CP, Emanuelsson H, Held C, et al. Ticagrelor versus clopidogrel in patients with acute coronary syndromes. N Engl J Med. 2009;361(11):1045–57.

15. Mehran R, Baber U, Sharma SK, Cohen DJ, Angiolillo DJ, Briguori C, et al. Ticagrelor with or without aspirin in high-risk patients after PCI. N Engl J Med. 2019;381(21):2032–42.

16. Lee MS, Kapoor N, Jamal F, Czer L, Aragon J, Forrester J, et al. Comparison of coronary artery bypass surgery with percutaneous coronary intervention with drug-eluting stents for unprotected left main coronary artery disease. J Am Coll Cardiol. 2006;47(4):864–70.

17. Makikallio TH, Niemela M, Kervinen K, Jokinen V, Laukkanen J, Ylitalo I, et al. Coronary angioplasty in drug eluting stent era for the treatment of unprotected left main stenosis compared to coronary artery bypass grafting. Ann Med. 2008;40(6):437–43.

18. Chieffo A, Magni V, Latib A, Maisano F, Ielasi A, Montorfano M, et al. 5-year outcomes following percutaneous coronary intervention with drug-eluting stent implantation versus coronary artery bypass graft for unprotected left main coronary artery lesions the Milan experience. JACC Cardiovasc Interv. 2010;3(6):595–601.

19. Chieffo A, Tanaka A, Giustino G, Briede I, Sawaya FJ, Daemen J, et al. The DELTA 2 registry: a multicenter registry evaluating percutaneous coronary intervention with new-generation drug-eluting stents in patients with obstructive left Main coronary artery disease. JACC Cardiovasc Interv. 2017;10(23):2401–10.

20. Park DW, Seung KB, Kim YH, Lee JY, Kim WJ, Kang SJ, et al. Long-term safety and efficacy of stenting versus coronary artery bypass grafting for unprotected left Main coronary artery disease: 5-year results from the MAIN-COMPARE (revascularization for unprotected left main coronary artery stenosis: comparison of percutaneous coronary angioplasty versus surgical revascularization) registry. J Am Coll Cardiol. 2010;56(2):117–24.

21. Serruys PW, Morice MC, Kappetein AP, Colombo A, Holmes DR, Mack MJ, et al. Percutaneous coronary intervention versus coronary-artery bypass grafting for severe coronary artery disease. N Engl J Med. 2009;360(10):961–72.

22. Morice MC, Serruys PW, Kappetein AP, Feldman TE, Stahle E, Colombo A, et al. Five-year outcomes in patients with left main disease treated with either percutaneous coronary intervention or coronary artery bypass grafting in the synergy between percutaneous coronary intervention with taxus and cardiac surgery trial. Circulation. 2014;129(23):2388–94.

23. Sianos G, Morel MA, Kappetein AP, Morice MC, Colombo A, Dawkins K, et al. The SYNTAX score: an angiographic tool grading the complexity of coronary artery disease. EuroIntervention. 2005;1(2):219–27.

24. Thuijs D, Kappetein AP, Serruys PW, Mohr FW, Morice MC, Mack MJ, et al. Percutaneous coronary intervention versus coronary artery bypass grafting in patients with three-vessel or left main coronary artery disease: 10-year follow-up of the multicentre randomised controlled SYNTAX trial. Lancet. 2019;394(10206):1325–34.

25. Park SJ, Kim YH, Park DW, Yun SC, Ahn JM, Song HG, et al. Randomized trial of stents versus bypass surgery for left main coronary artery disease. N Engl J Med. 2011;364(18):1718–27.

26. Ahn JM, Roh JH, Kim YH, Park DW, Yun SC, Lee PH, et al. Randomized trial of stents versus bypass surgery for left Main coronary artery disease: 5-year outcomes of the PRECOMBAT study. J Am Coll Cardiol. 2015;65(20):2198–206.

27. Cavalcante R, Sotomi Y, Lee CW, Ahn JM, Farooq V, Tateishi H, et al. Outcomes after percutaneous coronary intervention or bypass surgery in patients with unprotected left Main disease. J Am Coll Cardiol. 2016;68(10):999–1009.

28. Boudriot E, Thiele H, Walther T, Liebetrau C, Boeckstegers P, Pohl T, et al. Randomized comparison of percutaneous coronary intervention with sirolimus-eluting stents versus coronary artery bypass grafting in unprotected left main stem stenosis. J Am Coll Cardiol. 2011;57(5):538–45.

29. Buszman PE, Kiesz SR, Bochenek A, Peszek-Przybyla E, Szkrobka I, Debinski M, et al. Acute

and late outcomes of unprotected left main stenting in comparison with surgical revascularization. J Am Coll Cardiol. 2008;51(5):538–45.

30. Buszman PE, Buszman PP, Banasiewicz-Szkrobka I, Milewski KP, Zurakowski A, Orlik B, et al. Left Main stenting in comparison with surgical revascularization: 10-year outcomes of the (left Main coronary artery stenting) LE MANS trial. JACC Cardiovasc Interv. 2016;9(4):318–27.

31. Stone GW, Kappetein AP, Sabik JF, Pocock SJ, Morice MC, Puskas J, et al. Five-year outcomes after PCI or CABG for left Main coronary disease. N Engl J Med. 2019;381(19):1820–30.

32. Thygesen K, Alpert JS, Jaffe AS, Chaitman BR, Bax JJ, Morrow DA, et al. Fourth universal definition of myocardial infarction (2018). J Am Coll Cardiol. 2018;72(18):2231–64.

33. Holm NR, Makikallio T, Lindsay MM, Spence MS, Erglis A, Menown IBA, et al. Percutaneous coronary angioplasty versus coronary artery bypass grafting in the treatment of unprotected left main stenosis: updated 5-year outcomes from the randomised, non-inferiority NOBLE trial. Lancet. 2020;395(10219):191–9.

34. Christiansen EH, Makikallio T, Holm NR. Everolimus-eluting stents or bypass surgery for left Main coronary disease. N Engl J Med. 2017;376(11):1088–9.

35. Giacoppo D, Colleran R, Cassese S, Frangieh AH, Wiebe J, Joner M, et al. Percutaneous coronary intervention vs coronary artery bypass grafting in patients with left Main coronary artery stenosis: a systematic review and meta-analysis. JAMA Cardiol. 2017;2(10):1079–88.

36. Dangas G, Roumeliotis A, Giustino G. Invasive or conservative strategy for stable coronary disease. N Engl J Med. 2020;383(10):e66.

37. Stone GW, Sabik JF, Serruys PW, Simonton CA, Genereux P, Puskas J, et al. Everolimus-eluting stents or bypass surgery for left Main coronary artery disease. N Engl J Med. 2016;375(23):2223–35.

38. Neumann FJ, Sousa-Uva M, Ahlsson A, Alfonso F, Banning AP, Benedetto U, et al. 2018 ESC/EACTS Guidelines on myocardial revascularization. Eur Heart J. 2019;40(2):87–165.

39. Levine GN, Bates ER, Blankenship JC, Bailey SR, Bittl JA, Cercek B, et al. 2011 ACCF/AHA/SCAI guideline for percutaneous coronary intervention: a report of the American College of Cardiology Foundation/American Heart Association task force on practice guidelines and the Society for Cardiovascular Angiography and Interventions. Circulation. 2011;124(23):e574–651.

40. Holmes DR Jr, Rich JB, Zoghbi WA, Mack MJ. The heart team of cardiovascular care. J Am Coll Cardiol. 2013;61(9):903–7.

41. Nashef SA, Roques F, Sharples LD, Nilsson J, Smith C, Goldstone AR, et al. EuroSCORE II. Eur J Cardiothorac Surg 2012;41(4):734–44; discussion 44–5.

42. Biancari F, Vasques F, Mikkola R, Martin M, Lahtinen J, Heikkinen J. Validation of EuroSCORE II in patients undergoing coronary artery bypass surgery. Ann Thorac Surg. 2012;93(6):1930–5.

43. Chalmers J, Pullan M, Fabri B, McShane J, Shaw M, Mediratta N, et al. Validation of EuroSCORE II in a modern cohort of patients undergoing cardiac surgery. Eur J Cardiothorac Surg. 2013;43(4):688–94.

44. Shahian DM, O'Brien SM, Filardo G, Ferraris VA, Haan CK, Rich JB, et al. The Society of Thoracic Surgeons 2008 cardiac surgery risk models: part 1--coronary artery bypass grafting surgery. Ann Thorac Surg. 2009;88(1 Suppl):S2–22.

45. Head SJ, Milojevic M, Daemen J, Ahn JM, Boersma E, Christiansen EH, et al. Mortality after coronary artery bypass grafting versus percutaneous coronary intervention with stenting for coronary artery disease: a pooled analysis of individual patient data. Lancet. 2018;391(10124):939–48.

46. Capodanno D, Miano M, Cincotta G, Caggegi A, Ruperto C, Bucalo R, et al. EuroSCORE refines the predictive ability of SYNTAX score in patients undergoing left main percutaneous coronary intervention. Am Heart J. 2010;159(1):103–9.

47. Garg S, Sarno G, Garcia-Garcia HM, Girasis C, Wykrzykowska J, Dawkins KD, et al. A new tool for the risk stratification of patients with complex coronary artery disease: the clinical SYNTAX score. Circ Cardiovasc Interv. 2010;3(4):317–26.

48. Capodanno D, Caggegi A, Miano M, Cincotta G, Dipasqua F, Giacchi G, et al. Global risk classification and clinical SYNTAX (synergy between percutaneous coronary intervention with TAXUS and cardiac surgery) score in patients undergoing percutaneous or surgical left main revascularization. JACC Cardiovasc Interv. 2011;4(3):287–97.

49. Valgimigli M, Malagutti P, Rodriguez-Granillo GA, Garcia-Garcia HM, Polad J, Tsuchida K, et al. Distal left main coronary disease is a major predictor of outcome in patients undergoing percutaneous intervention in the drug-eluting stent era: an integrated clinical and angiographic analysis based on the rapamycin-eluting stent evaluated at Rotterdam cardiology Hospital (RESEARCH) and Taxus-stent evaluated at Rotterdam cardiology Hospital (T-SEARCH) registries. J Am Coll Cardiol. 2006;47(8):1530–7.

50. Biondi-Zoccai GG, Lotrionte M, Moretti C, Meliga E, Agostoni P, Valgimigli M, et al. A collaborative systematic review and meta-analysis on 1278 patients undergoing percutaneous drug-eluting stenting for unprotected left main coronary artery disease. Am Heart J. 2008;155(2):274–83.

51. Naganuma T, Chieffo A, Meliga E, Capodanno D, Park SJ, Onuma Y, et al. Long-term clinical outcomes after percutaneous coronary intervention for ostial/mid-shaft lesions versus distal bifurcation lesions in unprotected left main coronary artery: the DELTA registry (drug-eluting stent for left main coronary artery disease): a multicenter registry evaluating percutaneous coronary intervention versus coronary artery bypass grafting for left main treatment. JACC Cardiovasc Interv. 2013;6(12):1242–9.

52. Lefevre T, Girasis C, Lassen JF. Differences between the left main and other bifurcations. EuroIntervention. 2015;11(Suppl V):V106–10.

53. Gershlick AH, Kandzari DE, Banning A, Taggart DP, Morice MC, Lembo NJ, et al. Outcomes after left Main percutaneous coronary intervention versus coronary artery bypass grafting according to lesion site: results from the EXCEL trial. JACC Cardiovasc Interv. 2018;11(13):1224–33.

54. Kini AS, Dangas GD, Baber U, Vengrenyuk Y, Kandzari DE, Leon MB, et al. Influence of final kissing balloon inflation on long-term outcomes after PCI of distal left Main bifurcation lesions: analysis from the EXCEL trial. EuroIntervention. 2019;16:218–24.

55. Bangalore S, Guo Y, Samadashvili Z, Blecker S, Xu J, Hannan EL. Everolimus-eluting stents or bypass surgery for multivessel coronary disease. N Engl J Med. 2015;372(13):1213–22.

56. Wald DS, Morris JK, Wald NJ, Chase AJ, Edwards RJ, Hughes LO, et al. Randomized trial of preventive angioplasty in myocardial infarction. N Engl J Med. 2013;369(12):1115–23.

57. Gershlick AH, Khan JN, Kelly DJ, Greenwood JP, Sasikaran T, Curzen N, et al. Randomized trial of complete versus lesion-only revascularization in patients undergoing primary percutaneous coronary intervention for STEMI and multivessel disease: the CvLPRIT trial. J Am Coll Cardiol. 2015;65(10):963–72.

58. Engstrom T, Kelbaek H, Helqvist S, Hofsten DE, Klovgaard L, Holmvang L, et al. Complete revascularisation versus treatment of the culprit lesion only in patients with ST-segment elevation myocardial infarction and multivessel disease (DANAMI-3-PRIMULTI): an open-label, randomised controlled trial. Lancet. 2015;386(9994):665–71.

59. Smits PC, Abdel-Wahab M, Neumann FJ, Boxma-de Klerk BM, Lunde K, Schotborgh CE, et al. Fractional flow reserve-guided multivessel angioplasty in myocardial infarction. N Engl J Med. 2017;376(13):1234–44.

60. Mehta SR, Wood DA, Storey RF, Mehran R, Bainey KR, Nguyen H, et al. Complete revascularization with multivessel PCI for myocardial infarction. N Engl J Med. 2019;381(15):1411–21.

61. Garcia S, Sandoval Y, Roukoz H, Adabag S, Canoniero M, Yannopoulos D, et al. Outcomes after complete versus incomplete revascularization of patients with multivessel coronary artery disease: a meta-analysis of 89,883 patients enrolled in randomized clinical trials and observational studies. J Am Coll Cardiol. 2013;62(16):1421–31.

62. Ahn JM, Park DW, Lee CW, Chang M, Cavalcante R, Sotomi Y, et al. Comparison of stenting versus bypass surgery according to the completeness of revascularization in severe coronary artery disease: patient-level pooled analysis of the SYNTAX, PRECOMBAT, and BEST trials. JACC Cardiovasc Interv. 2017;10(14):1415–24.

63. Farooq V, Serruys PW, Bourantas CV, Zhang Y, Muramatsu T, Feldman T, et al. Quantification of incomplete revascularization and its association with five-year mortality in the synergy between percutaneous coronary intervention with taxus and cardiac surgery (SYNTAX) trial validation of the residual SYNTAX score. Circulation. 2013;128(2):141–51.

64. O'Neill WW, Kleiman NS, Moses J, Henriques JP, Dixon S, Massaro J, et al. A prospective, randomized clinical trial of hemodynamic support with Impella 2.5 versus intra-aortic balloon pump in patients undergoing high-risk percutaneous coronary intervention: the PROTECT II study. Circulation. 2012;126(14):1717–27.

65. Puskas JD, Halkos ME, DeRose JJ, Bagiella E, Miller MA, Overbey J, et al. Hybrid coronary revascularization for the treatment of multivessel coronary artery disease: a multicenter observational study. J Am Coll Cardiol. 2016;68(4):356–65.

66. Benjamin EJ, Virani SS, Callaway CW, Chamberlain AM, Chang AR, Cheng S, et al. Heart disease and stroke Statistics-2018 update: a report from the American Heart Association. Circulation. 2018;137(12):e67–e492.

67. Farkouh ME, Domanski M, Sleeper LA, Siami FS, Dangas G, Mack M, et al. Strategies for multivessel revascularization in patients with diabetes. N Engl J Med. 2012;367(25):2375–84.

68. Abizaid A, Costa MA, Centemero M, Abizaid AS, Legrand VM, Limet RV, et al. Clinical and economic impact of diabetes mellitus on percutaneous and surgical treatment of multivessel coronary disease patients: insights from the arterial revascularization therapy study (ARTS) trial. Circulation. 2001;104(5):533–8.

69. Bypass Angioplasty Revascularization Investigation (BARI) Investigators. Comparison of coronary bypass surgery with angioplasty in patients with multivessel disease. N Engl J Med. 1996;335(4):217–25.

70. Kappetein AP, Head SJ, Morice MC, Banning AP, Serruys PW, Mohr FW, et al. Treatment of complex coronary artery disease in patients with diabetes: 5-year results comparing outcomes of bypass surgery and percutaneous coronary intervention in the SYNTAX trial. Eur J Cardiothorac Surg. 2013;43(5):1006–13.

71. Cavalcante R, Sotomi Y, Mancone M, Whan Lee C, Ahn JM, Onuma Y, et al. Impact of the SYNTAX scores I and II in patients with diabetes and multivessel coronary disease: a pooled analysis of patient level data from the SYNTAX, PRECOMBAT, and BEST trials. Eur Heart J. 2017;38(25):1969–77.

72. Milojevic M, Serruys PW, Sabik JF 3rd, Kandzari DE, Schampaert E, van Boven AJ, et al. Bypass surgery or stenting for left Main coronary artery disease in patients with diabetes. J Am Coll Cardiol. 2019;73(13):1616–28.

73. Esper RB, Farkouh ME, Ribeiro EE, Hueb W, Domanski M, Hamza TH, et al. SYNTAX Score in Patients With Diabetes Undergoing Coronary Revascularization in the FREEDOM Trial. J Am Coll Cardiol. 2018;72(23 Pt A):2826–37.

74. Velazquez EJ, Lee KL, Deja MA, Jain A, Sopko G, Marchenko A, et al. Coronary-artery bypass surgery in patients with left ventricular dysfunction. N Engl J Med. 2011;364(17):1607–16.

75. Kang SH, Ahn JM, Lee CH, Lee PH, Kang SJ, Lee SW, et al. Differential event rates and independent predictors of long-term major cardiovascular events and death in 5795 patients with unprotected left Main coronary artery disease treated with stents, bypass surgery, or medication: insights from a large international multicenter registry. Circ Cardiovasc Interv. 2017;10(7):e004988.

76. Thuijs D, Milojevic M, Stone GW, Puskas JD, Serruys PW, Sabik JF 3rd, et al. Impact of left ventricular ejection fraction on clinical outcomes after left main coronary artery revascularization: results from the randomized EXCEL trial. Eur J Heart Fail. 2020;22(5):871–9.

77. Nadim MK, Forni LG, Bihorac A, Hobson C, Koyner JL, Shaw A, et al. Cardiac and vascular surgery-associated acute kidney injury: the 20th international consensus conference of the ADQI (acute disease quality initiative). Group J Am Heart Assoc. 2018;7(11):e008834.

78. Mehran R, Dangas GD, Weisbord SD. Contrast-associated acute kidney injury. N Engl J Med. 2019;380(22):2146–55.

79. Baber U, Farkouh ME, Arbel Y, Muntner P, Dangas G, Mack MJ, et al. Comparative efficacy of coronary artery bypass surgery vs. percutaneous coronary intervention in patients with diabetes and multivessel coronary artery disease with or without chronic kidney disease. Eur Heart J. 2016;37(46):3440–7.

80. Milojevic M, Head SJ, Mack MJ, Mohr FW, Morice MC, Dawkins KD, et al. The impact of chronic kidney disease on outcomes following percutaneous coronary intervention versus coronary artery bypass grafting in patients with complex coronary artery disease: five-year follow-up of the SYNTAX trial. EuroIntervention. 2018;14(1):102–11.

81. Giustino G, Mehran R, Serruys PW, Sabik JF 3rd, Milojevic M, Simonton CA, et al. Left Main revascularization with PCI or CABG in patients with chronic kidney disease: EXCEL trial. J Am Coll Cardiol. 2018;72(7):754–65.

82. Valgimigli M, Costa F, Lokhnygina Y, Clare RM, Wallentin L, Moliterno DJ, et al. Trade-off of myocardial infarction vs. bleeding types on mortality after acute coronary syndrome: lessons from the thrombin receptor antagonist for clinical event reduction in acute coronary syndrome (TRACER) randomized trial. Eur Heart J. 2017;38(11):804–10.

83. Urban P, Mehran R, Colleran R, Angiolillo DJ, Byrne RA, Capodanno D, et al. Defining high bleeding risk in patients undergoing percutaneous coronary intervention: a consensus document from the academic Research consortium for high bleeding risk. Eur Heart J. 2019;40(31):2632–53.

84. Dangas G, Baber U, Sharma S, Giustino G, Mehta S, Cohen DJ, et al. Ticagrelor with or without aspirin after complex PCI. J Am Coll Cardiol. 2020;75(19):2414–24.

CABG Should Be the First Option for Left Main Disease: A Cardiac Surgeon's Perspective

5

Guido Gelpi, Claudia Romagnoni, and Irene Binaco

Abbreviations

ACS	Acute coronary syndrome
CABG	Coronary artery bypass grafting
CAD	Coronary artery disease
ISR	Intra-stent restenosis
LAD	Left anterior descending
LM	Left main
MACCE	Major adverse cardiac and cerebro-vascular event
MI	Myocardial infarction
PCI	Percutaneous coronary intervention
SSII	Syntax score II
STS	Society of thoracic surgery
UDMI	Universal definition of myocardial infarction
ULM	Unprotected left main

G. Gelpi (✉)
Cardiac Surgery Department, Fondazione IRCCS Cà Granda Ospedale Maggiore Policlinico, Milan, Italy

Dipartimento di Elettronica, Informazione e Bioingegneria, Politecnico di Milano, Milan, Italy
e-mail: guido.gelpi@policlinico.mi.it

C. Romagnoni · I. Binaco
Cardiac Surgery Department, Fondazione IRCCS Cà Granda Ospedale Maggiore Policlinico, Milan, Italy
e-mail: claudia.romagnoni@policlinico.mi.it;
irene.binaco@policlinico.mi.it

© Springer Nature Switzerland AG 2022
B. Cortese (ed.), *Left Main Coronary Revascularization*,
https://doi.org/10.1007/978-3-031-05265-1_5

5.1 Introduction

The treatment of the left main (LM) disease must be surgical.

This statement has been for a long time, one of the few certainties in the cardiovascular field and one of the most powerful weapons in the hands of cardiac surgeons in their struggle against cardiologists.

Surgeon's self-confidence in stating that was mainly based on some important pathophysiological features that mitigate against the success of percutaneous coronary intervention (PCI) in left main lesions:

1. LM supplies a large area of jeopardized myocardium with a very high ischemic risk.
2. Up to 80% of left main disease involves bifurcation, which is known to be at higher risk of restenosis (Fig. 5.1).
3. Up to 80% of left main patients also have multivessel coronary artery disease, where coronary artery bypass grafting (CABG) offers a survival advantage independent of the presence of LM disease [1–3].

Moreover, compared to percutaneous stenosis treatment, surgical bypass allows to protect longer tracts of coronary artery vessels from the possible subsequent appearance of new proximal stenosis (Fig. 5.2) and in situ left internal mammary artery grafting has been demonstrated to be able to adjust blood flow in case of stenosis worsening [4].

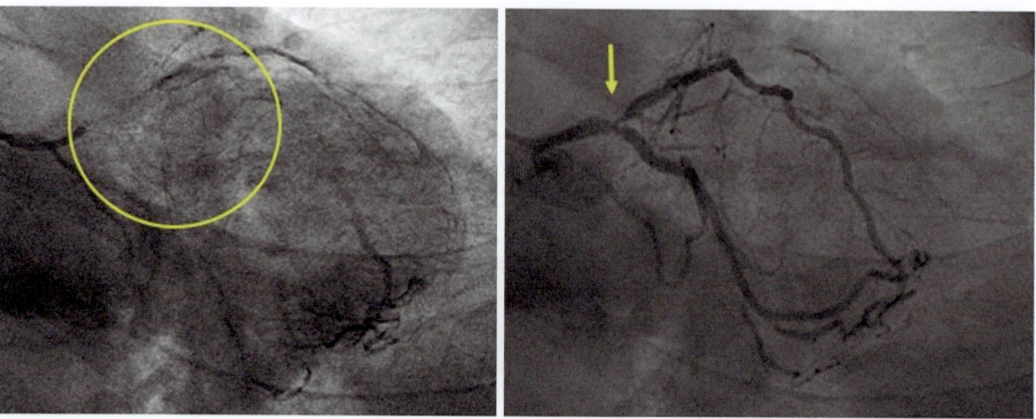

Fig. 5.1 Left main bifurcation intra-stent restenosis; on the left LM bifurcation stent (yellow circle), on the right intra-stent restenosis in the same patient (yellow arrow)

These are some of the reasons why left main pathology has been prerogative of the cardiac surgeon for a long time and both 2018 European [5] and 2011 American [6] guidelines strongly recommend (Class I) CABG as the treatment of choice for unprotected left main disease (ULM) while PCI could be considered as an alternative only depending on the anatomical complexity of the coronary artery disease and the surgical risk of the patients (Table 5.1).

These recommendations were based mainly on the results of the LM subgroup analysis of the 5 years results of the SYNTAX trial (Synergy Between Percutaneous Coronary Intervention with TAXUS and Cardiac Surgery) [7, 8] where no significant differences have been highlighted in rates of major adverse cardiac and cerebrovascular event (MACCE; 37% vs. 31%), mortality (13% vs. 15%) or myocardial infarction (MI) (8% vs. 5%) between PCI and CABG. However, the 5 years rate of repeat revascularization was higher in the PCI group (27% vs. 16%). In a stratified analysis based on baseline SYNTAX score, the rate of MACCE was similar between PCI and CABG in the lower 2 SYNTAX score tertiles (0–32) (31% vs. 32%). In contrast, in the group with high SYNTAX scores (≥33), MACCE occurred significantly more commonly in the PCI than in the CABG group (47% vs. 30%).

As in almost all areas, technologies improvement has, nowadays, called this dogma into question. The necessity to be competitive and less invasive in order to reduce the impact on patient's life and to reduce the hospital stay led to the development of always new drug-eluting stents (DES), technique and antithrombotic strategies with unexpected results, and many different studies have been designed comparing PCI and CABG with the aim of demonstrating the equivalence of these two techniques.

However, the results of the two landmark clinical trials conducted with the second-generation DES, the Evaluation of XIENCE Everolimus Eluting Stent Versus Coronary Artery Bypass Surgery for Effectiveness of Left Main Revascularization (EXCEL) and the Nordic-Baltic-British Left Main Revascularization Study (NOBLE), appear contradictory [9, 10]. Despite different inclusion criteria (NOBLE did not adopt a baseline SYNTAX score as a prespecified inclusion criteria but, instead, excluded patients with more than three additional non-complex coronary lesions or complex additional coronary lesions) and different primary composite endpoint (EXCEL adopted the clinically "harder" endpoint of all-cause death, MI, or stroke, while NOBLE adopted MACCE including all-cause death, non-procedural MI, stroke, or repeat revascularization), EXCEL reported that PCI is noninferior to CABG while NOBLE reported that CABG is superior to PCI. Careful interpretation of these data is required. Differences in results could be explained by many factors as the specific expertise of the interventional cardiologists and cardiac surgeons who performed the procedures or the different stent platform used

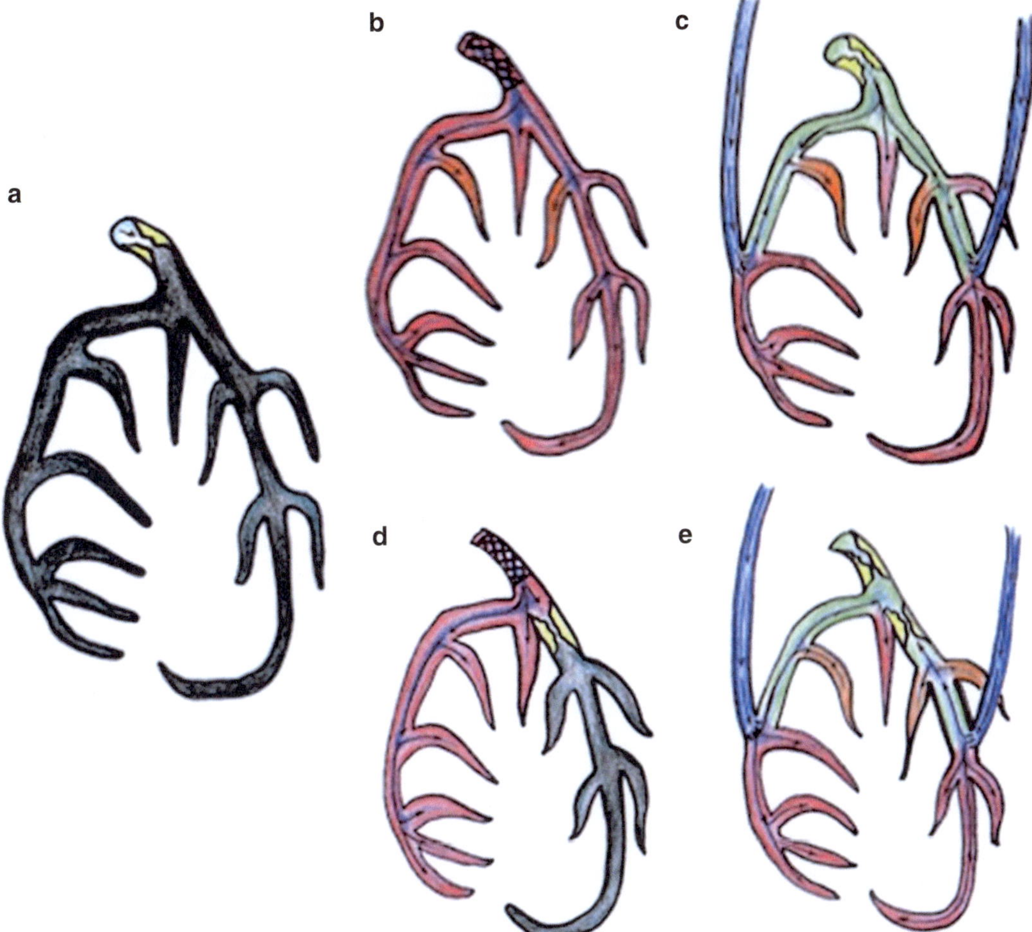

Fig. 5.2 Drawing showing how surgical bypass protects a major tract of coronary artery from the subsequent appearance of new stenosis: left main disease (**a**) treated with stent implantation (**b**) or double coronary artery bypass (**c**); new proximal anterior descending artery stenosis in the above patients treated with PTCA (**d**) and CABG (**e**). In gray the coronary arteries not supplied by full flow in case of coronary stenosis; in red, the tract of coronary artery non-protected, and, in green, the tract protected from the subsequent appearance of new proximal stenosis by the two different techniques; in orange, the branches usually not treated (acute margin and septal branches). Black arrows show the blood flow (blue) direction

Table 5.1 Summary table of 2018 ESC/EACTS recommendations for left main myocardial revascularization in patients with stable coronary artery disease

Left main disease	CABG	PCI
Left main disease with syntax score 0–22	I A	I A
Left main disease with syntax score 23–32	I A	II A
Left main disease with syntax score > 32	I A	IIIB

for the PCI but recently some shades are rising over the 5 years results of the EXCEL trial [11].

In December 2019, an unprecedented event happened: the European Association for Cardio-Thoracic Surgery withdrew its support for the left main disease recommendation exposed in the 2018 ESC-EACTS Myocardial Revascularization Guidelines.

Such a heavy choice was mainly due to a more complete understanding of the 3 years data from EXCEL [9], compared to the scientific evidence present at the time of 2018 guidelines draft: using the standard definition of a myocardial infarction the perceived advantage/non-inferiority of PCI compared with CABG for LM disease was reversed; moreover, the 5 years EXCEL data [11] have demonstrated a significant survival advantage for CABG over PCI for this group of patients.

Obviously, this move promoted a hard debate between surgeons and cardiologists represented, respectively, by D. Taggart and G. Stone.

The core of the controversy mainly concerned:

1. The rate of MI.

   Trial authors have not published the rate of MI, identified, according to the Universal Definition of Myocardial Infarction (UDMI), by a troponin (or, in alternative, CK-MB) increase despite it was listed in the study protocol as secondary endpoint. EXCEL authors tried to uphold this choice stating that troponin assessment was optional and infrequently performed; an attempt was made to assess UDMI rates using troponins in some patients and CK-MB measures in others (the latter having been collected with high compliance) but this was not scientifically sound given the different sensitivities of the two biomarkers. However, the study was not amended to reflect the decision not to publish this data and this represents a breach of the consolidated standards of reporting trials and good clinical practice guidelines

2. The all-cause mortality data was not strongly enough emphasized.

   When UDMI is used, PCI is associated with substantially worse outcomes at 3 years with a significantly higher risk of MI than CABG (HR 1.79, 95% CI 1.25–2.57; P = 0.002) and a 40% increased risk for all-cause death and stroke (HR 1.40, 95% CI 1.09–1.81; P = 0.009). This analysis is predictive of the published 5-year EXCEL results which show a 35% increased risk of death in the PCI group (Odds Ratio 1.38, 95% CI 1.03–1.85). Trial authors replied that while there were more deaths in the PCI arm, the study was not powered for mortality and the modest difference noted between groups was not adjusted for multiplicity so it was statistically uncertain; moreover, the difference was largely due to non-cardiovascular causes (especially cancer and infections), occurring several years after the index procedure.

3. Trial investigators downplayed concerns from the data and safety monitoring board about an increased mortality for the PCI group

   This kind of information would have led to a different conversation around the choice of guideline recommendation. Clearly, EXCEL leadership adamantly denied, stating that the board recommended that the study continue as planned without modifications.

4. Alleged conflicts of interest.

   Public concerns have arisen over potential commercial conflicts of interests but to state that hundreds of investigators, including cardiologists, surgeons, statisticians, and entire academic research organizations conspired to change definitions or withhold important study findings would perhaps be excessive.

Beyond the controversy, we must keep in mind that, up to date, the EXCEL trial finally defines only the non-inferiority of PCI compared to CABG for the patients with left main disease, that the limited follow-up could have penalized the CABG group and that the rate of repeated revascularization is higher in case of PCI (16.9 vs 10%). This doesn't mean that CABG is always the right choice in the case of LM disease but that overall comparative results should be interpreted with caution and cannot be considered definitively clinically directive. Probably, despite the need for operative guidelines, the most reasonable approach calls for a heart team that could evaluate every single case, considering patient's age, frailty, anatomical features, surgical risk, and clinical presentation.

5.2 When PCI Is the Better Choice?

For several decades, CABG was regarded as the standard of care for significant left main disease in patients eligible for surgery, particularly when the proximal left anterior descending (LAD) coronary artery was involved.

However, the innovation of second-generation stents and the development of cross-stenting techniques have implemented the effectiveness of PCI even for the treatment of left main disease [12].

In fact, many trials in the last 10 years have shown equal efficacy of PCI and CABG in the treatment of obstructive coronary artery disease. PCI and CABG have demonstrated equivalent results, in the medium term, for risk of mortality, stroke, and recurrence of symptoms; however, most clinical studies demonstrate a higher incidence of need for new revascularization in patients undergoing PCI; this evidence is prevalent in patients with left main disease and multivessel coronary artery disease (CAD) with high syntax score [3, 10, 11, 13]. Therefore, current European guidelines recommend both CABG and PCI for the treatment of left main coronary artery stenosis in patients with overall low to intermediate complexity of coronary artery disease while CABG is the first choice for all patients with left main disease or CAD with high syntax score [5]. As cardiac surgeons, we obviously agree with this CABG supremacy but, even for us, there are some cases in which we think that surgical intervention is not the best option and PCI should be preferred.

While in patients with stable angina and recurrence of symptoms despite optimal drug therapy there is general consensus in favoring the indication for surgical revascularization, especially in the presence of multivessel coronary artery disease with involvement of left main [3, 5, 14], the indication in acute coronary syndrome (ACS) is more debated. It is proven, in fact, that in acute coronary syndromes, the time of ischemia represents an important factor for the patient's prognosis. In these cases an early risk stratification is important in order to identify patients at high immediate risk for death and cardiovascular events.

In high-risk patients (refractory angina, severe heart failure, cardiogenic shock, or hemodynamic instability) early catheterization, followed by coronary intervention, reduces the risk of recurrent ACS and shortens hospital stay. Culprit lesion PCI is usually the first choice in most patients with ACS and multivessel disease. In the ACUITY (Acute Catheterization and Urgent Intervention Triage Strategy) trial, PCI-treated patients had lower rates of periprocedural stroke, MI, bleeding, and kidney injury, but significantly higher rates of unplanned revascularization at both 1 month and 1 year [15]. For this reason, when there is continuing or recurrent ischemia, hemodynamic instability, pulmonary edema, or total occlusion of the culprit coronary artery requiring urgent revascularization, PCI is reasonable and safe for the treatment of the culprit lesion. In these cases even the hybrid approach can be used thanks, above all, to the introduction of stents that need limited double antiplatelet therapy, allowing reduced time for the completion of the surgical revascularization. PCI can also be considered as a preferable option in patients at high risk for surgery due to elderly age, comorbidities, and previous cardiac surgery. PCI in these patients presents a lower risk of bleeding and periprocedural complications, promoting postoperative recovery and reducing hospital stay; however, it presents higher risk of necessity for repeat revascularization at medium term. In this highly comorbid population the choice of the best revascularization strategy should be based on patient surgical risk assessed by Society of Thoracic Surgery (STS) score or EuroSCORE II, frailty, life expectancy, and anatomical complexity measured by SYNTAX score.

Moreover, the management of recurring or persisting angina after coronary revascularization is challenging. Early and late graft failure are the major causes of resistant or recurrent angina after surgical revascularization. In a meta-analysis of nine studies of CABG, the rate of recurrent angina at 16 months was 8.9% with a repeat revascularization rate of 4.7% [16]. For these reasons it is reasonable to proceed with repeated revascularization in symptomatic patients with left main disease, three-vessel CAD or a patent left internal mammary artery to the left anterior descending artery and ischemia in the distribution of the right or left circumflex coronary arteries [17].

Progression of CAD can paradoxically lead to a lower likelihood of repeat surgical revascularization given the lack of adequate target vessels.

In these patients repeated cardiac surgery presents, also, a high risk of iatrogenic damage of the patent mammary artery graft during the new sternotomy. Repeat CABG is burden by a significant increase in morbidity and mortality so, in these patients PCI is often preferred for its lower invasiveness and periprocedural morbidity. However, due to procedural difficulties and incidence of complications, any attempt to treat the native artery should be done if feasible, considering that procedures may be required not only in the segment proximal to the graft insertion site but also distally [16].

5.3 When Surgery Is the Better Choice?

As already stated, based on the latest ESC/EACTS guidelines on myocardial revascularization, CABG is a well-established and proved, over long term, therapy for all patients with left main disease [5]. CABG is class I level A for all patients with left main disease independently on the anatomical coronary lesion defined by Syntax score. The decision to submit LM patient to surgery will be always the right one, supported by guidelines. Moreover, there are subgroups of patients with unprotected left main where surgery is still the only therapeutic option: patients with high Syntax score ($\geq$33) and patients with concomitant valve disease that need surgical correction.

The most recent randomized studies advocate non-inferior results of PCI compared to CABG; in the EXCEL trial the 4 years [18] primary composite major adverse cardiac event endpoint of death, myocardial infarction, or stroke was similar after PCI with everolimus-eluting stents and CABG. The same endpoint was independent of the baseline anatomic complexity or the extent of CAD. However, the relative and absolute hazard of major adverse cardiac or cerebrovascular events with PCI compared with CABG rose progressively with the Syntax Score, so coronary features of LM lesion is one of the most important characteristics that must be considered for treatment deci-

sion. For this reason, a patient with LM disease with intermediate Syntax Score (23–32), with low surgery risk should undergo surgery as the first choice. The new guidelines suggest, for this intermediate Syntax Score patient, PCI treatment as an alternative to surgery with a class IIA, suggesting that, whereas surgery is not feasible, PCI can be performed. For interventional cardiologists, anatomical complexity lesion of the left main has been the key point, particularly in the recent years, to drive the patient to surgery or to PCI regardless of the patient surgical risk score. In a recent meta-analysis, aggregate data from 6 trials totaling 4700 patients randomized to CABG or PCI were analyzed. At a mean follow-up ranging from 2.33 to 5 years, PCI was associated with a significantly higher risk of a composite of death/myocardial infarction/stroke/repeat revascularization. Data were analyzed also with meta-regression and, again, a higher mean SYNTAX score was associated with a higher risk of the primary outcome in the PCI group (p = 0.05) [19].

Coronary lesion in ULM patients is not the only characteristic that should be considered for the best treatment decision but also other aspects should be taken into account. In fact, it is well known that diabetic patients are more prone to develop more extensive multivessel coronary artery disease than non-diabetic patients and, as elucidated in the FREEDOM Follow-On study [20], CABG versus PCI has a significantly fewer death with a median follow-up of 7.5 years in patients with multivessel disease. For this reason, 2018 ESC/EACTS guidelines still advocate CABG for three-vessel CAD with diabetes mellitus independently on Syntax Score [5]. However, recent trials on ULM treatment didn't show any significant difference between PCI and CABG in the subgroup of diabetic patients [11]. Are these results biased by a too short follow-up or LM stenosis is a different coronary disease compared to multivessel CAD? In the EXCEL trial among both diabetic and non-diabetic patients, with LM disease and SYNTAX scores low-to-intermediate (<32), PCI using everolimus-eluting stent and CABG resulted in similar rates of the primary composite endpoint of death, stroke, or MI. Based on these results, many authors suggested that diabetic patients with LM disease and relatively non-complex coronary anatomy could benefit from PCI, whereas CABG could be considered for diabetic patients with more complex CAD [21]. However, although in the EXCEL trial design, randomization was stratified by diabetes status, and the diabetes subgroup analysis was pre-specified, the data presented were not powered to detect a difference in the primary endpoint of death, stroke, or MI between PCI and CABG in the diabetic cohort, and secondary outcome measures were not adjusted for multiple comparisons. Only in the limitation of the study authors pointed out that the results presented on these subgroup of EXCEL patients should be interpreted as hypothesis-generating only [21]. The paper conclusions drove to the non-inferiority of PCI compared to CABG, also in the subgroup of LM diabetic patients but this statement seems misleading. Moreover, patients with insulin-dependent diabetes mellitus appeared at higher risk of restenosis after PCI. Despite improvement in techniques and advance in the safety and efficacy profile of DES, this population is still burdened by high risk of repeated procedures, with an increase, although not significant, toward adverse prognosis. Interestingly, in a recent short report of a post hoc analysis from the large, international, multicenter DELTA-2 (Drug Eluting Stent for Left Main Coronary Artery) registry that investigates the outcomes associated with LM-PCI of intra-stent restenosis (ISR) compared with de novo lesions, highlighted that intra-stent restenosis patients were more likely to have diabetes (51.8% vs. 34.2%; p < 0.0001) [22]. Only further investigation in dedicated trials for diabetic patients will show if this subgroup with left main stenosis has similar progression and complexity of coronary artery disease as non-diabetic ULM ones. Recent trials for unprotected left main did not show any significant difference between PCI and CABG, also in the female gender group.

In the SYNTAX trial, sex had a significant interaction effect with revascularization strategy, and women had an overall higher mortality when treated with PCI than CABG; women undergoing PCI had a higher adjusted 4 years risk for mortality than men, whereas CABG outcomes were comparable between the sexes [23]. In the 3 years EXCEL trial women presented a lower SYNTAX scores related to an overall less anatomic complexity than men, with fewer left main bifurcation lesions, less concomitant multivessel disease, and a greater chance for a complete revascularization after PCI. However, the rate of PCI-related ischemic and hemorrhagic complications was more frequent in women than men; after 30 days and 3 years a significant interaction between treatment and sex for the outcome of myocardial infarction (MI) was present and the relative risk for MI (in particular periprocedural MI) tended to be higher after PCI in women [24]. The EXCEL trial demonstrated significantly higher all-cause mortality in women undergoing PCI than in women undergoing CABG and men treated with either PCI or CABG. However, in EXCEL, sex was not independently related to mortality and revascularization strategy. In the conclusions, the authors pointed out that in selected patients with ULM disease and low and intermediate SYNTAX scores undergoing revascularization, women had a higher prevalence of clinical risk factors but less coronary anatomic burden and complexity than men. Women had more PCI-related complications than men and the highest rate of all-cause death, stroke, and MI at 30 days [24]. The 5 years data are not yet available for this subgroup but, as for diabetic patients, previous trial, with longer follow-up, have shown robust evidence in favor of CABG.

Despite the limits of PCI in the treatment of LM disease, the daily practice is nowadays leading to the increasing widespread of this treatment therefore we expect to see an increase also in the number of restenosis (Fig. 5.3).

The overall incidence of LM restenosis and target lesion restenosis showed a wide variation ranging respectively between 0.9%–19% and 2%–16.1%, depending on the methodology used, as pointed out analyzing 18 studies (nearly 6000 pts) by De Caterina et al. [25]. When a LM restenosis is discovered, there is little room for a conservative approach, because a significant stenosis in this segment is associated with poor outcome.

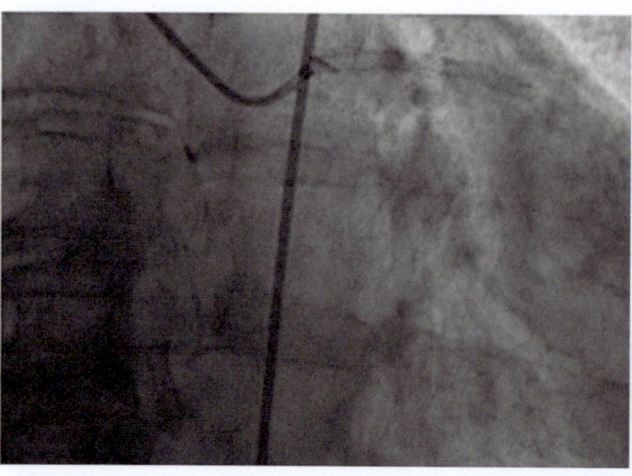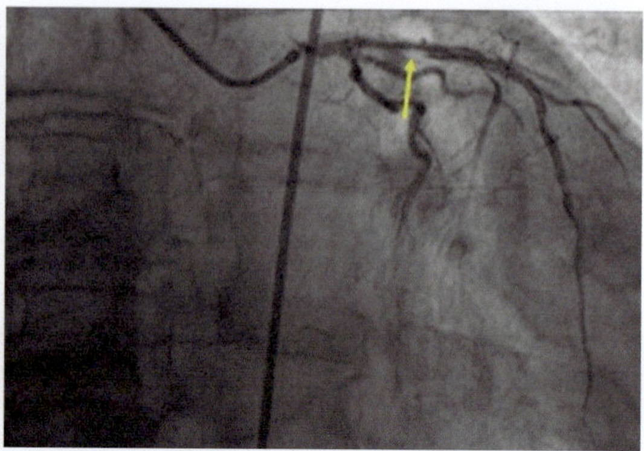

Fig. 5.3 Example of left main intrastent restenosis involving the origin of left anterior descending artery. On the left the stent, on the right the intra-stent restenosis in the same patient (yellow arrow)

ISR after DES implantation for unprotected LM lesions continues to occur, with such lesions being more clinically problematic compared with other coronary lesions. In addition, the incidence of ISR after DES implantation for unprotected LM disease has not been sufficiently evaluated in large numbers of studies, and the long-term prognosis of such patients has not been explored.

There are currently available limited data on the optimal management of LM restenosis, and the few available, all driven by interventional cardiologists, seem to indicate a good outcome with the implantation of second-generation DES [25]. Moreover, adding further metal struts to an often-complex bifurcation seems not an attractive solution for the problem. The choice of treatment strategy (medical therapy, repeated PCI, or CABG) for left main ISR lesions depends on several clinical and angiographic factors. In this regard, young patients presenting with LM stenosis should deserve a particular consideration. It is true that this group of patients is more prone to have single LM coronary lesion, rarely associated with multiple coronary lesions, that could achieve complete revascularization with PCI. However, the risk of restenosis after PCI for LM, as previously described, is not negligible and young patients usually do not have comorbidities that contraindicate or add risk to a surgical revascularization. In particular, in case of single LM lesion, young patients can benefit, in our opinion, from complete arterial revascularization with in situ double internal mammary arteries.

5.4 Conclusions

In summary, coronary artery bypass graft is still the gold standard therapy for patients with LM disease and intra-stent restenosis. CABG is the optimal therapeutic solution for LM patient due to the chance, for the surgeon, to perform a complete revascularization of major myocardial territories giving to the patient the best coronary flow to the ischemic myocardial area. In the last decade, cardiac surgeons have implemented the use of the so-called "off-pump" technique to perform CABG avoiding the possible side effects of cardiopulmonary bypass. The increase of the use of all arterial grafts (double mammary arteries or radial artery) for CABG has also guaranteed a better long-term surgical outcome. In particular, as outlined by EXCEL trial data, the 3 years rates of MACCE after surgical revascularization for LM coronary lesion improved between the performance of the SYNTAX and EXCEL trials. This improvement underlies why the relative outcomes of CABG versus PCI for the treatment of LM disease remained consistent over time despite the use of superior PCI devices and technique in the EXCEL trial compared with the SYNTAX trial. Moreover, in the EXCEL trial, the improvement of CABG procedures for LM coronary disease is supported by a primary outcome lower compared with the SYNTAX trial despite a significantly larger number of patients undergoing either emergent or urgent procedures (that can carry a worse prognosis [26].

Another key point for optimal patient outcome is operator volume, both for surgical and endovascular treatment. A single-center study of 1948 patients who underwent unprotected LM PCI, performed by 25 operators over a 7-year period, showed reduced 30 days and 3 years mortality for patients who had their PCI performed by a high-volume operator (defined as $\geq$15 LM PCI/year; mean 25/year) vs. a low-volume operator (<15 LM PCI/year) [27]. In this regard, the 2018 EACTS/ESC guidelines have added a new suggestion, with class IIa level C to consider that PCI for LM should be performed by trained operators with an annual volume of $\geq$25 LM PCI cases per year. Moreover, guidelines suggest that it should be considered that non-emergency high-risk PCI procedures, such as for LM disease, should be only performed by adequately experienced operators at centers that have access to circulatory support and intensive care treatment. These new suggestions highlight once more the importance to drive LM patients in high-volume hospitals where the heart team is available on site and the best treatment option can be chosen.

The heart team approach is vital to guide the management of patients with LM disease, when there is obvious clinical equipoise and a mandate for complete revascularization. The selection between the two alternatives should thus rely on assessment of the patient's comorbidities and anatomic characteristics, as well as physician and patient preferences, through a comprehensive heart team discussion. With an aging and increasing co-morbid patient population, clinical equipoise may not always be obvious, making extrapolation of clinical trial results to the "real world" difficult [28]. In this context, the need for a comprehensive patient evaluation method is evident but the TAVI (Transcatheter Aortic Valve Implantation) experience already highlighted the lack of an appropriate risk score, able to combine patient frailty, life expectancy, and comorbidities with anatomical characteristics and procedural features. The same problem subsists for the left main disease. Euroscore and STS scores mainly focus on surgical risk while the Syntax score deals with coronary anatomy in a percutaneous treatment perspective. Probably the perfect score doesn't exist because of too many variables to be considered but, for the moment, a good compromise seems to be the Syntax Score II (SSII), which combines both anatomical and clinical data. SSII proved to be superior to the syntax score in predicting long-term outcomes associated with left main PCI in the FAILS-2 registry and non-compliance with SSII CABG treatment recommendations was associated with higher 4 years all-cause mortality in the excel trial [29–31]. Waiting for an improved score, the heart team could benefit from the SSII use for the evaluation of every single patient in order to choose the best-tailored treatment option for each one conscious that only a full and true cooperation between the interventional cardiologist and the cardiac surgeon will provide the optimal therapeutic strategies for the more and more complex left main patients.

References

1. Park SJ, Kim YH, Park DW, Yun SC, Ahn JM, Song HG, Lee JY, Kim WJ, Kang SJ, Lee SW, Lee CW, Park SW, Chung CH, Lee JW, Lim DS, Rha SW, Lee SG, Gwon HC, Kim HS, Chae IH, Jang Y, Jeong MH, Tahk SJ, Seung KB. Randomized trial of stents vs. bypass surgery for left main coronary artery disease. N Engl J Med. 2011;364(18):1718–27.
2. Taggart DP, Kaul S, Boden WE, Ferguson TB Jr, Guyton RA, Mack MJ, Sergeant PT, Shemin RJ, Smith PK, Yusuf S. Revascularization for unprotected left main stem coronary artery stenosis stenting or surgery. J Am Coll Cardiol. 2008;51(9):885–92.
3. Morice MC, Serruys PW, Kappetein AP, Feldman TE, Stahle E, Colombo A, Mack MJ, Holmes DR, Choi JW, Ruzyllo W, Religa G, Huang J, Roy K, Dawkins KD, Mohr F. Five-year outcomes in patients with left Main disease treated with either percutaneous coronary intervention or coronary artery bypass grafting in the SYNTAX trial. Circulation. 2014;129: 2388–94.
4. Höltgen R, Krijne R, Heinrich KW, Sons H, Krian A. Internal mammary artery bypass grafting in left main stenosis. Cardiology. 1993;82(5):343–6.
5. Neumann FJ, Sousa-Uva M, Ahlsson A, Alfonso F, Banning AP, Benedetto U, Byrne RA, Collet JP, Falk V, Head SJ, Jüni P, Kastrati A, Koller A, Kristensen SD, Niebauer J, Richter DJ, Seferovic PM, Sibbing D, Stefanini GG, Windecker S, Yadav R, Zembala MO, ESC Scientific Document Group. 2018 ESC/EACTS Guidelines on myocardial revascularization. Eur Heart J. 2019;40(2):87–165.

6. Hillis LD, Smith PK, Anderson JL, Bittl JA, Bridges CR, Byrne JG, et al. 2011 ACCF/AHA guideline for coronary artery bypass graft surgery. A report of the American College of Cardiology Foundation/American Heart Association task force on practice guidelines. Developed in collaboration with the American Association for Thoracic Surgery, Society of Cardiovascular Anesthesiologists, and Society of Thoracic Surgeons. J Am Coll Cardiol. 2011;58:e123–210.

7. Morice MC, Serruys PW, Kappetein AP, et al. Outcomes in patients with de novo left main disease treated with either percutaneous coronary intervention using paclitaxel-eluting stents or coronary artery bypass graft treatment in the synergy between percutaneous coronary intervention with TAXUS and cardiac surgery (SYNTAX) trial. Circulation. 2010;121:2645–53.

8. Morice MC, Serruys PW, Kappetein AP, et al. Five-year outcomes in patients with left main disease treated with either percutaneous coronary intervention or coronary artery bypass grafting in the synergy between percutaneous coronary intervention with taxus and cardiac surgery trial. Circulation. 2014;129:2388–94.

9. Stone GW, Sabik JF, Serruys PW, et al. Everolimus-eluting stents or bypass surgery for left Main coronary artery disease. N Engl J Med. 2016;375:2223–35.

10. Makikallio T, Holm NR, Lindsay M, et al. Percutaneous coronary angioplasty versus coronary artery bypass grafting in treatment of unprotected left main stenosis (NOBLE): a prospective, randomised, open-label, non-inferiority trial. Lancet. 2016;388:2743–52.

11. Stone GW, Kappetein AP, Sabik JF, Pocock SJ, Morice M-C, Puskas J, Kandzari DE, et al. Five-year outcomes after PCI or CABG for left main coronary disease. N Engl J Med. 2019;381:1820–30.

12. Morris PD, Iqbal J, Chiastra C, Wu W, Migliavacca F, Gunn JP. Simultaneous kissing stents to treat unprotected left main stem coronary artery bifurcation disease; stent expansion, vessel injury, hemodynamics, tissue healing, restenosis, and repeat revascularization. Catheter Cardiovasc Interv. 2018;92(6):E381–92.

13. Giacoppo D, Colleran R, Cassese S, Frangieh AH, Wiebe J, Joner M, Schunkert H, Kastrati A, Byrne RA. Percutaneous coronary intervention vs coronary artery bypass grafting in patients with left Main coronary artery stenosis. A Systematic Review and Meta-analysis. JAMA Cardiol. 2017;2(10):1079–88.

14. Lancaster TS, Schill MR, Greenberg JW, Ruaengsri C, Schuessler RB, Lawton JS, Maniar HS, Pasque MK, Moon MR, Damiano RJ Jr, Melby SJ. Long-term survival prediction for coronary artery bypass grafting: validation of the ASCERT model compared with the Society of Thoracic Surgeons predicted risk of mortality. Ann Thorac Surg. 2018;105(5):1336–43.

15. Meadows ES, Bae JP, Zagar A, Sugihara T, Ramaswamy K, McCracken R, Heiselman D. Rehospitalization following percutaneous coronary intervention for commercially insured patients with acute coronary syndrome: a retrospective analysis. BMC Res Notes. 2012;5:342.

16. Abbate A, Biondi-Zoccai GGL, Agostoni P, Lipinski MJ, Vetrovec JV. Recurrent angina after coronary revascularization: a clinical challenge. Eur Heart J. 2007;28:1057–65.

17. Locker C, Greiten LE, Bell MR, Frye RL, Lerman A, Daly RC, Greason KL, Said SM, Lahr BD, Stulak JM, Dearani JA, Schaff HV. Repeat coronary bypass surgery or percutaneous coronary intervention after previous surgical revascularization. Mayo Clin Proc. 2019;94(9):1743–52.

18. Shlofmits E, Généreux P, Chen S, Dressler O, Ben-Yehuda O, Morice MC, Puskas JD, Taggart DP, Kandzari DE, Crowley A, Redfors B, Mehdipoor G, Kappetein AP, Sabik JF III, Serruys PW, Stone GW. Left main coronary artery disease revascularization according to the SYNTAX score. Circ Cardiovasc Interv. 2019;12(9):e008007.

19. Rahouma M, Abouarab A, Di Franco A, Leonard JR, Lau C, Kamel M, Ohmes LB, Girardi LN, Gaudino M. Percutaneous coronary intervention versus coronary bypass surgery for unprotected left main disease: a meta-analysis of randomized controlled trials. Ann Cardiothorac Surg. 2018;7(4):454–62.

20. Farkouh ME, Domanski M, Dangas GD, Godoy LC, Mack MJ, Siami FS, Hamza TH, Shah B, Stefanini GG, Sidhu MS, Tanguay JF, Ramanathan K, Sharma SK, French J, Hueb W, Cohen DJ, Fuster V. FREEDOM follow-on study investigators. Long-term survival following multivessel revascularization in patients with diabetes: the FREEDOM follow-on study. J Am Coll Cardiol. 2019;73(6):629–38.

21. Milojevic M, Serruys PW, Sabik JF 3rd, Kandzari DE, Schampaert E, van Boven AJ, Horkay F, Ungi I, Mansour S, Banning AP, Taggart DP, Sabaté M, Gershlick AH, Bochenek A, Pomar J, Lembo NJ, Noiseux N, Puskas JD, Crowley A, Kosmidou I, Mehran R, Ben-Yehuda O, Généreux P, Pocock SJ, Simonton CA, Stone GW, Kappetein AP. Bypass surgery or stenting for left Main coronary artery disease in patients with diabetes. J AM Col Cardiol. 2019;73(13):1616–28.

22. Giustino G, Tanaka A, Erglis A, Morice MC, Van Mieghem NM, Meliga E, D'Ascenzo F, Stefanini GG, Capodanno D, Chieffo A. DELTA-2 investigators. New-generation drug-eluting stents for left Main in-stent restenosis: the DELTA-2 registry. JACC Cardiovasc Interv. 2018;11(23):2438–40.

23. Farooq V, Serruys PW, Bourantas C, Vranckx P, Diletti R, Garcia Garcia HM, Holmes DR, Kappetein AP, Mack M, Feldman T, Morice MC, Colombo A, Morel MA, de Vries T, van Es GA, Steyerberg EW, Dawkins KD, Mohr FW, James S, Ståhle E. Incidence and multivariable correlates of long-term mortality in patients treated with surgical or percutaneous revascularization in the synergy between percutaneous coronary intervention with Taxus and cardiac surgery (SYNTAX) trial. Eur Heart J. 2012;33:3105–13.

24. Serruys PW, Cavalcante R, Collet C, Kappetein AP, Sabik JF 3rd, Banning AP, Taggart DP, Sabaté M, Pomar J, Boonstra PW, Lembo NJ, Onuma Y, Simonton CA, Morice MC, McAndrew T, Dressler O, Stone GW. Outcomes after coronary stenting or bypass surgery for men and women with unprotected left Main disease the EXCEL trial. JACC Cardiovasc Interv. 2018;11(13):1234–43.

25. De Caterina AR, Cuculi F, Banning AP. Incidence, predictors and management of left main coronary artery stent restenosis: a comprehensive review in the era of drug- eluting stents. EuroIntervention. 2013;8:1326–34.

26. Modolo R, Chichareon P, Kogame N, Dressler O, Crowley A, Ben-Yehuda O, Puskas J, Banning A, Taggart DP, Kappetein AP, Sabik JA, Onuma Y, Stone GW, Serruys PW. Contemporary outcomes following coronary artery bypass graft surgery for left Main disease. J Am Coll Cardiol. 2019;73(15):1877–86.

27. Xu B, Redfors B, Yang Y, Qiao S, Wu Y, Chen J, Liu H, Chen J, Xu L, Zhao Y. Outcomes after left main coronary artery percutaneous coronary intervention. JACC Cardiovasc Interv. 2016;9:2086–93.

28. Kassimis G, Raina T, Kontogiannis N, Krasopoulos G, Gunn J. Percutaneous or surgical revascularization for left main stem disease: NOBLE ideas, but do they EXCEL? Expert Rev Cardiovasc Ther. 2019;17(5):361–8.

29. Yang H, Zhang L, Xu CH. Use of the SYNTAX score II to predict mortality in interventional cardiology: a systematic review and meta-analysis. Medicine (Baltimore). 2019;98(2):e14043.

30. Cerrato E, Barbero U, Quadri G, Ryan N, D'Ascenzo F, Tomassini F, Quirós A, Bellucca S, Conrotto F, Ugo F, Kawamoto H, Rolfo C, Pavani M, Mejia-Renteria H, Gili S, Iannaccone M, Debenedictis M, Baldassarre D, Biondi-Zoccai G, Colombo A, Varbella F, Escaned J. Prediction of long-term patient outcome after contemporary left main stenting using the SYNTAXand SYNTAX II scores: A comparative analysis from the FAIL-II multicenter registry (failure in left main study with 2nd generation stents-Cardiogroup III study). Catheter Cardiovasc Interv. 2019; https://doi.org/10.1002/ccd.28468. [Epub ahead of print]

31. Modolo R, Chichareon P, van Klaveren D, Dressler O, Zhang Y, Sabik JF, Onuma Y, Kappetein AP, Stone GW, Serruys PW. Impact of non-respect of SYNTAX score II recommendation for surgery in patients with left main coronary artery disease treated by percutaneous coronary intervention: an EXCEL sub-study. Eur J Cardiothorac Surg. 2019; https://doi.org/10.1093/ejcts/ezz274. [Epub ahead of print]. pii: ezz274

PCI Should Be the First Option for All Left Main Disease? An Interventional Cardiologist's Perspective

Daniel A. Jones, Anthony Mathur, and Andreas Baumbach

6.1 Introduction

Revascularization for significant left main stem (LMS) coronary artery disease (CAD) has been the standard of care for more than 30 years. Coronary artery bypass grafting (CABG) has traditionally been considered the gold standard therapy for LMS disease due to historical data, the technical challenges (calcium, major bifurcation, burden of atherosclerotic disease), and the excellent results achieved using the left internal mammary artery graft to the left anterior descending artery. However, percutaneous coronary intervention (PCI) is being increasingly performed as an alternative. Advances in stent technology, use of intravascular imaging, mechanical support and potent anti-platelet agents have improved outcomes and levelled the playing field between PCI and CABG. PCI is now an established safe and effective option for LMS disease, and in certain circumstances could and should be the first option. This chapter will discuss these circumstances evaluating current evidence, and its limitations alongside PCI technique, strategy and advances.

6.2 Not all LMS Disease is the Same

LMS disease is associated with a poor prognosis with medical therapy, given the large myocardial territory at risk (ranging from 75–100% of the myocardium depending on the coronary dominance) LMS disease is therefore a challenging subset for PCI, although this is dependent on the anatomical location with mid-shaft lesions reasonably straightforward to treat, but are typically uncommon. Instead, disease more typically involves the aorto-ostium with heavy calcification, or most frequently the distal bifurcation. This is associated with the technical challenges of any bifurcation lesion but with the added risk that the "side branch" is a major epicardial vessel, a particular problem in left-dominant circulations. Consequently, the large mass of myocardium subtended by the LMS may cause haemodynamic collapse during intervention.

D. A. Jones (✉)
Department of Cardiology, Barts Heart Centre, St Bartholomew's Hospital, London, UK

Centre for Cardiovascular Medicine and Devices, William Harvey Research Institute, Queen Mary University of London, London, UK
e-mail: dan.jones8@nhs.net

A. Mathur · A. Baumbach
Department of Cardiology, Barts Heart Centre, St Bartholomew's Hospital, London, UK

Centre for Cardiovascular Medicine and Devices, William Harvey Research Institute, Queen Mary University of London, London, UK

Yale School of Medicine, Yale University, New Haven, CT, USA

© Springer Nature Switzerland AG 2022
B. Cortese (ed.), *Left Main Coronary Revascularization*,
https://doi.org/10.1007/978-3-031-05265-1_6

Furthermore, the size difference between LMS and LAD/Cx can be a challenge for balloon expandable stents. All of these factors need to be considered when undertaking PCI for LMS disease.

6.3 The Evidence

To date, randomized trial comparisons between the two strategies for LMS disease have not demonstrated a conclusive winner. Six randomized clinical trials have compared PCI with CABG in the setting of LMS disease, but only two of them—EXCEL and NOBLE—were conducted in the era of second-generation drug-eluting stents (DES) [1] [2], with three of them (SYNTAX [3], NOBLE [4], and EXCEL [5]) now publishing longer-term follow-up results. In these cases, long-term follow-up is essential to determine the true effects of each treatment strategy and better inform therapeutic decision-making. There are clear advantages to PCI upfront (radial procedures, early ambulation, with minimal hospital stay), and therefore longer f/u is important to truly provide a fair comparison with cardiac surgery.

6.4 Longer Term Outcomes PCI vs CABG

There are 3 large randomised controlled studies with long term outcome data (5–10 year f/u).

1. The SYNTAX (Synergy Between Percutaneous Coronary Intervention With TAXUS and Cardiac Surgery) trial was a large randomized study comparing PCI and CABG for patients with complex CAD and included a subset of 705 patients with LMS disease (357 patients underwent PCI, 348 underwent CABG). The PCI arm underwent treatment with the paclitaxel-eluting Taxus stent system (Boston Scientific Corporation). Reported 5-year outcome data for patients with a SYNTAX score > 33 had lower mortality and lower rates of repeat revascularization with CABG com-

pared with PCI, thus establishing CABG as the preferred revascularization method for patients with LMS disease and high SYNTAX scores. Interestingly, the subgroup with low-to-intermediate SYNTAX scores (0–32) had a lower mortality and stroke rate with PCI with no difference in the rate of repeat revascularization. The longer-term 10-year data is now available and demonstrated there was no difference in all-cause mortality between the PCI group and the CABG group (26% vs 28%), despite the use of the earlier generation Taxus stent in the PCI arm [3].

2. In the EXCEL trial, 1905 patients with LMS disease were randomized to PCI with DES (using the everolimus-eluting Xience stent system, Abbott) or CABG. The primary outcome measure was a composite of all-cause death, stroke, and myocardial infarction (MI). This composite measure was not different at 5 years between the 2 groups (22% PCI vs 19.2% CABG, P = 0.13). All-cause mortality was statistically significantly greater with PCI (13% vs 9.9% with CABG), but the trial was not powered for this endpoint. There were no significant differences in cardiac death or myocardial infarction between the two groups.

3. The NOBLE trial randomized 1201 patients with LMS disease to PCI or CABG. Most patients in the PCI arm were treated with the umirolimus-eluting BioMatrix stent system (Biosensors International). The primary outcome measure was different to the EXCEL study with a composite of all-cause mortality, nonprocedural MI, repeat revascularization, and stroke used. This measure occurred more frequently with PCI than CABG (28% vs 19%; HR, 1.58; 95% CI, 1.24–2.01; p = 0.0002). All-cause mortality was the same in the two groups (9% in each arm; HR, 1.08; 95% CI, 0.74–1.59; p = 0.68). Similarly, there was no difference in cardiac death (4% in each arm; HR, 0.99; 95% CI, 0.57–1.73; p = 0.99).

Importantly while the 5-year data from the NOBLE trial showed superiority for CABG over PCI in patients with low or intermediate syntax scores, it was driven primarily by the need for repeat revascularization and non-fatal MI, while peri-procedural MI – which was in favour of PCI in the EXCEL trial – was not included in the event analysis. *Importantly, the incidence of cardiovascular mortality and stroke in both landmark trials was similar between PCI and CABG.*

Meta-analyses There are several meta-analyses [6–10] which have combined the RCTs looking at LMS revascularization. The 2 most recent of which include the long-term data from EXCEL and NOBLE, and as such produce similar results, although differences between them are seen. Zhang et al. [10] assessed the long-term outcome so only include trials with over 5 years of outcome data (excludes Boudriot et al. [11]), whilst Ahmad et al. do not [9], and they have different primary endpoints. Ahmad et al. in total included five eligible trials in which 4612 patients were randomized [9]. The weighted mean follow-up duration was 67.1 months. There were no significant differences between PCI and CABG for the risk of all-cause mortality (RR:1.03, 95% CI 0.81–1.32; P = 0.779) or cardiac death (RR 1.03, 95% CI 0.79–1.34; P = 0.817). There were also no significant differences in the risk of stroke (RR 0.74, 95% CI 0.35–1.50; P = 0.400) or MI (RR 1.22, 95% CI 0.96–1.56; P = 0.110). There was an increased risk of unplanned revascularization (RR 1.73, 95% CI 1.49–2.02; P < 0.001) seen with PCI [9].

The second review (Zhang et al. [10]) included 4 RCTS and 4394 patients distributed randomly into PCI (n = 2197) and CABG (n = 2197) groups. In comparison to CABG, PCI showed non-inferiority concerning a composite of death, MI, and stroke (HR 1.22, 95% CI 0.84–1.75), death (HR 1.06, 95% CI 0.81–1.40) and stroke (HR 0.80, 95% CI 0.42–1.53). Regarding major adverse cardiac or cerebrovascular events (MACCE) rate, both strategies show clinical equipoise in patients with a low-to-intermediate SYNTAX score (HR 1.20, 95% CI 0.85–1.70), while CABG had an advantage over PCI in those with a high SYNTAX score (HR 1.64, 95% CI 1.20–2.24).

Overall depending on trials and f/u included, meta-analyses show similar outcomes and equipoise between PCI and CABG in patients with LMS disease and low to intermediate SYNTAX scores. However, when it comes to revascularization of anatomically complex LMS disease (High Syntax score) CABG appears superior to PCI, although this superiority is driven by repeat revascularization. This data has driven the recommendations of European guidelines which were only recently updated to recommend PCI as an appropriate alternative to CABG in LMS disease with low-to-intermediate anatomical complexity (class I recommendation for low SYNTAX scores and class IIa for intermediate SYNTAX scores; but against PCI [class III] for high SYNTAX scores) [12]. Importantly these authors suggest that there are limitations to the trials performed and evidence available to date with considerable scope for improvement in PCI technology, technique and strategy which could mean PCI becomes even more equivalent.

6.5 Limitations of Trials to Date

Choice of Endpoint The primary outcome measures of all trials performed to date are composite endpoints, which although necessary from a sample size and practicality perspective lead to difficulties in data interpretation, especially when these vary in terms of composition or definition between studies. Firstly, each trial does not have a uniform definition of the composite endpoint it uses as its primary outcome. For example; the NOBLE trial included the endpoint of repeat revascularization as part of the primary composite endpoint, whereas EXCEL did not. Thus, conflicting primary results between the EXCEL and NOBLE trials were mainly driven by this differing definition. Secondly, the individual components may have varied definitions which can be important, i.e. the prognostic impact of MI is dependent on the definition used. Finally, each component is given equal weighting, which can be debated. It has been long debated whether the risk of repeat revascularization can be equally balanced against the risk of death, MI, or stroke.

Previous data from the SYNTAX trial showed that increased repeat revascularization with PCI as compared with CABG did not seem to translate into a significant overall increase in the rate of death or MI [13], although more recent analysis from EXCEL does suggest that repeat revascularization after either PCI or CABG is associated with 3-year mortality [14].

Interventional Technique and Stent Technology To date only 2 of the RCTs performed have used newer or second-generation DES (NOBLE and EXCEL), now considered the standard of care for coronary intervention. However, even in those trials, there were key differences in the platforms used. EXCEL used a thin-strut, fluoropolymer-based cobalt chromium, everolimus-eluting stent, which has been shown to be associated with the lowest risk of stent thrombosis of all available DES [15]. In contrast, NOBLE used first-generation, thicker-strut, stainless steel, sirolimus-eluting Cypher stents in 11% or the biolimus-eluting Biomatrix Flex stent in the rest (89%). There was a substantial difference in rates of definite stent thrombosis seen between the studies (0.7% in the EXCEL and 3% in the NOBLE); as a result, the rate of definite stent thrombosis or symptomatic graft occlusion was much higher after CABG than after PCI (5.4% versus 0.7%) in EXCEL, but similar (4% versus 3%) in NOBLE. This in part may have contributed to differences in the study outcomes and reflect the importance of stent choice. Further support for possible improvements in outcome with later or newer generation stents is provided when assessing the absolute differences in rates of repeat revascularization between PCI and CABG in the EXCEL trial, which are lower than those reported in the SYNTAX trial, which admittedly may reflect the lower anatomical complexity of the EXCEL population but also the improved properties of new-generation metallic everolimus-eluting stent compared to that used in SYNTAX.

Intravascular Imaging Intravascular imaging was not mandatory in any of the studies assessing PCI vs CABG for LMS intervention performed to date. NOBLE and EXCEL had usage rates of 47% pre/72% post and 77% post respectively. The implementation of mandated intra-coronary imaging resulted in significantly lower cumulative outcomes after PCI in the single-arm SYNTAX II trial when compared with the original SYNTAX I PCI cohort (13.2% vs. 21.9%) [16]. Moreover, equipoise was also observed when the same contemporary cohort was compared with the original SYNTAX CABG cohort, albeit in patients with three-vessel CAD and not LMS disease (13.2% vs. 21.9%). This would suggest that imaging is crucial to improving outcomes further in this group, a matter discussed further later in this chapter.

Anti-platelets There is increasing data to support the benefit of utilizing more potent P2Y12 inhibitors (i.e. ticagrelor) or longer duration of DAPT in patients who have undergone complex PCI (normally defined as bifurcation stenting, CTO stenting, stenting of long segments, or deploying more ≥3 stents). A recent trial PRECISE-DAPT [17] concluded that complex PCI had higher risk of ischaemic burden and therefore higher ischaemic events and benefitted from long-duration DAPT therapy in absence of any bleeding risk [17]. LMS PCI is a risk criterion for extended treatment with a second anti-thrombotic agent in recent guidelines [18]. With clopidogrel being the primary choice of P2Y12 inhibitor used in LMS studies to date, utilizing more potent and effective anti-platelets would logically improve ischaemic outcomes in this patient group, although naturally tailored against bleeding risk.

Syntax Scores Current guidelines and consensus is the higher the syntax score, the greater the benefit from CABG. European guidelines were updated to recommend PCI as an appropriate alternative to CABG in LMS disease with low-to-intermediate anatomic complexity (class I recommendation for low SYNTAX scores and class IIa for intermediate SYNTAX scores; but against PCI [class III] for high SYNTAX scores) [12]. However, in trials when you exclude high SYNTAX scores and more complex diseases, the role of the SYNTAX score is no longer clear. In EXCEL, there was a discrepancy between the site-designated and core laboratory-designated SYNTAX scores. In fact, 24% of patients had high scores (>33) by core laboratory, and yet the population overall still did well with PCI. Subgroup analysis in the EXCEL trial based on SYNTAX score did not reveal differences in outcome. In NOBLE, outcomes did not relate to SYNTAX score, and low scores did better with CABG. It therefore suggests that other factors, potentially patient or technical, are important.

6.6 PCI Technique and Strategy

LMS disease is a challenging subset for PCI. Although the LMS can be considered "just" another bifurcation, the unique technical complexities (large mass of myocardium supplied by LMS, side-branch is a major epicardial vessel, calcification, burden of atherosclerotic disease) and the proven efficacy of CABG in this situation means there is no room for error with PCI. It is essential that when performed, every effort to ensure a perfect final PCI result that is as good or better than CABG, i.e. optimal and complete revascularization is required. This requires experience, careful rigorous procedural planning and application of the best available technology (i.e. stent technology, adjunctive techniques and intravascular imaging techniques).

Experience The first aspect of LMS PCI relates to understanding the importance of the above. Patients treated by experienced operators (e.g. operators who performed at least 15 LMCA PCIs per year for at least 3 consecutive years) have better short- and long-term outcomes compared with LMS patients treated by operators who are less experienced [19]. This suggests that sufficient experience should be available for the procedure either as first or second operator in 2 consultant cases.

Strategy In the field of percutaneous LMS treatment, defining the optimal stenting technique depends on the anatomical location of the dis-

ease, with the LM bifurcation affected in the majority of patients [20] and PCI of the distal LMS bifurcation having been associated with worse outcomes compared PCI on isolated ostial/midshaft lesions [21]. This was seen in the EXCEL study where repeat revascularization rates after PCI during follow-up were greater for lesions in the distal LM bifurcation but were similar to CABG for disease isolated to the LM ostium or shaft [22]. Despite the LMS ostium or shaft being technically less challenging to treat percutaneously adjunctive modification techniques, i.e. rotational atherectomy or intravascular lithotripsy (IVL) may well be needed and should be considered upfront and based on intravascular imaging if uncertainty exists.

With respect to the optimal treatment strategy of the LMS bifurcation, controversy exists on the optimal stenting strategy, especially after good clinical benefits revealed by double-kissing (DK) crush two-stent strategy [16, 23]. The European Bifurcation Club (EBC) recommends a "provisional" side branch (SB) stenting strategy when feasible for the treatment of the vast majority of bifurcation lesions, but a two-stent strategy may be required in cases of extensive SB disease [24]. In slight contrast, the recently published ESC guidelines "strongly suggest" the use of DK-crush in the treatment of LM bifurcations (class IIb, LOE B) [12], following the results of the DKCRUSH-V trial, where provisional stenting was associated with significantly higher ST rate (3.3%) than DK-crush (0.4%) [16]. However, it is important to consider that in the DK-CRUSH-V trial, one-half of the patients in the provisional group received a second stent mainly due to complications during the procedure and the operators performing the DK-CRUSH technique were experts in the technique. As such, the DK-crush technique has emerged as a preferred approach for true distal LMS bifurcation lesions, although this technique is technically challenging and should be performed by expert operators. A 2-stent strategy is also supported by the recently published DEFINITION II study [25] which documented that the systematic use of a two-stent strategy was associated with a significant improvement in clinical outcomes compared with provisional stenting in complex bifurcation lesions. In this study, 653 patients with complex bifurcation lesions were randomly assigned to undergo the systematic two-stent technique or provisional stenting. At the 1-year follow-up, TLF occurred in 37 (11.4%) and 20 (6.1%) patients in the provisional and two-stent groups, respectively (HR 0.52, 95% CI:0.30–0.90; P = 0.019), largely driven by increased target vessel MI (7.1%, HR 0.43, 95% CI 0.20–0.90; P = 0.025) and clinically driven TLR (5.5%, HR 0.43, 95% CI 0.19–1.00; P = 0.049) in the provisional group. Although not a dedicated LMS bifurcation study, 30% of patients in both groups had distal LMS bifurcation lesions and 77.8% of the two-stent strategies were DK-CRUSH, adding so-called fuel to the fire.

Therefore, it appears important to select individualized treatment based on anatomy with implantation of a second stent following a failed provisional approach potentially associated with worse prognosis. Consistently expert opinion would recommend choosing treatment strategy before the procedure, with optimal preparation before stenting coupled with kissing balloon inflations followed by a final proximal optimization technique [26]. Simultaneous kissing stents may be considered for the haemodynamically unstable patient, although this approach has fallen out of favour because of the creation of a new carina and side branch access issues. There are several ongoing randomized studies assessing provisional versus two-stent strategies for distal LMS disease including that of the European Bifurcation Club, the EBC MAIN study [27] NCT02497014 which will provide more evidence. Therefore, whilst awaiting the results of ongoing randomized trials, current evidence suggests aligning the stenting strategy with an individual patient's coronary anatomy and clinical condition, with an imperative of meticulously planning and performing two-stent techniques within the experience limits of an individual operator, with currently DK-CRUSH appearing the optimal strategy when feasible. Examples of two-stent and provisional strategies are shown in Figs. 6.1 and 6.2, chosen based on anatomy and clinical presentation.

Evolution of Stent Technology The evolution from balloon angioplasty to bare-metal stents to first and later generation DES has resulted in progressively reduced rates of restenosis and clinically driven revascularization after PCI [28, 29]. Nonetheless, recent meta-analyses confirm that even in the DES-era, CABG results in fewer unplanned revascularization procedures than PCI. This finding may be attributed to bypass grafts protecting long diseased segments that are likely to progress over time, a mechanism that may also contribute to the lower risk of very late MI after CABG compared with PCI. However, potentially the use of longer more potent antithrombotic therapies, i.e. ticagrelor as per PEGASUS [30] or rivaroxaban as per COMPASS [31] could also reduce rates of further revascularization in suitable patients. Additionally, suitable targets for revascularization are less likely to be found after CABG than PCI due to accelerated proximal disease progression after bypass, with health status deterioration notably greater before and after repeat revascularization after CABG compared with PCI.

Newer stent technologies now exist such as the Synergy stent (Boston Scientific, Marlborough, MA, USA) which is a new-generation everolimus-eluting stent with a biodegradable polymer coating, presenting several features that have the potential to reduce acute and long-term thrombogenicity and the subsequent need for DAPT. In a series of patients undergoing complex PCI (high rates of CTO, bifurcation and 25% of patients turned down for surgery (LMS and 3VD), there were excellent event rates at 1 year (0% ST and 1.2% TLR at 1 year), suggesting its potential in this patient group [32].

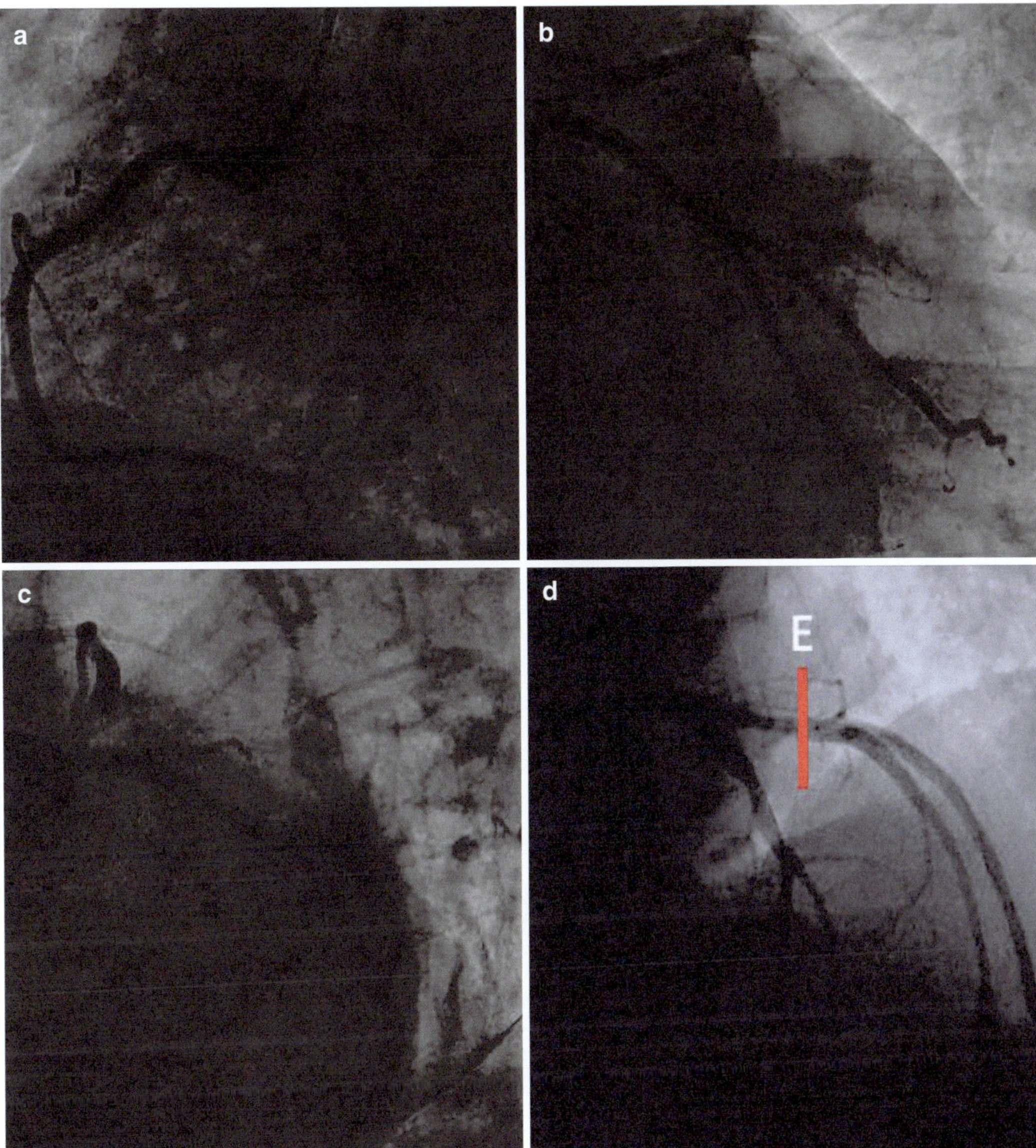

Fig. 6.1 Provisional stenting strategy in ACS. A 52-year-old gentleman presented with a Wellens ECG, and ongoing chest pain. He was sent for emergency angiography. Panel A shows a dominant unobstructed RCA. Panel B and C show a distal LMS stenosis extending into a thrombus laden critical ostial LAD stenosis. The Cx is unaffected. This was treated with a provisional stenting strategy. A 4 by 28 mm XIENCE Sierra DES was directly placed in LMS-LAD and optimized with a 5.0 by 12 mm NC balloon to POT. Panel D and F display the final angiographic result. Panel E shows the IVUS of distal stented segment with Panel G showing the final LMS result on IVUS

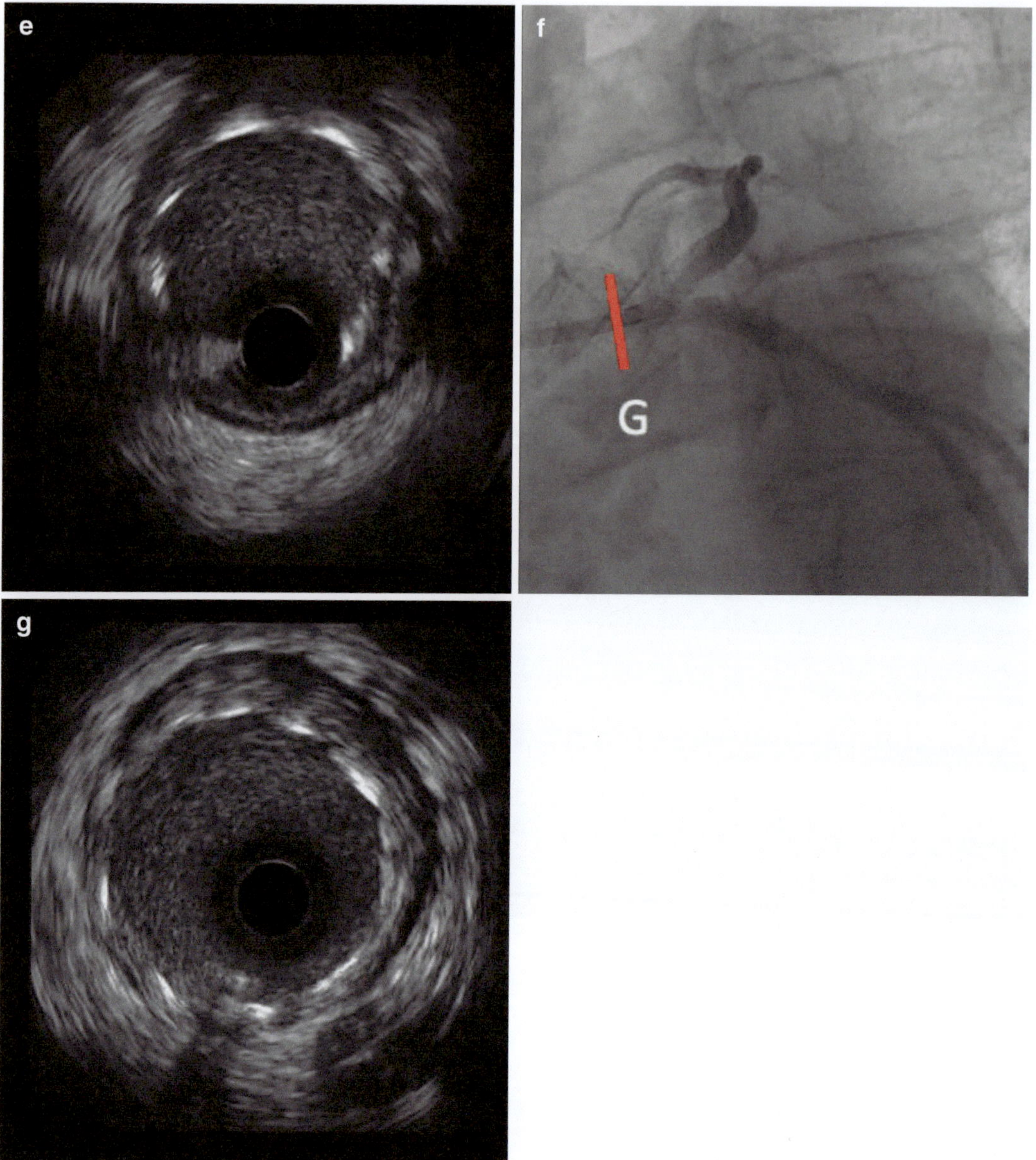

Fig. 6.1 (continued)

Size mismatch between the LMS and the proximal vessel (i.e. LAD) is a technical challenge of LMS PCI. Self-expanding stents (i.e. Xposition S self-apposing stent), which reduce the need for proximal optimization and bridge large diameter differences, were trialled however despite promising observational series [33], they never were tested in a randomized fashion and are currently now not available. Further advancements of the SYNERGY stent range have recently been added with the introduction of the Synergy Megatron bioabsorbable polymer coronary stent for this purpose. This is designed for large proximal vessels, including left main, bifurcations and ostial lesions and boasts increased radial strength and the ability to accommodate tapered vessels. To date, there is limited data in the literature with outcome data although a recent retrospective study from two UK centres showed excellent results [34] although further study is needed.

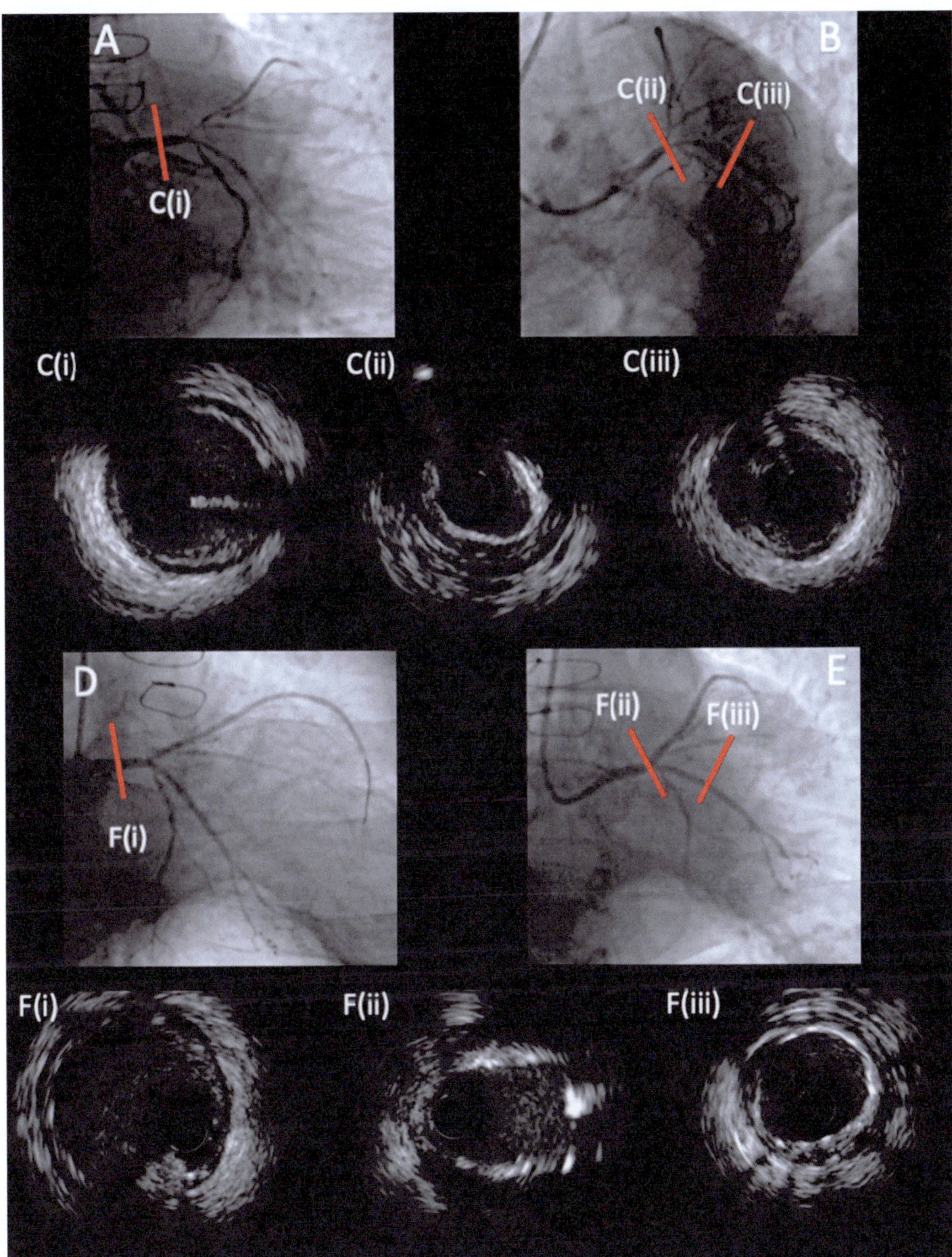

Fig. 6.2 Cullotte stenting strategy in high-risk ACS. A 67-year-old male presented with ACS. Angiography demonstrated severe distal LMS disease (Panel A) with confirmed LV impairment (35–40%). In view of ACS presentation, impaired LV function and history of pericardectomy he was listed for PCI. This was performed unsupported from the RRA (7F). Panel B demonstrates the LAO Caudal view highlighting the diseased segments in the distal LMS, LAD and Cx with corresponding IVUS images (c(ii) and c(iiii). Fig. D and E show the final angiographic result of Cullotte stenting prstrategy (3 x 28 mm XIENCE Sierra DES LMS-Cx and 3 by 48 mm LMS-LAD, optimized with 4.5 mm by 12 NC Balloon). Final angiographic result (Panel D and E) demonstrated well-expanded stents with TIMI III flow in all vessels. Post-procedure IVUS demonstrated well-expanded stents in both LMS (F(i) and F(ii) and LAD and LCx (Fiii) with no obvious dissection

Adjunctive Technology Heavy calcification of coronary stenoses, particularly in the setting of the LMS is a major factor in making PCI complex and unfavourable. The immediate mechanical result of PCI has a strong influence on outcomes with data supporting a direct correlation between final minimum stent area (MSA) and outcome (ST and TLR). However, for many patients, achieving adequate stent deployment remains a major issue owing to the presence of calcification. Typically rotational atherectomy is used to modify calcified lesions and debulk plaque; however, technical considerations exist in terms of being able to protect a major epicardial side-branch with a coronary guidewire and the potential for distal embolization/procedural MI. Intravascular lithotripsy (IVL; Shockwave Medical, Santa Clara, CA, USA) is a novel device that uses sonic waves at the target site to deliver pulsatile lithotripsy, which selectively fractures intimal and medial layer calcium. The DISRUPT CAD I, II and III trials [35, 36] have demonstrated the utility of IVL in patients with calcific non-LM coronary disease. Observational series support the use of IVL in LMS stenoses of both ostial, shaft and importantly distal disease [37, 38]. The largest series from 3 UK centres involving 31 patients has recently demonstrated the effective use of IVL in distal LMS stenoses achieving high mean MSAs in each of the distal LM segments, including the LCX ostium, with only two patients failing to meet accepted target values in all treated vessels [37]. The mean distal MSAs were 12.9mm^2 comparing favourably to that achieved in RCTs (EXCEL 9.8mm^2 and 12.5 mm^2 in NOBLE) [37]. The addition of IVL to the armoury of the interventional cardiologist has the potential to improve stent results and outcomes potentially challenging the TLR issue that hampers PCI in complex anatomical disease.

Imaging Guidance The role of imaging in LMS intervention is increasingly recognized with accumulating observational data to support its use. Imaging is performed to assess the vessel diameter, to understand plaque morphology (? Need for adjunctive debulking), to determine the extent of the atherosclerosis—whether distal bifurcation and ostia of LAD and LCX are involved—and finally to optimize the stent expansion and identify complications (e.g. dissection). Importantly just the use post procedure can ensure adequate expansion and apposition of stents, which improves clinical outcomes following LM PCI, particularly in patients with distal LM lesions and those treated with a two-stent strategy [39, 40].

Although there are no large randomized clinical trials to assess ad hoc whether intravascular imaging-guided LMS PCI is associated with better long-term clinical outcomes, convincing data from large registries suggest a long-term mortality benefit in patients undergoing IVUS-guided compared with angio-guided LMS PCI. Observational data from 11,264 unprotected LMS PCI procedures from the UK (2007–2014) demonstrated lower rates of coronary complications, lower in-hospital major adverse cardiac events (OR: 0.47; 95% CI: 0.37–0.59; p < 0.001), and improved 30-day (OR: 0.54; 95% CI: 0.43–0.68; p < 0.001) and 12-month (OR: 0.66; 95% CI: 0.57–0.77; p < 0.001) mortality were observed with imaging use compared with no imaging use. In logistic regression modelling, imaging use was associated with improved 12-month survival [41]. Greater mortality reductions were observed with higher operator LMS PCI volume supporting the need for experience present during these procedures.

Further data is provided by a sub-study of the NOBLE trial which investigated the association between the use and findings of IVUS with clinical outcomes in the study [42]. Of 603 patients treated by PCI, 435 (72%) underwent post-PCI IVUS assessment. At 5 years, the composite of MACCE was 18.9% if post-PCI IVUS was performed versus 25.0% if it was not performed (p = 0.45, after adjustment). Overall repeat revascularization was not reduced (10.6% vs 16.5%, p = 0.11); however, LMS TLR was (5.1% vs 11.6%, p = 0.01) if IVUS was used. Rates of repeat revascularization and LMS TLR were associated with tertile of stent expansion (LMS MLA) at the end of the case [42]. Impressively, in this cohort, none of the patients who had a minimum stent area (MSA) greater than 13.4 mm^2 post PCI required TLR at 5-year follow-up. This would suggest that IVUS guidance and optimization for LMS PCI have a direct effect on TLR (the predominant endpoint that drives the superiority of CABG in trials), but has not been mandated in all patients randomized in previous trials to date.

Stent optimization is the main indication for IVUS in LMS PCI, and in our opinion at least a post-stenting IVUS should always be performed when it is safe to do so. This use to prevent stent under-expansion in LMS PCI is likely to improve outcomes but in the absence of randomized controlled trial data this is currently based on observational data and expert opinion (ESC Level IIa Class B) [12]. In this regard, the OPTIMA (OPtimizaTIon of Left MAin PCI With Intravascular Ultrasound) study (NCT04111770), recruiting 800 patients will be the first randomized powered study to answer this.

Although a large proportion of the PCI techniques and evolving techniques are speculative there are data that with the implementation of coronary physiology, and mandated intra-coronary imaging optimization, that cumulative outcomes after PCI are better. In the single-arm SYNTAX II trial outcomes after PCI were significantly lower when compared with the original SYNTAX I PCI cohort (13.2% vs. 21.9%) [43]. Moreover, equipoise was also observed when the same contemporary cohort was compared with the original SYNTAX CABG cohort, albeit in patients with three-vessel CAD and not LMS CAD (13.2% vs. 21.9%). This suggests and supports the theory that the above techniques and advancing technology will significantly improve PCI outcomes further (noting that syntax II did not involve newer stent technology, anti-platelets or IVL).

6.7   PCI in the Emergency Setting

Unprotected LMS occlusion is a relatively uncommon presentation with rates of 0.6–5% in STEMI registries [44–46] but typically presents with cardiogenic shock and is associated with higher risks of major cardiac adverse events and higher mortality even if treated with reperfusion therapy in time [45–47]. In these situations, prompt early reperfusion is crucial, potentially reversing arrhythmic and hemodynamic instability. CABG can be considered but delays to reperfusion, which may take an hour or longer during off-peak hours to establish cardiopulmonary bypass, can be catastrophic in this situation. PCI has been shown in registries and prior series to have clinical outcomes comparable to that of CABG in these circumstances, with formal randomized study difficult to perform for obvious reasons [48, 49]. An example of emergency PCI in an unstable patient is shown in Fig. 6.3.

Hence, in the emergency setting, we advocate the consideration of PCI as a preferred alternative to CABG, when PCI can be performed in a timely fashion by experienced operators [5]: when (1) LMS occlusion with Thrombolysis In Myocardial Infarction (TIMI) flow grade <3; (2) cardiogenic shock and/or life-threatening arrhythmias; or (3) coexisting illnesses or conditions that pose excessive risk of CABG-related complications. In more stable circumstances, i.e. TIMI flow grade 3, stable haemodynamics and time is less critical, the decision regarding PCI versus CABG can be made based on similar criteria to the stable setting (location of disease, co-existent coronary disease and patient co-morbidities).

Mechanical Support The advent of minimally invasive, potent, and rapidly deployable percutaneous left ventricular assist devices, such as the Impella heart pump, can help interventional cardiologists to safely and effectively treat patients presenting with LMS disease with associated high-risk features for haemodynamic instability and periprocedural complications [50]. In patients with LMS disease, who present acutely (acute coronary syndromes, haemodynamic instability) or with known severe left ventricular dysfunction or co-existent anatomical features (e.g. chronically occluded RCA), mechanical circulatory support devices can help unload the left ventricle during the procedure, augmenting cardiac output sufficiently to maintain myocardial flow and end-organ perfusion. IABP is the most

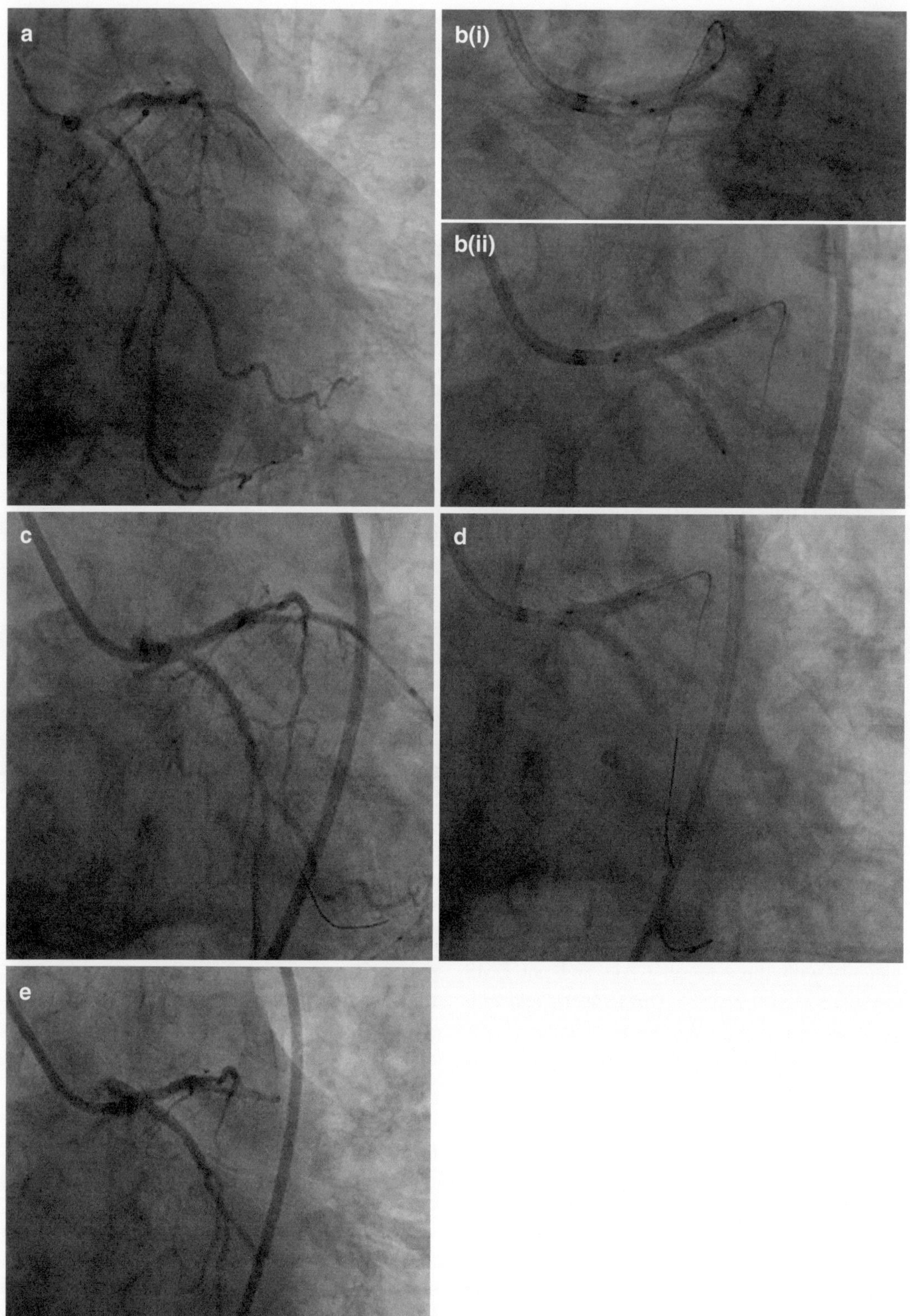

commonly available device with easy and expeditious insertion, but is associated with low efficacy to augment cardiac output. It may be useful in pre-shock/shock patients, electively or during emergency crash situations during LM PCI. Newer more effective devices, such as Impella (Abiomed), provide higher cardiac output and may be considered, supported by observational studies and registry data. Currently, Impella CP is not commissioned for use in complex, high-risk, and indicated PCI by the National Institute of Health and Clinical Excellence (NICE) or National Health Service England, but both European (European Society of Cardiology) [12] and U.S. (American College of Cardiology) [51] guidelines advise mechanical circulatory support in high-risk percutaneous coronary intervention (i.e. LMS) as a Class IIb indication.

In our practice, we recognize that a subset of patients may benefit from the use of mechanical circulatory support during LMS PCI (Poor LV, bystander RCA CTO, haemodynamic instability). We advocate that if needed it is crucial to plan the device strategy and place the device prior to the commencement of LMS intervention.

6.8 Unanswered Questions

Future trials, mandating intra-coronary imaging, adjunctive techniques where indicated (calcium modification (IVL or rotational atherectomy), mechanical support), contemporary anti-platelet regimes and coronary physiology within protocols, are necessary to determine the optimal strategy for treating LMS disease. Ideally, these trials should implement consistent and homogenous endpoint definitions and provide long-term follow-up. Sufficient power to assess sub-groups, i.e. diabetes mellitus, elderly, emergent presentations and renal failure would be desirable. If the main driver behind CABG superiority in this group is related to unplanned revascularization, this may not be a large deterrent compared to PCI (radial, day case procedures) when offset against the initial impact of undergoing CABG and therefore assessment of patient-reported outcome measures (PROMS) and quality of life both in the short- and long-term are needed.

6.9 Conclusion

Despite certain controversies, current contemporary and long-term trial data supports the safety and efficacy of PCI for the treatment of LMS disease. Advances in stent technology, use of adjunctive techniques (IVL) and mechanical support alongside the mandated intravascular imaging, and appropriate prescription of potent anti-platelet agents are only likely to improve outcomes further, specifically rates of TLR and stent thrombosis, the achilles heel of PCI compared to CABG. Arguably for selected patient cohorts (low-intermediate syntax score, emergency presentations, frail, co-morbidities), PCI should be the first-line strategy; however, involvement of local Heart teams is crucial in selecting appropriate patients given the complexities of this cohort.

Conflict of Interest No conflicts of interest, nothing to disclose.

Fig. 6.3 ShotGun stenting strategy for emergency PCI. An 87-year-old gentleman presented with an ACS with an ECG demonstrating anterior ST depression, and ST elevation in AVR. Angiography demonstrated a chronic ostial occlusion of the RCA and critical distal LMS disease (Fig. 6.3a). LV ventriculography demonstrated mod-severe LV impairment (LVEDP 30 mmHg). He was therefore treated with PCI (ongoing ischaemia, co-morbidity, impaired LV Function). IABP was inserted for support. Upgraded to 8F femoral system. Panel B (i). Shows kissing pre-dilatation with (2.5 by 15 mm Non-compliant balloons in LAD and Cx). Panel B (ii) demonstrates the shotgun stenting strategy (3.0 by 24 mm SYNERGY LAD, 2.75 by 24 mm SYNERGY Cx). Panel C: Angiographic images post Panel D: Kissing post stenting (Kissing Balloon 3.0 by 15 mm NC (LAD and Cx) Panel E shows the Final angiographic result

References

1. Stone GW, Sabik JF, Serruys PW, Simonton CA, Généreux P, Puskas J, Kandzari DE, Morice MC, Lembo N, Brown WM, Taggart DP, Banning A, Merkely B, Horkay F, Boonstra PW, van Boven AJ, Ungi I, Bogáts G, Mansour S, Noiseux N, Sabaté M, Pomar J, Hickey M, Gershlick A, Buszman P, Bochenek A, Schampaert E, Pagé P, Dressler O, Kosmidou I, Mehran R, Pocock SJ, Kappetein AP, T. I. EXCEL. Everolimus-eluting stents or bypass surgery for left Main coronary artery disease. N Engl J Med. 2016;375:2223–35.

2. Mäkikallio T, Holm NR, Lindsay M, Spence MS, Erglis A, Menown IB, Trovik T, Eskola M, Romppanen H, Kellerth T, Ravkilde J, Jensen LO, Kalinauskas G, Linder RB, Pentikainen M, Hervold A, Banning A, Zaman A, Cotton J, Eriksen E, Margus S, Sørensen HT, Nielsen PH, Niemelä M, Kervinen K, Lassen JF, Maeng M, Oldroyd K, Berg G, Walsh SJ, Hanratty CG, Kumsars I, Stradins P, Steigen TK, Fröbert O, Graham AN, Endresen PC, Corbascio M, Kajander O, Trivedi U, Hartikainen J, Anttila V, Hildick-Smith D, Thuesen L, Christiansen EH, S. I. NOBLE. Percutaneous coronary angioplasty versus coronary artery bypass grafting in treatment of unprotected left main stenosis (NOBLE): a prospective, randomised, open-label, non-inferiority trial. Lancet. 2016;388:2743–52.

3. Thuijs DJFM, Kappetein AP, Serruys PW, Mohr FW, Morice MC, Mack MJ, Holmes DR, Curzen N, Davierwala P, Noack T, Milojevic M, Dawkins KD, da Costa BR, Jüni P, Head SJ, E. S. I. SYNTAX. Percutaneous coronary intervention versus coronary artery bypass grafting in patients with three-vessel or left main coronary artery disease: 10-year follow-up of the multicentre randomised controlled SYNTAX trial. Lancet. 2019;394: 1325–34.

4. Holm NR, Mäkikallio T, Lindsay MM, Spence MS, Erglis A, Menown IBA, Trovik T, Kellerth T, Kalinauskas G, Mogensen LJH, Nielsen PH, Niemelä M, Lassen JF, Oldroyd K, Berg G, Stradins P, Walsh SJ, Graham ANJ, Endresen PC, Fröbert O, Trivedi U, Anttila V, Hildick-Smith D, Thuesen L, Christiansen EH, I. NOBLE. Percutaneous coronary angioplasty versus coronary artery bypass grafting in the treatment of unprotected left main stenosis: updated 5-year outcomes from the randomised, non-inferiority NOBLE trial. Lancet. 2020;395:191–9.

5. Stone GW, Kappetein AP, Sabik JF, Pocock SJ, Morice MC, Puskas J, Kandzari DE, Karmpaliotis D, Brown WM, Lembo NJ, Banning A, Merkely B, Horkay F, Boonstra PW, van Boven AJ, Ungi I, Bogáts G, Mansour S, Noiseux N, Sabaté M, Pomar J, Hickey M, Gershlick A, Buszman PE, Bochenek A, Schampaert E, Pagé P, Modolo R, Gregson J, Simonton CA, Mehran R, Kosmidou I, Généreux P, Crowley A, Dressler O, Serruys PW, T. I. EXCEL. Five-year outcomes after PCI or CABG for left Main coronary disease. N Engl J Med. 2019;381:1820–30.

6. Nerlekar N, Ha FJ, Verma KP, Bennett MR, Cameron JD, Meredith IT, Brown AJ. Percutaneous coronary intervention using drug-eluting stents versus coronary artery bypass grafting for unprotected left Main coronary artery stenosis: A meta-analysis of randomized trials. Circ Cardiovasc Interv. 2016;9:e004729.

7. Upadhaya S, Baniya R, Madala S, Subedi SK, Khan J, Velagapudi RK, Bachuwa G. Drug-eluting stent placement versus coronary artery bypass surgery for unprotected left main coronary artery disease: A meta-analysis of randomized controlled trials. J Card Surg. 2017;32:70–9.

8. Sardar P, Giri J, Elmariah S, Chatterjee S, Kolte D, Kundu A, Nairooz R, Aronow WS, Owan T, Mukherjee D, Feldman DN, Abbott JD. Meta-analysis of drug-eluting stents versus coronary artery bypass grafting in unprotected left Main coronary narrowing. Am J Cardiol. 2017;119:1746–52.

9. Ahmad Y, Howard JP, Arnold AD, Cook CM, Prasad M, Ali ZA, Parikh MA, Kosmidou I, Francis DP, Moses JW, Leon MB, Kirtane AJ, Stone GW, Karmpaliotis D. Mortality after drug-eluting stents vs. coronary artery bypass grafting for left main coronary artery disease: a meta-analysis of randomized controlled trials. Eur Heart J. 2020;41:3228–35.

10. Zhang J, Jiang T, Hou Y, Chen F, Yang K, Sang W, Wu H, Ma Y, Xu F, Chen Y. Five-year outcomes comparing percutaneous coronary intervention with drug-eluting stents versus coronary artery bypass grafting in patients with left main coronary artery disease: A systematic review and meta-analysis. Atherosclerosis. 2020;308:50–6.

11. Boudriot E, Thiele H, Walther T, Liebetrau C, Boeckstegers P, Pohl T, Reichart B, Mudra H, Beier F, Gansera B, Neumann FJ, Gick M, Zietak T, Desch S, Schuler G, Mohr FW. Randomized comparison of percutaneous coronary intervention with sirolimus-eluting stents versus coronary artery bypass grafting in unprotected left main stem stenosis. J Am Coll Cardiol. 2011;57:538–45.

12. Neumann FJ, Sousa-Uva M, Ahlsson A, Alfonso F, Banning AP, Benedetto U, Byrne RA, Collet JP, Falk V, Head SJ, Jüni P, Kastrati A, Koller A, Kristensen SD, Niebauer J, Richter DJ, Seferovic PM, Sibbing D, Stefanini GG, Windecker S, Yadav R, Zembala MO, S. D. G. ESC. 2018 ESC/EACTS Guidelines on myocardial revascularization. Eur Heart J. 2019;40:87–165.

13. Parasca CA, Head SJ, Milojevic M, Mack MJ, Serruys PW, Morice MC, Mohr FW, Feldman TE, Colombo A, Dawkins KD, Holmes DR, Kappetein PA, I. SYNTAX. Incidence, characteristics, predictors, and outcomes of repeat revascularization after percutaneous coronary intervention and coronary artery bypass grafting: the SYNTAX trial at 5 years. JACC Cardiovasc Interv. 2016;9:2493–507.

14. Giustino G, Serruys PW, Sabik JF, Mehran R, Maehara A, Puskas JD, Simonton CA, Lembo NJ,

Kandzari DE, Morice MC, Taggart DP, Gershlick AH, Ragosta M, Kron IL, Liu Y, Zhang Z, McAndrew T, Dressler O, Généreux P, Ben-Yehuda O, Pocock SJ, Kappetein AP, Stone GW. Mortality after repeat revascularization following PCI or CABG for left Main disease: the EXCEL trial. JACC Cardiovasc Interv. 2020;13:375–87.

15. Palmerini T, Biondi-Zoccai G, Della Riva D, Stettler C, Sangiorgi D, D'Ascenzo F, Kimura T, Briguori C, Sabatè M, Kim HS, De Waha A, Kedhi E, Smits PC, Kaiser C, Sardella G, Marullo A, Kirtane AJ, Leon MB, Stone GW. Stent thrombosis with drug-eluting and bare-metal stents: evidence from a comprehensive network meta-analysis. Lancet. 2012;379:1393–402.

16. Chen SL, Zhang JJ, Han Y, Kan J, Chen L, Qiu C, Jiang T, Tao L, Zeng H, Li L, Xia Y, Gao C, Santoso T, Paiboon C, Wang Y, Kwan TW, Ye F, Tian N, Liu Z, Lin S, Lu C, Wen S, Hong L, Zhang Q, Sheiban I, Xu Y, Wang L, Rab TS, Li Z, Cheng G, Cui L, Leon MB, Stone GW. Double kissing crush versus provisional stenting for left Main distal bifurcation lesions: DKCRUSH-V randomized trial. J Am Coll Cardiol. 2017;70:2605–17.

17. Costa F, Van Klaveren D, Feres F, James S, Räber L, Pilgrim T, Hong MK, Kim HS, Colombo A, Steg PG, Bhatt DL, Stone GW, Windecker S, Steyerberg EW, Valgimigli M, S. I. PRECISE-DAPT. Dual antiplatelet therapy duration based on ischemic and bleeding risks after coronary stenting. J Am Coll Cardiol. 2019;73:741–54.

18. Collet J-P, Thiele H, Barbato E, Barthélémy O, Bauersachs J, Bhatt DL, Dendale P, Dorobantu M, Edvardsen T, Folliguet T. 2020 ESC guidelines for the management of acute coronary syndromes in patients presenting without persistent ST-segment elevationThe task force for the management of acute coronary syndromes in patients presenting without persistent ST-segment elevation of the European Society of Cardiology (ESC). Eur Heart J. 2020;42(14):1289–367.

19. Xu B, Redfors B, Yang Y, Qiao S, Wu Y, Chen J, Liu H, Chen J, Xu L, Zhao Y, Guan C, Gao R, Généreux P. Impact of operator experience and volume on outcomes after left Main coronary artery percutaneous coronary intervention. JACC Cardiovasc Interv. 2016;9:2086–93.

20. Chieffo A, Tanaka A, Giustino G, Briede I, Sawaya FJ, Daemen J, Kawamoto H, Meliga E, D'Ascenzo F, Cerrato E, Stefanini GG, Capodanno D, Mangiameli A, Templin C, Erglis A, Morice MC, Mehran R, Van Mieghem NM, Nakamura S, De Benedictis M, Pavani M, Varbella F, Pisaniello M, Sharma SK, Tamburino C, Tchetche D, Colombo A, I. DELTA. The DELTA 2 registry: A multicenter registry evaluating percutaneous coronary intervention with new-generation drug-eluting stents in patients with obstructive left Main coronary artery disease. JACC Cardiovasc Interv. 2017;10:2401–10.

21. Naganuma T, Chieffo A, Meliga E, Capodanno D, Park SJ, Onuma Y, Valgimigli M, Jegere S, Makkar RR, Palacios IF, Costopoulos C, Kim YH, Buszman PP, Chakravarty T, Sheiban I, Mehran R, Naber C, Margey R, Agnihotri A, Marra S, Capranzano P, Leon MB, Moses JW, Fajadet J, Lefevre T, Morice MC, Erglis A, Tamburino C, Alfieri O, Serruys PW, Colombo A. Long-term clinical outcomes after percutaneous coronary intervention for ostial/mid-shaft lesions versus distal bifurcation lesions in unprotected left main coronary artery: the DELTA registry (drug-eluting stent for left main coronary artery disease): a multicenter registry evaluating percutaneous coronary intervention versus coronary artery bypass grafting for left main treatment. JACC Cardiovasc Interv. 2013;6:1242–9.

22. Gershlick AH, Kandzari DE, Banning A, Taggart DP, Morice MC, Lembo NJ, Brown WM, Banning AP, Merkely B, Horkay F, van Boven AJ, Boonstra PW, Dressler O, Sabik JF, Serruys PW, Kappetein AP, Stone GW. Outcomes after left Main percutaneous coronary intervention versus coronary artery bypass grafting according to lesion site: results from the EXCEL trial. JACC Cardiovasc Interv. 2018;11:1224–33.

23. Chen X, Li X, Zhang JJ, Han Y, Kan J, Chen L, Qiu C, Santoso T, Paiboon C, Kwan TW, Sheiban I, Leon MB, Stone GW, Chen SL, I. DKCRUSH-V. 3-year outcomes of the DKCRUSH-V trial comparing DK crush with provisional stenting for left Main bifurcation lesions. JACC Cardiovasc Interv. 2019;12:1927–37.

24. Burzotta F, Lassen JF, Banning AP, Lefèvre T, Hildick-Smith D, Chieffo A, Darremont O, Pan M, Chatzizisis YS, Albiero R, Louvard Y, Stankovic G. Percutaneous coronary intervention in left main coronary artery disease: the 13th consensus document from the European bifurcation Club. EuroIntervention. 2018;14:112–20.

25. Zhang JJ, Ye F, Xu K, Kan J, Tao L, Santoso T, Munawar M, Tresukosol D, Li L, Sheiban I, Li F, Tian NL, Rodríguez AE, Paiboon C, Lavarra F, Lu S, Vichairuangthum K, Zeng H, Chen L, Zhang R, Ding S, Gao F, Jin Z, Hong L, Ma L, Wen S, Wu X, Yang S, Yin WH, Zhang J, Wang Y, Zheng Y, Zhou L, Zhou L, Zhu Y, Xu T, Wang X, Qu H, Tian Y, Lin S, Liu L, Lu Q, Li Q, Li B, Jiang Q, Han L, Gan G, Yu M, Pan D, Shang Z, Zhao Y, Liu Z, Yuan Y, Chen C, Stone GW, Han Y, Chen SL. Multicentre, randomized comparison of two-stent and provisional stenting techniques in patients with complex coronary bifurcation lesions: the DEFINITION II trial. Eur Heart J. 2020;41:2523–36.

26. Banning AP, Lassen JF, Burzotta F, Lefèvre T, Darremont O, Hildick-Smith D, Louvard Y, Stankovic G. Percutaneous coronary intervention for obstructive bifurcation lesions: the 14th consensus document from the European bifurcation Club. EuroIntervention. 2019;15:90–8.

27. Chieffo A, Hildick-Smith D. The European bifurcation Club left Main study (EBC MAIN): rationale and design of an international, multicentre, randomised comparison of two stent strategies for the treatment of left main coronary bifurcation disease. EuroIntervention. 2016;12:47–52.

28. Sarno G, Lagerqvist B, Fröbert O, Nilsson J, Olivecrona G, Omerovic E, Saleh N, Venetzanos D, James S. Lower risk of stent thrombosis and restenosis with unrestricted use of 'new-generation' drug-eluting stents: a report from the nationwide Swedish coronary angiography and angioplasty registry (SCAAR). Eur Heart J. 2012;33:606–13.

29. Stefanini GG, Holmes DR. Drug-eluting coronary-artery stents. N Engl J Med. 2013;368:254–65.

30. Bonaca MP, Bhatt DL, Cohen M, Steg PG, Storey RF, Jensen EC, Magnani G, Bansilal S, Fish MP, Im K, Bengtsson O, Oude Ophuis T, Budaj A, Theroux P, Ruda M, Hamm C, Goto S, Spinar J, Nicolau JC, Kiss RG, Murphy SA, Wiviott SD, Held P, Braunwald E, Sabatine MS, S. C. A. I. PEGASUS-TIMI. Long-term use of ticagrelor in patients with prior myocardial infarction. N Engl J Med. 2015;372:1791–800.

31. Eikelboom JW, Connolly SJ, Bosch J, Dagenais GR, Hart RG, Shestakovska O, Diaz R, Alings M, Lonn EM, Anand SS, Widimsky P, Hori M, Avezum A, Piegas LS, Branch KRH, Probstfield J, Bhatt DL, Zhu J, Liang Y, Maggioni AP, Lopez-Jaramillo P, O'Donnell M, Kakkar AK, Fox KAA, Parkhomenko AN, Ertl G, Störk S, Keltai M, Ryden L, Pogosova N, Dans AL, Lanas F, Commerford PJ, Torp-Pedersen C, Guzik TJ, Verhamme PB, Vinereanu D, Kim JH, Tonkin AM, Lewis BS, Felix C, Yusoff K, Steg PG, Metsarinne KP, Cook Bruns N, Misselwitz F, Chen E, Leong D, Yusuf S, COMPASS. I. Rivaroxaban with or without aspirin in stable cardiovascular disease. N Engl J Med. 2017;377:1319–30.

32. Noad RL, Hanratty CG, Walsh SJ. Initial experience of bioabsorbable polymer Everolimus-eluting Synergy stents in high-risk patients undergoing complex percutaneous coronary intervention with early discontinuation of dual-antiplatelet therapy. J Invasive Cardiol. 2017;29:36–41.

33. Briguori C, Tamburino C, Jessurun GAJ, Meyer-Geßner M, Reczuch K, Cortese B, Maillard L, Anthonio RL, La Manna A, Morice MC, Bouchez D, Balland A, Huynh VP, Baumbach A. Prospective evaluation of drug eluting self-apposing stent for the treatment of unprotected left main coronary artery disease: 1-year results of the TRUNC study. Catheter Cardiovasc Interv. 2020;96:E142–8.

34. Mailey JA, Ahmed M, Hogg M, Cosgrove C, Murphy JC, McNeice AH, Spratt JC, Spence MS, Walsh SJ. Initial experiences of percutaneous coronary intervention using a new-generation everolimus-eluting stent platform. Invasive Cardiol. 2021;33(10):E784–90.

35. Blachutzik F, Honton B, Escaned J, Hill JM, Werner N, Banning AP, Lansky AJ, Schlattner S, De Bruyne B, Di Mario C, Dörr O, Hamm C, Nef HM. Safety and effectiveness of coronary intravascular lithotripsy in eccentric calcified coronary lesions: a patient-level pooled analysis from the Disrupt CAD I and CAD II studies. Clin Res Cardiol. 2020;

36. Hill JM, Kereiakes DJ, Shlofmitz RA, Klein AJ, Riley RF, Price MJ, Herrmann HC, Bachinsky W, Waksman R, Stone GW. Intravascular lithotripsy for treatment of severely calcified coronary artery disease: the Disrupt CAD III study. J Am Coll Cardiol. 2020;76(22):2635–46.

37. Cosgrove CS, Wilson SJ, Bogle R, Hanratty CG, Williams R, Walsh SJ, McEntegart M, Spratt JC. Intravascular lithotripsy for lesion preparation in patients with calcific distal left main disease. EuroIntervention. 2020;16:76–9.

38. Wong B, El-Jack S, Khan A, Newcombe R, Glenie T, Cicovic A, Armstrong G. Treatment of heavily calcified unprotected left Main disease with lithotripsy: the first case series. J Invasive Cardiol. 2019;31:E143–7.

39. de la Torre Hernandez JM, Baz Alonso JA, Gómez Hospital JA, Alfonso Manterola F, Garcia Camarero T, Gimeno de Carlos F, Roura Ferrer G, Recalde AS, Martínez-Luengas IL, Gomez Lara J, Hernandez Hernandez F, Pérez-Vizcayno MJ, Cequier Fillat A, Perez de Prado A, Gonzalez-Trevilla AA, Jimenez Navarro MF, Mauri Ferre J, Fernandez Diaz JA, Pinar Bermudez E, Zueco Gil J, S. S. IVUS-TRONCO-ICP. Clinical impact of intravascular ultrasound guidance in drug-eluting stent implantation for unprotected left main coronary disease: pooled analysis at the patient-level of 4 registries. JACC Cardiovasc Interv. 2014;7:244–54.

40. Park S-J, Kim Y-H, Park D-W, Lee S-W, Kim W-J, Suh J, Yun S-C, Lee CW, Hong M-K, Lee J-H. Impact of intravascular ultrasound guidance on long-term mortality in stenting for unprotected left main coronary artery stenosis. Circ Cardiovasc Interv. 2009;2:167–77.

41. Kinnaird T, Johnson T, Anderson R, Gallagher S, Sirker A, Ludman P, de Belder M, Copt S, Oldroyd K, Banning A. Intravascular imaging and 12-month mortality after unprotected left main stem PCI: an analysis from the British cardiovascular intervention society database. J Am Coll Cardiol Intv. 2020;13:346–57.

42. Ladwiniec A, Walsh SJ, Holm NR, Hanratty CG, Mäkikallio T, Kellerth T, Hildick-Smith D, Mogensen LJH, Hartikainen J, Menown IBA, Erglis A, Eriksen E, Spence MS, Thuesen L, Christiansen EH. Intravascular ultrasound to guide left main stem intervention: a NOBLE trial substudy. EuroIntervention. 2020;16:201–9.

43. Serruys PW, Kogame N, Katagiri Y, Modolo R, Buszman PE, Íñiguez-Romo A, Goicolea J, Hildick-Smith D, Ochala A, Dudek D, Piek JJ, Wykrzykowska JJ, Escaned J, Banning AP, Farooq V, Onuma Y. Clinical outcomes of state-of-the-art percutaneous coronary revascularisation in patients with three-vessel disease: two-year follow-up of the SYNTAX II study. EuroIntervention. 2019;15:e244–52.

44. Pappalardo A, Mamas MA, Imola F, Ramazzotti V, Manzoli A, Prati F, El-Omar M. Percutaneous coronary intervention of unprotected left main coronary artery disease as culprit lesion in patients with acute myocardial infarction. JACC Cardiovasc Interv. 2011;4:618–26.

45. Pedrazzini GB, Radovanovic D, Vassalli G, Sürder D, Moccetti T, Eberli F, Urban P, Windecker S, Rickli H, Erne P, P. I. AMIS. Primary percutaneous coronary intervention for unprotected left main disease in patients with acute ST-segment elevation myocardial infarction the AMIS (acute myocardial infarction in Switzerland) plus registry experience. JACC Cardiovasc Interv. 2011;4:627–33.

46. Patel N, De Maria GL, Kassimis G, Rahimi K, Bennett D, Ludman P, Banning AP. Outcomes after emergency percutaneous coronary intervention in patients with unprotected left main stem occlusion: the BCIS national audit of percutaneous coronary intervention 6-year experience. J Am Coll Cardiol Intv. 2014;7:969–80.

47. Quigley RL, Milano CA, Smith LR, White WD, Rankin JS, Glower DD. Prognosis and management of anterolateral myocardial infarction in patients with severe left main disease and cardiogenic shock. The left main shock syndrome. Circulation. 1993;88:II65-70.

48. Montalescot G, Brieger D, Eagle KA, Anderson FA, FitzGerald G, Lee MS, Steg PG, Avezum A, Goodman SG, Gore JM, I. GRACE. Unprotected left main revascularization in patients with acute coronary syndromes. Eur Heart J. 2009;30:2308–17.

49. Caggegi A, Capodanno D, Capranzano P, Chisari A, Ministeri M, Mangiameli A, Ronsivalle G, Ricca G, Barrano G, Monaco S, Di Salvo ME, Tamburino C. Comparison of one-year outcomes of percutaneous coronary intervention versus coronary artery bypass grafting in patients with unprotected left main coronary artery disease and acute coronary syndromes (from the CUSTOMIZE registry). Am J Cardiol. 2011;108:355–9.

50. O'Neill WW, Kleiman NS, Moses J, Henriques JP, Dixon S, Massaro J, Palacios I, Maini B, Mulukutla S, Dzavík V, Popma J, Douglas PS, Ohman M. A prospective, randomized clinical trial of hemodynamic support with Impella 2.5 versus intra-aortic balloon pump in patients undergoing high-risk percutaneous coronary intervention: the PROTECT II study. Circulation. 2012;126:1717–27.

51. Levine GN, Bates ER, Blankenship JC, Bailey SR, Bittl JA, Cercek B, Chambers CE, Ellis SG, Guyton RA, Hollenberg SM. 2011 ACCF/AHA/SCAI guideline for percutaneous coronary intervention: executive summary: a report of the American College of Cardiology Foundation/American Heart Association task force on practice guidelines and the Society for Cardiovascular Angiography and Interventions. Catheter Cardiovasc Interv. 2012;79:453–95.

Which Interventional Device for Left Main PCI? A Description of Available Stents

Vinayak Nagaraja and Samir Kapadia

Key Points

- Left main coronary artery provides blood supply to a large mass of the myocardium.
- It is crucial to have a stent platform that would match long-term outcomes of surgical revascularization.
- The published literature so far provides robust evidence to support the use of the current generation stents in left main intervention.
- Among the contemporary stents, third drug eluting generation stents (Xience, Synergy, and Biomatrix) have the maximum evidence in the left main arena.

7.1 Introduction

The left main coronary artery (LMCA) is pivotal for survival and provides blood supply to a large mass of the myocardium [1]. Based on intravascular imaging studies, the dimensions of the left main coronary artery are around 5 mm in diameter (range 3.5–6.5 mm) and 10 mm in length [2, 3]. It has an oval orifice with a curvilinear course

[3]. The term "reverse tapering" has been often used to describe the LMCA [4]. The LMCA ostium is smaller in dimensions compared to the distal LMCA bifurcation [4–6]. The atherosclerotic burden involves the lateral walls of the left main and extends into the left anterior descending artery (LAD) and left circumflex artery (LCx) [7]. The left main bifurcation is frequently diseased with a large angle (70–80°) however, quite variable [3]. In at least one-fourth of the instances, a left main trifurcation is encountered with a large intermediate artery [8]. In uncomplicated left main disease, drug-eluting stents provide a durable result similar to CABG [9]. The event rates post LMCA PCI are similar to multivessel coronary artery intervention [10] and the risk of stroke at 1 year post LMCA PCI is significantly lower than CABG [11]. The published data so far suggests that second-generation drug-eluting stents are far superior to first-generation drug-eluting stents in unprotected left main stenosis [12–16]. The SYNTAX trial [17], LE MANS trial [18, 19], PRECOMBAT trial [20], and Boudriot et al. [21] were randomized trials that compared percutaneous coronary intervention (PCI) and coronary artery bypass grafting (CABG) in individuals with severe left main disease. However, the stents used in these trials were older generation stents like TAXUS and CYPHER. Nevertheless, it has been observed that PCI and CABG were similar long-term primary composite endpoint. However, CABG was

V. Nagaraja · S. Kapadia (✉)
Department of Cardiovascular Medicine, Cleveland Clinic Foundation, Cleveland, OH, USA
e-mail: kapadis@ccf.org

© Springer Nature Switzerland AG 2022
B. Cortese (ed.), *Left Main Coronary Revascularization*,
https://doi.org/10.1007/978-3-031-05265-1_7

superior to PCI in patients with diabetes and complex coronary disease (SYNTAX score >32) [17] with lower rates of ischemia-driven target lesion revascularization [20]. These trials laid the foundation for EXCEL and NOBLE that assessed contemporary drug-eluting stents in this arena [22, 23]. There has been a heated debate regarding left main revascularization especially after EXCEL [23] and NOBLE [24] trials. It is crucial to have a stent platform that would match long-term outcomes of surgical revascularization. This chapter covers the contemporary stent platforms and the evidence supporting their use in the LMCA arena.

7.1.1 Xience (Abbott Vascular, Santa Clara, CA, USA)

Xience V® is a cobalt-chromium everolimus embedded stent (strut thickness of 81 μm) that has a 7.6 μm thick coating of polyvinylidene fluoride co-hexafluoropropylene. Everolimus ($C_{53}H_{83}NO_{14}$, molecular weight 958 Da) is a derivative of sirolimus and has a hydroxyl group on the C40 position of sirolimus, which is replaced with a 2-hydroxyethyl group. Everolimus is more lipophilic than sirolimus and better absorbed by the vessel wall. It is also less inflammatory compared to sirolimus or paclitaxel [25]. With the Xience V® platforms the elution of everolimus occurs over 4 months. Xience PRIME™ is the next version of Xience V® with an enhanced delivery system making it more flexible and deliverable. The stent balloon has a shorter taper reducing-edge dissection. Xience Prime was closely followed by Xpedition™/Alpine/Sierra/PRO. These versions had subsequent improvements making them more deliverable. Xience Pro also offers a 48 mm platform. The Xience series of stents are fluorinated polymer-coated stents with good expansible capacity. The bench testing [26] suggests a 3.5–4.0 mm XIENCE stent can over-expanded to 6 mm.

The best evidence regarding the role of Xience as a stent platform in LMCA PCI comes from the EXCEL trial [23]. The EXCEL non-inferiority trial [23] randomly assigned nearly 1900 individuals with the left main disease and a SYNTAX score of 32 or lower to CABG and PCI. The drug-eluting stents used were fluoropolymer-based cobalt-chromium everolimus-eluting stents manufactured by Xience, Abbott Vascular. These stents included Xience PRIME™/V®/Xpedition™/PRO. At 5 years, the primary composite endpoint consisting of death from any cause, stroke, or MI was similar in both cohorts (hazard ratio (HR) 1.19, 95% confidence interval (CI): 0.95–1.50) [27]. However, ischemia-driven revascularization was substantially higher in the PCI cohort at 5 years with a hazard ratio of 1.84 (95% CI: 1.39 to 2.44) [27]. The outcomes were no different irrespective of the presentation (acute coronary syndromes versus stable angina) [28] nor diabetes [29]. The utility of FFR/IVUS was 86.2% in the PCI cohort [30, 31] and this trial's post hoc analysis demonstrated an upfront 2-stent strategy had inferior outcomes compared to the provisional approach in patients outside the realm of true bifurcations [31]. The 5-year stent thrombosis rates in the EXCEL trial was 1.8% [27] far superior to the TAXUS stent (SYNTAX trial) with stent thrombosis rates of nearly 5% at 5 years [32, 33].

DKCRUSH-III and V trials [34–37] evaluated double kissing crush stenting against culotte and provisional stenting in unprotected true distal left main bifurcation PCI (Medina 1,1,1 or 0,1,1), respectively. These trials have made the double kissing crush stenting the new gold standard double stent strategy in true distal left main bifurcation disease management [35–38]. The DKCRUSH-V trial used Xience Prime (Abbott Vascular, Santa Clara, California) and Resolute (Medtronic, Santa Rosa, California) stents, whereas DKCRUSH-III trial utilized Firebird-2 Sirolimus-eluting-Eluting Coronary CoCr Stent (Microport Co., Shanghai, China) and Xience V (Abbott Vascular, Irvine, California). In the DKCRUSH-V trial, target lesion failure was observed in 8.3% along with a 0.4% rate of definite or probable stent thrombosis at 3 years in patients undergoing the DKCRUSH strategy [35]. In the DKCRUSH-III trial, target vessel revascularization was observed in 5.8% along with no definite or probable stent thrombosis at 3 years in patients undergoing the DKCRUSH strategy [37].

7.1.2 Xience Vs Synergy

Synergy stent (Boston Scientific, Natick, MA, USA) is a platinum chromium everolimus-eluting stent with a strut thickness of 74 μm. The abluminal surface consists of bioerodable poly lactic-co-glycolic acid polymer coating (4 μm thickness) and everolimus. The 3.0- and 3.5-mm platforms can be post-dilated to 4.25 mm. Whereas, the 4.0 mm platform can be post-dilated to 5.75 mm. To accommodate large vessels, the Synergy Megatron platform was launched as the next iteration of the Synergy stent. The Synergy Megatron platform is currently available in Europe and can expand from 3.5 mm to 6.0 mm.

The IDEAL-LM was an investigator-initiated all-comers trial that compared Xience and Synergy platforms in patients undergoing LMCA PCI (NCT02303717) [39]. The IDEAL-LM trial was enrolled 799 patients undergoing left main PCI across multiple centers in Europe. The intervention arms of this non-inferiority trial included Synergy stent implantation along with 4 months of dual antiplatelet therapy (DAPT) and Xience stent implantation along with 12 months of DAPT. After 2 years, major adverse cardiovascular events (MACE) that included all-cause mortality, myocardial infarction, and ischemia-driven target vessel revascularization were similar across the two cohorts and achieved non-inferiority (Synergy 14.6% vs Xience 11.4%). The incidence of definite/probable stent thrombosis in the Synergy cohort was 2.7% and the Xience cohort was 1.3% (P value: 0.21). The Synergy cohort had numerically higher ischemic events, this was largely driven by myocardial infarction and ischemia-driven target vessel revascularization rates.

7.1.3 Biomatrix ™ Stent

The Biomatrix ™ stent (Biosensors International PTE LTD, Singapore) consists of a Biolimus A9 (semi-synthetic sirolimus analogue) and a poly-lactic acid (PLA) biodegradable polymer. The Biomatrix ™ stent has thick struts measuring 112 μm. Biolimus A9 is a semi-synthetic siroli-mus analogue which is highly lipophilic. An alkoxy-alkyl group replaces hydrogen at the 42-O position. The drug along with the biodegradable, PLA polymer at a concentration of 15.6 mg/cm^2 is coated on the abluminal surface of the stent. Nobori™ stent (Terumo, Japan) is the first iteration of the BioMatrix stent and utilizes the S-Stent platform. Nobori™ stent does not use the automated autopipette proprietary technology for coating the biodegradable, PLA polymer like the BioMatrix stent.

The Nordic-Baltic-British left main revascularization (NOBLE) trial [22] was an open-label, non-inferiority trial that randomized 1201 patients with left main coronary artery disease with SYNTAX scores <32 to PCI or CABG. At 5 years PCI was inferior to CABG in terms of major adverse cardiac and cerebrovascular events with an HR of 1.58 (95% CI: 1.24–2.01). The definite stent thrombosis rate at 5 years was 2% [40]. The NOBLE trial had a similar FFR/IVUS utility of 74% compared to the EXCEL trial [23]. The heterogeneity between EXCEL and the NOBLE trial was significant with a lower representation of diabetes and acute coronary syndrome in the NOBLE trial as well as differences in protocol definition for endpoints [41]. When compared to the real-world data [41], the EXCEL trial was far more generalizable. The contradictory results of the EXCEL and NOBLE trial probably also highlight the different stent platforms Xience and Biomatrix (89% of the NOBLE trial). Table 7.1 summarizes all the left main PCI trials.

7.1.4 Resolute Onyx

Resolute Onyx (Medtronic, CA, USA) is a zotarolimus drug-eluting stent. Zotarolimus ($C_{52}H_{79}N_5O_{12}$, molecular weight 966 Da) is an equipotent sirolimus analogue. Zotarolimus is derived from sirolimus to reduce restenosis where the C40 position is altered by a tetrazole ring and hence a shorter circulating half-life. Zotarolimus has improved penetration of cell membranes courtesy its lipophilic nature. Zotarolimus is packed on the Biolinx polymer

Table 7.1 Outcomes from randomized trials in LMCA percutaneous revascularization

Study ID	Stent platform	Mortality outcomes [event/participants] (%)			Individual outcomes [event/participants] (%)		
		Outcome	Events in PCI	Follow-up	Outcome	Events in PCI	Follow-up
LE MANS trial [18, 19]	BMS, first-generation drug-eluting stents	Death	0/52	30 days	Nonfatal MI	1/52 (1.92)	30 days
		Death	1/52(1.92)	1 year	Nonfatal MI	1/52(1.92)	1 year
		Death	11/52(21.15)	10 years	MI	5/52(9.62)	10 years
					Major bleeding	0/52	30 days
					Major bleeding	0/52	1 year
					Stroke	0/52	30 days
					Stroke	0/52	1 year
					Stroke/TIA	2/52(3.84)	10 years
					Revascularization	1/52(1.92)	30 days
					Revascularization	15/52 (28.84)	1 year
					Revascularization	14/52 (26.92)	10 years
SYNTAX trial [17, 63, 64]	TAXUS	Death	26/357(7.28)	3 years	Stroke	4/357(1.12)	3 years
		Death	45/357(12.6)	5 years	Stroke	5/357(1.4)	5 years
		Cardiac death	30/357(8.4)	5 years	MI	25/357 (7)	3 years
					MI	28/357(7.84)	5 years
					Revascularization	71/357 (19.9)	3 years
					Revascularization	90/357(25.21)	5 years
					Stent thrombosis	17/357(4.76)	5 years
Boudriot et al. [21]	CYPHER	Death	2/100(2)	1 year	MI	3/100(3)	30 days
					MI	3/100 (3)	1 year
					Revascularization	1/100(1)	30 days
					Revascularization	14/100 (14)	1 year
PRECOMBAT trial [20, 65, 66]	CYPHER	Death	6/300(2)	1 year	MI	4/300	1 year
		Death	7/300(2.34)	2 years	MI	5/300(1.67)	2 years
		Death	17/300(5.67)	5 years	MI	6/300(2)	5 years
		Death	42 (14.5)	10 years	MI	9 (3.2)	10 years
		Cardiac death	3/300(1)	2 years	Stroke	0/300	1 year
		Cardiac death	11/300(3.67)	5 years	Stroke	1/300(0.34)	2 years
		Cardiac death	22 (7.8)	10 years	Stroke	2/300(0.67)	5 years
					Stroke	5 (1.9)	10 years
					Revascularization	18/300(6)	1 year
					Revascularization	26/300 (8.67)	2 years
					Revascularization	38/300(12.67)	5 years
					Revascularization	59 (21.3)	10 years
					Stent thrombosis	0/300	1 year
					Stent thrombosis	1/300	2 years
					Stent thrombosis	4 (1.4)	10 years
EXCEL trial [23, 27]	XIENCE	Death	9/948(0.95)	30 days	Stroke	6/948(0.63)	30 days
		Death	71/948(7.5)	3 years	Stroke	20/948(2.1)	3 years
		Death	119 (13.0)	5 years	Stroke	26 (2.9)	5 years
		Cardiac death	39/948(4.1)	3 years	MI	37/948(3.9)	30 days
		Cardiac death	61 (6.8)	5 years	MI	72/948(7.6)	3 years
					MI	95 (10.6)	5 years
					Revascularization	7/948(0.73)	30 days
					Revascularization	114/948(12)	3 years
					Revascularization	153 (17.2)	5 years
					Stent thrombosis	16 (1.8)	5 years

Table 7.1 (continued)

Study ID	Stent platform	Mortality outcomes [event/participants] (%)			Individual outcomes [event/participants] (%)		
		Outcome	Events in PCI	Follow-up	Outcome	Events in PCI	Follow-up
NOBLE trial [22]	BioMatrix and other drug-eluting stents	Death	2/592(0.33)	30 days	MI	3/592(0.5)	30 days
		Death	9/592(1.52)	1 year	MI	11/592(1.86)	1 year
		Death	36/592(6.08)	5 years	MI	29/592(4.9)	5 years
		Cardiac death	2/592(0.33)	30 days	Revascularization	7/592(1.18)	30 days
		Cardiac death	8/592 (1.35)	1 year	Revascularization	32/592(5.4)	1 year
		Cardiac death	14/592 (2.4)	5 years	Revascularization	71/592(12)	5 years
		Cardiac death			Stent thrombosis	1/592(0.17)	30 days
		Cardiac death			Stent thrombosis	2/592(0.33)	1 year
					Stent thrombosis	9/592(1.52)	5 years
					Stroke	0/592	30 days
					Stroke	2/592(0.33)	1 year
					Stroke	16/592(2.7)	5 years

MI Myocardial infarction, *BARC* Bleeding Academic Research Consortium, *TIA* Transient ischemic attack, *TIMI* Thrombolysis in myocardial infarction, *PCI* percutaneous coronary intervention

coating that facilitates fast drug release and at 2 months 85% of the drug is released. The platform has a strut thickness of 81 μm, consists of a single sinusoidal shaped continuous wire that is helically wrapped. The metal consists of a cobalt alloy shell and a platinum-iridium core. Thin strut design provides good deliverability, flexibility and lowers thrombogenicity. Platinum-iridium core provides great radial strength and makes it radiopaque. The 4.5 mm and 5.0 mm stent platforms can be post-dilated to 5.75 mm, whereas the 3.5 mm and 4.0 mm stent platforms can only be post-dilated to 4.75 mm. The Rolex Registry (Rolex) NCT03316833 is a European multicenter, prospective registry that will enroll 450 patients undergoing unprotected left main coronary artery disease PCI with Resolute onyx. This would shed more light on the efficacy and long-term outcomes of zotarolimus drug-eluting stent in this arena.

7.1.5 Orsiro Sirolimus-Eluting Stent

Orsiro (Biotronik, Germany) is a cobalt-chromium sirolimus-eluting stent made of ultra-thin stent struts (60 or 80 μm). The stent surface is completely covered with hydrogen-rich silicon carbide, sirolimus, and PLLA polymer. Sirolimus ($C_{51}H_{79}NO_{13}$, molecular weight 914 Da) is a highly lipophilic drug and elutes over 100 days from the polymer. The asymmetric polymer matrix results in a greater drug concentration on the abluminal than the luminal side. Orsiro has been implanted in the LMCA; however, granular data regarding the stent specific have not been published [42, 43]. A large conglomerate of 3, multicenter, prospective registries (IRIS-DES registry, IRIS-MAIN registry, and PRECOMBAT study) that included 2692 patients undergoing left main intervention evaluated different stent platforms [44]. This study compared cobalt-chromium everolimus-eluting stent (CoCr-EES; Xience V, Prime, Xpedition, or Alpine model; Abbott Vascular, Santa Clara, California), the platinum chromium-EES (PtCr-EES) (Promus Element or Premier model; Boston Scientific, Natick, Massachusetts), the Resolute-zotarolimus-eluting stent (Re-ZES; Resolute Integrity model; Medtronic Inc., Santa Rosa, California), and the biodegradable polymer-biolimus-eluting stent (BP-BES; BioMatrix model; Biosensors, Newport Beach, California, and Nobori, Terumo Clinical Supply, Kakamigahara, Japan). The rates of target vessel failure at 3 years were numerically the highest in the PtCr-EES cohort (14.7% Re-ZES, 13.2% BP-BES, 16.7% CoCr-EES, 18.7% PtCr-EES) The 3-year stent thrombosis rates were less than <1% across all four stent platforms. No statisti-

Table 7.2 Commercially available drug-eluting stents

Stent	Strut thickness microns	Polymer	Polymer thickness	Drug	Alloy
Orsiro (Biotronik)	61	Bioabsorbable, circumferential	3.5 (7.5 on abluminal surface)	Sirolimus	Cobalt chromium
Synergy (Boston Scientific)	74	Bioabsorbable, abluminal	4	Everolimus	Platinum chromium
Ultimaster (Terumo)	80	Bioabsorbable, abluminal	15	Sirolimus	Cobalt chromium
Xience Prime (Abbott Vascular)	81	Permanent, circumferential	8	Everolimus	Cobalt chromium
Resolute Onyx (Medtronic)	81	Permanent, circumferential	6	Zotarolimus	Cobalt chromium with platinum chromium core wire
Biomatrix (Biosensors)	112	Bioabsorbable, abluminal	10	Biolimus A9	Stainless steel

cally significant differences were noted on propensity score analysis concerning major adverse cardiovascular events (all-cause death, any myocardial infarction, or any revascularization) rates at 3 years. When PtCr-EES and BP-BES were compared to each other, the rates of target vessel failure were statistically significantly higher in the PtCr-EES (HR: 1.60; 95% CI: 1.01 to 2.54).

7.1.6 Ultimaster™ Tansei™ Stent (Terumo Corporation, Tokyo, Japan)

The Ultimaster™ Tansei™ stent is a cobalt-chromium stent with a strut thickness of 80 μm. It is an open-cell platform with an abluminal biodegradable polymer consisting of poly-DL-lactic acid (PDLLA) and polycaprolactone copolymer that elutes sirolimus which degrades over 3–4 months. The Ultimaster Tansei has a "2-link" design that facilitates side branch access and the 3.5–4.0 mm stent platforms can be post-dilated to 5.8 mm. Its tapered tip design and exit port make it more deliverable with coaxial alignment. The e-Ultimaster registry (NCT02188355) presented at EURO PCR 2018 demonstrates favorable outcomes in left main disease with Ultimaster Tansei stent platform (n = 391). The stent thrombosis rate at 30 days was 0.5%. Long-term outcomes are awaited with the Ultimaster Tansei stent platform. Table 7.2 summarizes all the commercially available drug-eluting stents.

7.1.7 Xposition S Sirolimus-Eluting Stent (Stentys, Paris, France)

Xposition S sirolimus-eluting stent (1.4 μg/mm^2 of drug per surface) is a relatively new device that consists of a nickel-titanium (nitinol) stent which is fitted on a semi-compliant balloon and is restricted by a sheath that can split. To split the sheath and release the stent, the balloon is inflated at low pressure. After deflation of the balloon, the nitinol stent is apposed to the vessel wall. The width of the strut is 133 μm for larger platforms and has a polymer matrix consisting of polysulfone and polyvinylpyrrolidone (ProTeqtor R Hemoteq AG, Würselen, Germany). This stent platform is particularly useful in aneurysmal vessels and situations where the vessel dimension is hard to predict like STEMI. This device is 6 Fr compatible and has acquired the Conformit'e Europ'eenne (CE) mark. Xposition S sirolimus-eluting stent system has significantly thicker stent struts compared to modern drug-eluting stent platforms and can accommodate vessels from 3.5 to 6.0 mm in diameter. Its utility in the left main disease has been evaluated in a few studies [45–47]. A multicenter trial of 150 patients assessed the role of Xposition S in the left main disease [48]. After nearly one year of follow-up, MACE occurred in 9.3% patients, and target lesion revascularization occurred in 5.3% and 1.33% cases of definite stent thrombosis. The Xposition S sirolimus-eluting stent system (STENTYS, Paris, France) was also evaluated in a trial of 205 patients undergoing left main PCI [47]. Procedural success was 96.6% and the target lesion failure rate at one year was 8.3%. The rate of cardiac mortality was 2.0%, and the rate of target vessel myocardial infarction was 2.9%.

7.1.8 Dedicated Bifurcation Stent

There are a few commercially available dedicated bifurcation stents. The rationale behind using dedicated bifurcation stents is to facilitate side branch (SB) recrossing and allowing good apposition across the left main bifurcation. These stents include Tryton stent [49], BiOSS LIM C sirolimus-eluting cobalt-chromium bifurcation dedicated stent [50–52], and BiOSS Expert® [53, 54]. The Tryton stent is a dedicated bare-metal cobalt-chromium thin-strutted SB stent and has minimal evidence in the arena of the left main disease [49]. The BiOSS Expert/BiOSS LIM® is a stainless steel bifurcation dedicated stent (Balton, Poland) with a strut thickness of 120 μm. The BiOSS Expert has a biodegradable polymer as well as paclitaxel while the BiOSS LIM® is a bare-metal stent [53]. The latest generation BiOSS LIM C bifurcation dedicated stent is a sirolimus-eluting cobalt-chromium stent (strut thickness 70 μm) [52]. Dedicated bifurcation stent consists of two zones that are wider proximally and smaller distally. The ratio between proximal and distal zones ranges between 1.15 and 1.3. The stent is loaded on a tapered semi-compliant balloon (Bottle®, Balton, Warsaw, PL) with a nominal pressure of 10 atm. This rapid exchange delivery system is compatible with 0.014 guidewire and 5 Fr guide catheters. The sirolimus-eluting BiOSS LIM has been evaluated in just over one hundred patients with unprotected distal left main stenosis [52, 55, 56]. At one year the MACE rate was nearly 10%. There was no

cardiac mortality or definite stent thrombosis. The POLBOS LM study (NCT03508219) is currently recruiting patients to determine the non-inferiority of the BiOSS LIM C sirolimus-eluting cobalt-chromium bifurcation dedicated stent to the Xience stent in the distal left main bifurcations [50]. The primary endpoint for this trial is the composite of cardiac death, myocardial infarction (MI), and target lesion revascularization (TLR) at one year. This study would shed more light on the efficacy of the BiOSS LIM C sirolimus-eluting cobalt-chromium bifurcation dedicated stent in distal left main disease.

7.2 Conclusion

LMCA PCI warrants a stent that is first capable of dealing with a size disparity between the LMCA and LAD/LCx. The overexpansion capacity of the left main stent is crucial [26] along with acceptable longitudinal shortening as well as it is essential to have preserved drug-polymer. Stent recoil after post-dilation can be prevented by selecting an appropriate malleable alloy. Also, a fine balance must be maintained between thinner stent strut size along with lower thrombogenic potential and thicker struts that provide superior radial strength. Most operators prefer a provisional bailout strategy in the context of carina shift for a distal left main bifurcation and at times a medina 1, 1, 1 bifurcation warrants a two-stent bifurcation strategy like DK crush, nano crush, culotte, or TAP (Fig. 7.1). It is essential the stent has good overexpansion property and provides adequate side branch access. During a two-stent strategy, stent visibility is crucial during recrossing and ostial side branch stenting. Besides, during ostial LMCA stent deployment visibility is essential as stent protrusion can lead to increased risk of stent thrombosis. This is more pronounced during a chimney procedure for transcatheter aortic valve replacement [57]. On the other hand, lack of ostial LMCA coverage can potentially lead to longitudinal stent deformation of the proximal edge mainly due to guide catheter manipulation. Repeat revascularization after any form of revascularization (surgical or percutaneous) is an independent pre-

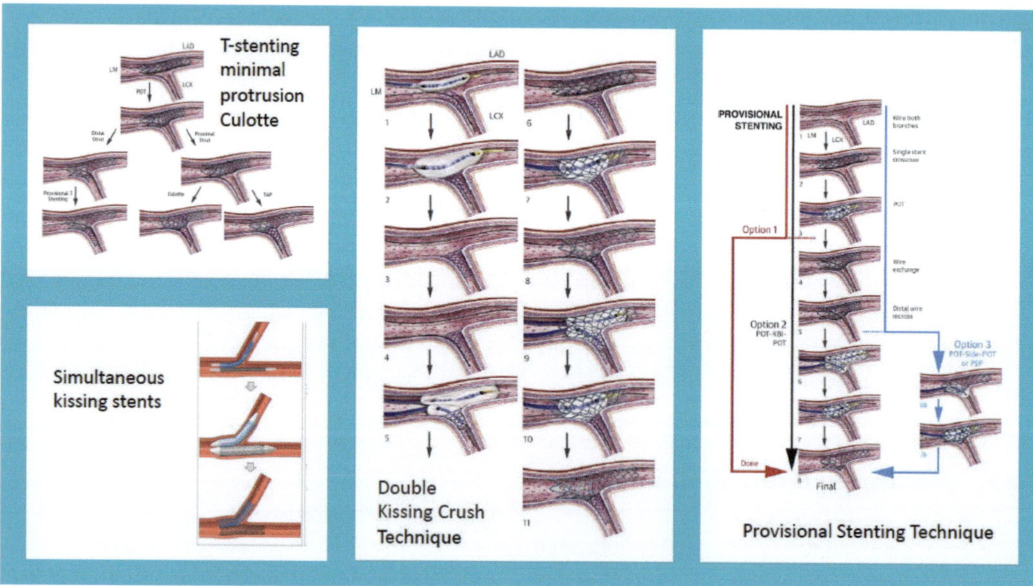

Fig. 7.1 Different bifurcation stenting techniques permission acquired [67, 68]

dictor of 3-year all-cause mortality [58] and unplanned revascularization was higher in the PCI cohort compared to the CABG cohort [59]. An ideal stent should also result in minimal repeat revascularization. Current generation stents have good data to support their use in the LMCA. There is strong evidence to suggest that intravascular ultrasound (IVUS) in LMCA PCI [60]. However, the utility of IVUS during LMCA PCI continues to be remarkably low. IVUS was not performed in nearly 75% of the unprotected LMCA PCI cases ($n = 2468$ patients) in the Swedish nationwide observational study [61]. The National Cardiovascular Data Registry [62] evaluation of 33,128 unprotected left main PCI cases stated nearly 40% IVUS use. Similarly, over the years (2007–2014) IVUS use ranged from 30% to 50% in the British Cardiovascular Intervention Society ($n = 11,264$ patients). The published literature so far provides robust evidence to support the use of the current generation stents especially the third drug eluting generation stents (Xience, Synergy and Biomatrix). To make the PCI outcomes better, intravascular ultrasound and appropriate bifurcation stent strategy are essential.

References

1. El-Menyar AA, Al Suwaidi J, Holmes DR Jr. Left main coronary artery stenosis: state-of-the-art. Curr Probl Cardiol. 2007;32(3):103–93.
2. van Zandvoort LJC, Tovar Forero MN, Masdjedi K, Lemmert ME, Diletti R, Wilschut J, et al. References for left main stem dimensions: a cross sectional intravascular ultrasound analysis. Catheter Cardiovasc Interv. 2019;93(2):233–8.
3. Pau M-G, John AO, Mark WIW, Susann B, Alistair Y, Chris E, et al. A computational atlas of normal coronary artery anatomy. EuroIntervention. 2016;12(7):845–54.
4. Wang P, Chen T, Ecabert O, Prummer S, Ostermeier M, Comaniciu D. Image-based device tracking for the co-registration of angiography and intravascular ultrasound images. Med Image Comput Comput Assist Interv. 2011;14(Pt 1):161–8.
5. Puri R, Kapadia SR, Nicholls SJ, Harvey JE, Kataoka Y, Tuzcu EM. Optimizing outcomes during left Main percutaneous coronary intervention with intravascular ultrasound and fractional flow reserve: the current state of evidence. J Am Coll Cardiol Intv. 2012;5(7):697–707.
6. Iyisoy A, Ziada K, Schoenhagen P, Tsutsui H, Kapadia S, Popovich J, et al. Intravascular ultrasound evidence of ostial narrowing in nonatherosclerotic left main coronary arteries. Am J Cardiol. 2002;90(7):773–5.
7. Oviedo C, Maehara A, Mintz GS, Araki H, Choi SY, Tsujita K, et al. Intravascular ultrasound classification of plaque distribution in left main coronary artery

bifurcations: where is the plaque really located? Circ Cardiovasc Interv. 2010;3(2):105–12.

8. Burzotta F, Lassen JF, Banning AP, Lefevre T, Hildick-Smith D, Chieffo A, et al. Percutaneous coronary intervention in left main coronary artery disease: the 13th consensus document from the European bifurcation Club. EuroIntervention. 2018;14(1):112–20.

9. Athappan G, Patvardhan E, Tuzcu ME, Ellis S, Whitlow P, Kapadia SR. Left main coronary artery stenosis: a meta-analysis of drug-eluting stents versus coronary artery bypass grafting. JACC Cardiovasc Interv. 2013;6(12):1219–30.

10. Agarwal S, Zaman T, Tuzcu EM, Shishehbor M, Lincoff AM, Whitlow PL, et al. Comparison of outcomes of unprotected left main versus multivessel coronary artery interventions. Am J Cardiol. 2011;108(1):15–20.

11. Athappan G, Chacko P, Patvardhan E, Gajulapalli RD, Tuzcu EM, Kapadia SR. Late stroke: comparison of percutaneous coronary intervention versus coronary artery bypass grafting in patients with multivessel disease and unprotected left main disease: a meta-analysis and review of literature. Stroke. 2014;45(1):185–93.

12. Rodriguez AE, Santaera O, Larribau M, Sarmiento R, Haiek C, Del Pozo JF, et al. Second vs. first-generation drug-eluting stents in complex lesions subsets: 3 years' follow-up of ERACI IV study. Minerva Cardioangiol. 2017;65(1):81–90.

13. Rodriguez AE. Second versus first generation DES in multiple vessel disease and unprotected left main stenosis: insights from ERACI IV study. Minerva Cardioangiol. 2015;63(4):317–27.

14. Park SJ, Ahn JM, Kim YH, Park DW, Yun SC, Yoon SH, et al. Temporal trends in revascularization strategy and outcomes in left main coronary artery stenosis: data from the ASAN medical center-left MAIN revascularization registry. Circ Cardiovasc Interv. 2015;8(3):e001846.

15. Chieffo A, Meliga E, Latib A, Park SJ, Onuma Y, Capranzano P, et al. Drug-eluting stent for left main coronary artery disease. The DELTA registry: a multicenter registry evaluating percutaneous coronary intervention versus coronary artery bypass grafting for left main treatment. JACC Cardiovasc Interv. 2012;5(7):718–27.

16. Anouska M, Neus S, Talal H, Olivier D, Nicolas B, Nicolas D, et al. Two-year outcomes of everolimus vs. paclitaxel-eluting stent for the treatment of unprotected left Main lesions: a propensity score matching comparison of patients included in the French left Main Taxus (FLM Taxus) and the LEft MAin Xience (LEMAX) registries. EuroIntervention. 2013;9(4):452–62.

17. Morice MC, Serruys PW, Kappetein AP, Feldman TE, Stahle E, Colombo A, et al. Outcomes in patients with de novo left main disease treated with either percutaneous coronary intervention using paclitaxel-eluting stents or coronary artery bypass graft treatment in the synergy between percutaneous coronary intervention with TAXUS and cardiac surgery (SYNTAX) trial. Circulation. 2010;121(24):2645–53.

18. Buszman PE, Kiesz SR, Bochenek A, Peszek-Przybyla E, Szkrobka I, Debinski M, et al. Acute and late outcomes of unprotected left main stenting in comparison with surgical revascularization. J Am Coll Cardiol. 2008;51(5):538–45.

19. Buszman PE, Buszman PP, Banasiewicz-Szkrobka I, Milewski KP, Zurakowski A, Orlik B, et al. Left Main stenting in comparison with surgical revascularization: 10-year outcomes of the (left Main coronary artery stenting) LE MANS trial. JACC Cardiovasc Interv. 2016;9(4):318–27.

20. Park SJ, Kim YH, Park DW, Yun SC, Ahn JM, Song HG, et al. Randomized trial of stents versus bypass surgery for left main coronary artery disease. N Engl J Med. 2011;364(18):1718–27.

21. Boudriot E, Thiele H, Walther T, Liebetrau C, Boeckstegers P, Pohl T, et al. Randomized comparison of percutaneous coronary intervention with sirolimus-eluting stents versus coronary artery bypass grafting in unprotected left main stem stenosis. J Am Coll Cardiol. 2011;57(5):538–45.

22. Makikallio T, Holm NR, Lindsay M, Spence MS, Erglis A, Menown IB, et al. Percutaneous coronary angioplasty versus coronary artery bypass grafting in treatment of unprotected left main stenosis (NOBLE): a prospective, randomised, open-label, non-inferiority trial. Lancet. 2016;388(10061):2743–52.

23. Stone GW, Sabik JF, Serruys PW, Simonton CA, Genereux P, Puskas J, et al. Everolimus-eluting stents or bypass surgery for left Main coronary artery disease. N Engl J Med. 2016;375(23):2223–35.

24. Mäkikallio T, Holm NR, Lindsay M, Spence MS, Erglis A, Menown IBA, et al. Percutaneous coronary angioplasty versus coronary artery bypass grafting in treatment of unprotected left main stenosis (NOBLE): a prospective, randomised, open-label, non-inferiority trial. Lancet. 2016;388(10061):2743–52.

25. Joner M, Nakazawa G, Finn AV, Quee SC, Coleman L, Acampado E, et al. Endothelial cell recovery between comparator polymer-based drug-eluting stents. J Am Coll Cardiol. 2008;52(5):333–42.

26. Nicolas F, Sayan S, Eduardo A, Ricardo P, Sukhjinder SN, Darrel PF, et al. Maximal expansion capacity with current DES platforms: a critical factor for stent selection in the treatment of left main bifurcations? EuroIntervention. 2013;8(11):1315–25.

27. Stone GW, Kappetein AP, Sabik JF, Pocock SJ, Morice MC, Puskas J, et al. Five-year outcomes after PCI or CABG for left Main coronary disease. N Engl J Med. 2019;381(19):1820–30.

28. Doucet S, Jolicoeur EM, Serruys PW, Ragosta M 3rd, Kron IL, Scholtz W, et al. Outcomes of left main revascularization in patients with acute coronary syndromes and stable ischemic heart disease: analysis from the EXCEL trial. Am Heart J. 2019;214:9–17.

29. Milojevic M, Serruys PW, Sabik JF 3rd, Kandzari DE, Schampaert E, van Boven AJ, et al. Bypass surgery or stenting for left Main coronary artery dis-

ease in patients with diabetes. J Am Coll Cardiol. 2019;73(13):1616–28.

30. Maehara A, Mintz G, Serruys P, Kappetein A, Kandzari D, Schampaert E, et al. Impact of final minimal stent area by IVUS on 3-year OUTCOME after PCI of left main coronary artery disease: the excel trial. J Am Coll Cardiol. 2017;69(11 Supplement):963.

31. Kandzari David E, Gershlick Anthony H, Serruys Patrick W, Leon Martin B, Morice M-C, Simonton Charles A, et al. Outcomes among patients undergoing distal left Main percutaneous coronary intervention. Circ Cardiovasc Interv. 2018;11(10):e007007.

32. Kappetein AP, Feldman TE, Mack MJ, Morice MC, Holmes DR, Stahle E, et al. Comparison of coronary bypass surgery with drug-eluting stenting for the treatment of left main and/or three-vessel disease: 3-year follow-up of the SYNTAX trial. Eur Heart J. 2011;32(17):2125–34.

33. Parasca CA, Head SJ, Milojevic M, Mack MJ, Serruys PW, Morice M-C, et al. Incidence, characteristics, predictors, and outcomes of repeat revascularization after percutaneous coronary intervention and coronary artery bypass grafting: the SYNTAX trial at 5 years. J Am Coll Cardiol Intv. 2016;9(24):2493–507.

34. Chen SL, Xu B, Han YL, Sheiban I, Zhang JJ, Ye F, et al. Comparison of double kissing crush versus Culotte stenting for unprotected distal left main bifurcation lesions: results from a multicenter, randomized, prospective DKCRUSH-III study. J Am Coll Cardiol. 2013;61(14):1482–8.

35. Chen X, Li X, Zhang JJ, Han Y, Kan J, Chen L, et al. 3-year outcomes of the DKCRUSH-V trial comparing DK crush with provisional stenting for left Main bifurcation lesions. JACC Cardiovasc Interv. 2019;12(19):1927–37.

36. Chen SL, Zhang JJ, Han Y, Kan J, Chen L, Qiu C, et al. Double kissing crush versus provisional stenting for left Main distal bifurcation lesions: DKCRUSH-V randomized trial. J Am Coll Cardiol. 2017;70(21):2605–17.

37. Chen SL, Xu B, Han YL, Sheiban I, Zhang JJ, Ye F, et al. Clinical Outcome after DK crush versus Culotte stenting of distal left Main bifurcation lesions: the 3-year follow-up results of the DKCRUSH-III study. JACC Cardiovasc Interv. 2015;8(10):1335–42.

38. Crimi G, Mandurino-Mirizzi A, Gritti V, Scotti V, Strozzi C, de Silvestri A, et al. Percutaneous coronary intervention techniques for bifurcation disease: network meta-analysis reveals superiority of double-kissing crush. Can J Cardiol. 2019;36(6):906–14.

39. Lemmert ME, Oldroyd K, Barragan P, Lesiak M, Byrne RA, Merkulov E, et al. Reduced duration of dual antiplatelet therapy using an improved drug-eluting stent for percutaneous coronary intervention of the left main artery in a real-world, all-comer population: rationale and study design of the prospective randomized multicenter IDEAL-LM trial. Am Heart J. 2017;187:104–11.

40. Holm NR, Makikallio T, Lindsay MM, Spence MS, Erglis A, Menown IBA, et al. Percutaneous coronary angioplasty versus coronary artery bypass grafting in the treatment of unprotected left main stenosis: updated 5-year outcomes from the randomised, non-inferiority NOBLE trial. Lancet (London, England). 2020;395(10219):191–9.

41. Lee PH, Kang SH, Han S, Ahn JM, Bae JS, Lee CH, et al. Generalizability of EXCEL and NOBLE results to a large registry population with unprotected left main coronary artery disease. Coron Artery Dis. 2017;28(8):675–82.

42. Rigatelli G, Zuin M, Vassilev D, Dinh H, Giatti S, Carraro M, et al. Culotte versus the novel nano-crush technique for unprotected complex bifurcation left main stenting: difference in procedural time, contrast volume and X-ray exposure and 3-years outcomes. Int J Cardiovasc Imaging. 2019;35(2):207–14.

43. Rigatelli G, Zuin M, Dinh H, Giatti S, Nguyen VT, Maddali N, et al. Long-term outcomes of left Main bifurcation double stenting in patients with STEMI and cardiogenic shock. Cardiovas Revascul Med. 2019;20(8):663–8.

44. Lee PH, Kwon O, Ahn JM, Lee CH, Kang DY, Lee JB, et al. Safety and effectiveness of second-generation drug-eluting stents in patients with left Main coronary artery disease. J Am Coll Cardiol. 2018;71(8):832–41.

45. Andrea S, Luca Nai F, Andrea P, Giuseppe T. Left main bifurcation PCI with the culotte technique using two self-apposing stents. EuroIntervention. 2020;15(16):1458–9.

46. Yew KL, Kang Z. First-in-man unprotected left main stenting with Stentys Xposition S self-apposing sirolimus eluting stent and optical coherence tomography guidance: the emerging panacea for left main intervention. Int J Cardiol. 2015;201:628–30.

47. Tamburino C, Carlo B, Jessurun GA, Meyer-Gessner M, Reczuch K, Cortese B, et al. TCT-389 prospective evaluation of the drug-eluting self-apposing stent for the treatment of unprotected left Main coronary artery disease: 2-year results of the TRUNC study. J Am Coll Cardiol. 2019;74(13 Supplement):B385.

48. Cortese B, Montefusco A, D'Ascenzo F, La Manna A, Ando G, Bisceglia T, et al. Clinical performance of a dedicated self-apposing stent for the treatment of left main stem disease. Results of the left Main AngioplasTy wIth a Self-apposing StEnt - the MATISSE study. Cardiovas Revascul Med. 2018;19(7 Pt B):831–6.

49. Neupane S, Edla S, Ambulgekar N, Zaitoun A, Torey J, Attallah A. Tryton dedicated bifurcation stent in treatment of unprotected distal left main bifurcation disease. Cardiovas Revascul Med. 2018;19(8s):60–4.

50. Asano T, Kogame N, Onuma Y, Modolo R, Chichareon P, Lefevre T, et al. Treatment with a dedicated bifurcation sirolimus-eluting cobalt-chromium stent for distal left main coronary artery disease: rationale and design of the POLBOS LM study. EuroIntervention. 2019;16(8):654–62.

51. Gil RJ, Bil J, Grundeken MJ, Kern A, Inigo Garcia LA, Vassilev D, et al. Regular drug-eluting stents versus the dedicated coronary bifurcation sirolimus-eluting BiOSS LIM(R) stent: the randomised, multicentre, open-label, controlled POLBOS II trial. EuroIntervention. 2016;12(11):e1404–e12.

52. Gil RJ, Bil J, Kern AK, Garcia LAI, Formuszewicz R, Dobrzycki S. Five-year clinical outcomes following drug-eluting stent implantation in left main trifurcations. Postepy Kardiol Interwencyjnej. 2019;15(1):116–9.

53. Bil J, Gil RJ, Vassilev D, Rzezak J, Kulawik T, Pawlowski T. Dedicated bifurcation paclitaxel-eluting stent BiOSS expert(R) in the treatment of distal left main stem stenosis. J Interv Cardiol. 2014;27(3):242–51.

54. Gil RJ, Bil J, Dzavik V, Vassilev D, Kern A, Formuszewicz R, et al. Regular drug-eluting stent vs dedicated coronary bifurcation BiOSS expert stent: multicenter open-label randomized controlled POLBOS I trial. Can J Cardiol. 2015;31(5):671–8.

55. Briguori C, Visconti G, Golino M, Focaccio A, Signoriello G. Sirolimus-eluting BiOSS LIM dedicated bifurcation stent in the treatment of unprotected distal left main stenosis. Catheter Cardiovas Intervent. 2019;94(3):323–31.

56. Gil RJ, Bil J, Vassiliev D, Inigo Garcia LA. First-in-man study of dedicated bifurcation sirolimus-eluting stent: 12-month results of BiOSS LIM(R) registry. J Interv Cardiol. 2015;28(1):51–60.

57. Chakravarty T, Sharma R, Abramowitz Y, Kapadia S, Latib A, Jilaihawi H, et al. Outcomes in patients with Transcatheter aortic valve replacement and left Main stenting: the TAVR-LM registry. J Am Coll Cardiol. 2016;67(8):951–60.

58. Giustino G, Serruys PW, Sabik JF 3rd, Mehran R, Maehara A, Puskas JD, et al. Mortality after repeat revascularization following PCI or CABG for left Main disease: the EXCEL trial. JACC Cardiovasc Interv. 2020;13(3):375–87.

59. Ahmad Y, Howard JP, Arnold AD, Cook CM, Prasad M, Ali ZA, et al. Mortality after drug-eluting stents vs. coronary artery bypass grafting for left main coronary artery disease: a meta-analysis of randomized controlled trials. Eur Heart J. 2020;41(34):3228–35.

60. Mintz GS, Lefevre T, Lassen JF, Testa L, Pan M, Singh J, et al. Intravascular ultrasound in the evaluation and treatment of left main coronary artery disease: a consensus statement from the European bifurcation Club. EuroIntervention. 2018;14(4):e467–e74.

61. Andell P, Karlsson S, Mohammad MA, Gotberg M, James S, Jensen J, et al. Intravascular ultrasound guidance is associated with better Outcome in patients undergoing unprotected left Main coronary artery stenting compared with angiography guidance alone. Circ Cardiovasc Interv. 2017;10(5):004813.

62. Valle JA, Tamez H, Abbott JD, Moussa ID, Messenger JC, Waldo SW, et al. Contemporary use and trends in unprotected left Main coronary artery percutaneous coronary intervention in the United States: an analysis of the National Cardiovascular Data Registry Research to practice initiative. JAMA Cardiol. 2019;4(2):100–9.

63. Serruys PW, Morice M-C, Kappetein AP, Colombo A, Holmes DR, Mack MJ, et al. Percutaneous coronary intervention versus coronary-artery bypass grafting for severe coronary artery disease. N Engl J Med. 2009;360(10):961–72.

64. Thuijs DJFM, Kappetein AP, Serruys PW, Mohr F-W, Morice M-C, Mack MJ, et al. Percutaneous coronary intervention versus coronary artery bypass grafting in patients with three-vessel or left main coronary artery disease: 10-year follow-up of the multicentre randomised controlled SYNTAX trial. Lancet. 2019;394(10206):1325–34.

65. Ahn JM, Roh JH, Kim YH, Park DW, Yun SC, Lee PH, et al. Randomized trial of stents versus bypass surgery for left Main coronary artery disease: 5-year outcomes of the PRECOMBAT study. J Am Coll Cardiol. 2015;65(20):2198–206.

66. Park D-W, Ahn J-M, Park H, Yun S-C, Kang D-Y, Lee Pil H, et al. Ten-year outcomes after drug-eluting stents versus coronary artery bypass grafting for left main coronary disease: extended follow-up of the PRECOMBAT trial. Circulation. 2020;141(18):1437–46.

67. Morris PD, Iqbal J, Chiastra C, Wu W, Migliavacca F, Gunn JP. Simultaneous kissing stents to treat unprotected left main stem coronary artery bifurcation disease; stent expansion, vessel injury, hemodynamics, tissue healing, restenosis, and repeat revascularization. Catheter Cardiovas Intervent. 2018;92(6):E381–E92.

68. Rab T, Sheiban I, Louvard Y, Sawaya FJ, Zhang JJ, Chen SL. Current interventions for the left main bifurcation. J Am Coll Cardiol Intv. 2017;10(9):849–65.

Antoinette Neylon and Thierry Lefèvre

8.1 Introduction

Vessel bifurcations are particularly susceptible to atheroma formation due to mechanical and sheer stress factors. The left main stem (LMS) is the most important bifurcation in the coronary tree subtending up to 75% of the myocardium. Significant LMS disease is associated with increased mortality and morbidity. For many years, coronary artery bypass grafting (CABG) was the gold-standard treatment for LMS disease. Over the last two decades or so advances in stent design, pharmacotherapy and an increasing body of evidence have seen the evolution of percutaneous techniques to rival this paragon. Randomized controlled trials and registry data have demonstrated similar outcomes to surgery in terms of cardiovascular mortality, albeit with higher needs for re-intervention. Such data have led to widespread guideline acceptance of this management strategy in selected cases.

The distribution of atheroma in the left main stem is highly heterogeneous ranging from the more straightforward ostial or mid-shaft disease to complex distal bifurcation plaque. Accordingly, more complex disease calls for more complex interventions to deal with two or even three diseased branches. While CABG can largely ignore such complexity the optimal technique for dealing with bifurcation disease still remains a matter of debate. In EXCEL, the largest trial to date of contemporary LMS PCI, almost a third of screen failures were due to LMS disease deemed too complex for PCI [1].

In this chapter, we aim to discuss the particularities of LMS disease and describe a fundamentally simple provisional side branch stenting technique that can be used as a foundation for dealing with the most complex disease. We will also discuss two-stent approaches and share some tips and tricks from our own clinical experience.

8.2 What Is Special About the Left Main Stem?

The amount of myocardium at risk sets the LMS apart from all other percutaneous coronary interventions (PCI). The clinical implications of suboptimal results or side branch (SB) loss are unforgiving and potentially devastating. In most LM bifurcations considering the circumflex as a SB may not be appropriate given the importance of the territory implicated. Consequently, the decision not to treat an ostial circumflex has much further reaching consequences than a "keep-it-open" strategy for a diagonal branch. Accordingly, the thresholds for an upfront

A. Neylon · T. Lefèvre (✉)
Institut Cardiovasculaire Paris Sud, Hopital privé
Jacques Cartier, Ramsay Générale de santé,
Massy, France
e-mail: t.lefevre@icps.com.fr

© Springer Nature Switzerland AG 2022
B. Cortese (ed.), *Left Main Coronary Revascularization*,
https://doi.org/10.1007/978-3-031-05265-1_8

two-stent approach or for a second stent in a provisional strategy are not comparable to non-LMS bifurcations.

Disease complexity and the associated technical challenge increase as we move from ostial to distal bifurcation disease. Ostial lesions occur more frequently in women and are associated with larger luminal areas and less calcification [2]. A relationship between the length of the LMS and the location of atheroma has been described with shorter LMS more prone to ostial disease. Histologically the ostial part of the LMS contains more elastic tissue making it more susceptible to elastic recoil. In rare cases, a second stent may be needed to correct recoil after the first stent implantation.

Outside of recoil, treatment of ostial disease has other particular technical challenges. Guide catheter choice and an angulated cranial angiographic working view are important. Judkins left guides are preferred as they are easier to align and maintain a stable position when extubated from the ostium for stent deployment. The less aggressive shape also facilitates guide control to avoid interaction with the stent and longitudinal distortion.

Registry data have shown that ostial and mid-shaft lesions treated with drug-eluting stents (DES) have similar outcomes to surgery; however, this lesion sub-set represents less than 20% of cases [3].

The majority of disease in the LMS involves the distal bifurcation because of flow disturbance at the level of the bifurcation. Low sheer stress areas at the lateral wall of the LAD and circumflex are particularly susceptible. High sheer stress at the level of the carina usually leaves it free of disease. IVUS studies on the plaque distribution show that plaque extends into the LAD in 90% of cases [4]. The circumflex is often angulated making re-access after main branch (MB) intervention challenging. To further complicate matters, trifurcation disease occurs in up to 20% of cases calling for specific strategies.

Unlike other coronary bifurcations, the distal LMS has a T-shaped configuration. The mean angle between the MB and SB in the SYNTAX trial was 95° in contrast with 60° angulation for the LAD-D1 bifurcation. Such acute angulation particularly when the side branch is stented can promote areas of low sheer stress. It may also lead to stent metal fatigue and subsequent fracture as well as areas of mal-apposition. These factors may be important in promoting the higher rate of restenosis noted in the circumflex ostium particularly in two-stent strategies.

The mean age of cohorts treated for LMS disease is 68 years and with this more advanced age comes more significant coronary calcification. Resistant calcified plaque may result in stent under expansion and mal apposition, factors that increase restenosis and stent thrombosis rates. Adjunctive intracoronary imaging and specific techniques therefore play a critical role.

Issues relating to under expansion because of significant calcification are more readily dealt with before stent implantation. At a minimum the presence of significant angiographic calcification should prompt lesion preparation with appropriately sized non-compliant balloons. In the case of resistant calcification cutting or scoring balloons can also be employed; however, the poor crossing profile can make delivery challenging.

In the case of resistant bulky calcifications, modification with the rotablator system (Boston Scientific, Natick, MA) is advocated. When using the rotablator, the SB wire must be given up; however, this generally is not an issue as access to the other branch is usually facilitated after debulking. Hence, this strategy can be a very useful advanced technique to facilitate difficult SB or even MB access.

Intracoronary lithotripsy with the Shockwave system (Shockwave Medical, Fremont, CA) is an attractive alternative that may decrease the risk of slow flow or no reflow in high-risk procedures. This technique has a very short learning curve and an excellent safety profile. It is of special interest in bifurcation lesions as the technique can be safely used after wiring both branches of the bifurcation or even with three wires in a trifurcation.

The LMS is the largest vessel with normal reference diameter of 4.5 ± 0.5 mm. In order to respect the fractal law of bifurcations as described by Murray and Finet, any stent chosen to treat the

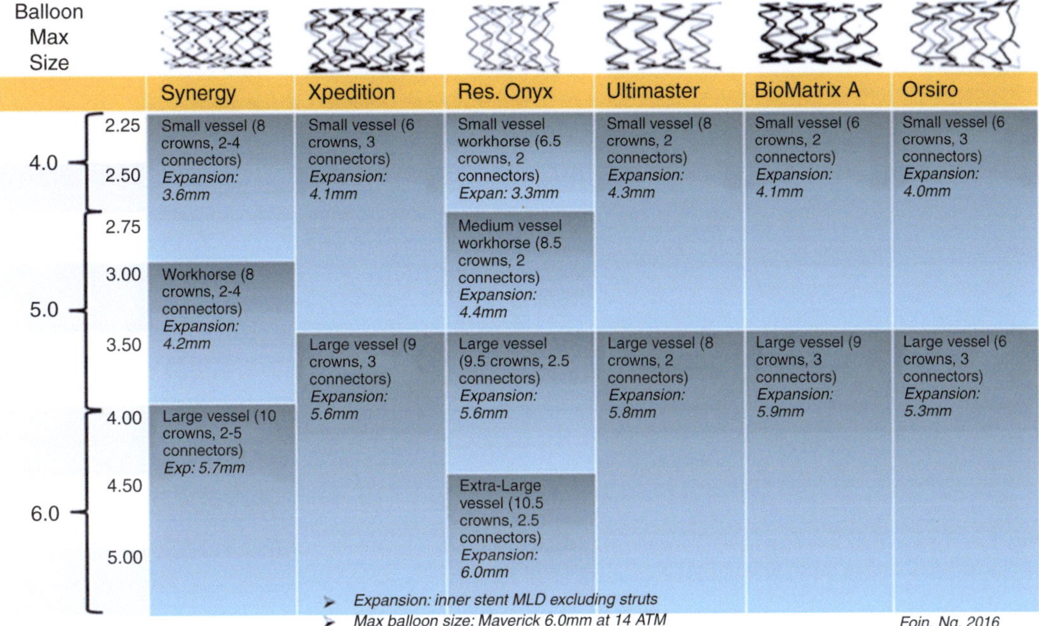

Fig. 8.1 Expansion capacity of different stents (Foin et al.)

bifurcation must be appropriately sized to the distal MB and have the capacity to be optimized to the proximal MB diameter (Fig. 8.1). Knowledge of the cut-off diameters between different stent models and sizes is therefore crucial in selecting the most suitable device. This avoids severe overstretching of the stent that could result in mal apposition and/or damage to the scaffolding and polymer [5]. In practice, this may require oversizing and under-deploying the distal MB stent in order to have the expansion capacity required to adequately perform proximal optimization technique (POT).

In general, it is not necessary to stent to the ostium if the proximal part of the LMS is free of atheroma. To avoid geographic miss when performing the POT there should be adequate stent coverage in the proximal main vessel. In practical terms, this depends on the shortest available balloon available in your cathlab (6, 8, or 10 mm). In the case of short LMS or diffuse LMS disease, coverage to the ostium is recommended. The need for ostial coverage requires careful positioning in an anteroposterior-cranial or left anterior oblique-cranial projection (Fig. 8.2), with special attention to guide control using left hand to avoid interaction between the guide and stent. This control is especially required when pulling back the jailed wire or removing a balloon that is not fully deflated (Fig. 8.3). Indeed, such concerns relating to longitudinal compression have prompted specific design features among certain manufacturers. The Boston Scientific Megatron (Boston Scientific, Natick, MA) is an evolution of the Synergy DES platform specifically adapted for LMS and ostial lesions. Changes in the platform architecture increase both axial and longitudinal strength with the ability to adapt to a LM diameter up to 6 mm (Fig. 8.4).

Equally important is the access to the SB. The positioning and efficacity of the POT (Fig. 8.5) is critical in terms of SB access; however, stent design also plays a role. The number of connectors and stent cell size has been shown to impact crossability [6]. Progressive improvements in design have led to a reduction in the number of connectors and advances in ring design have helped improve radial and longitudinal force [7].

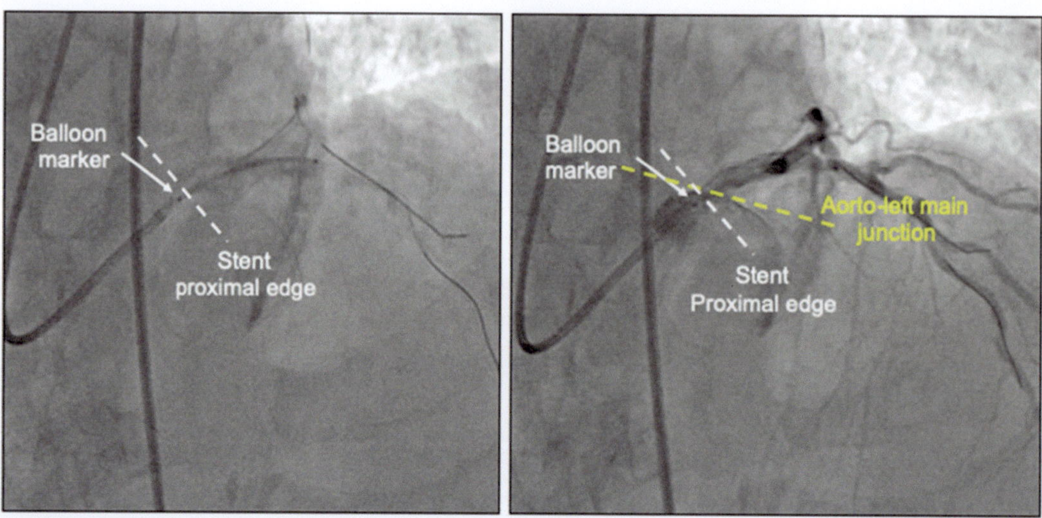

Fig. 8.2 Typical Rao 10°, cranial 40° view showing the relationship between the aorta and the LMS ostium. This view is crucial when ostium needs to be covered

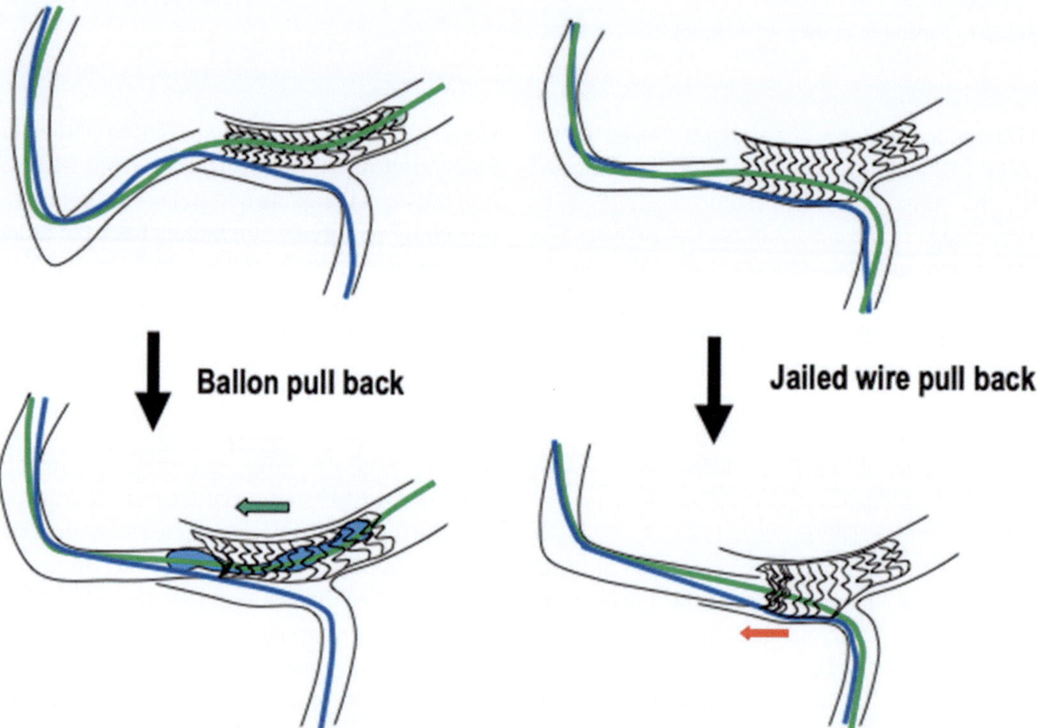

Fig. 8.3 Illustration of longitudinal compression mechanism and the role of "left-hand control". left panel: pulling-back the balloon after stent deployment to early. Right panel, pulling-back the jailed wire without control of the guiding catheter

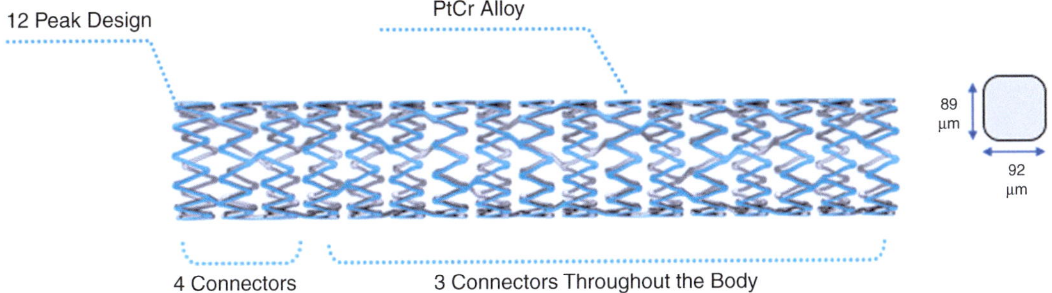

Fig. 8.4 Design of the Megatron stent from Boston scientific specifically designed for LM PCI and large and/or ostial coronary vessels. Note the high number of connectors at the proximal edge in order to decrease the risk of longitudinal compression and the high number of peaks for better expansion capacity

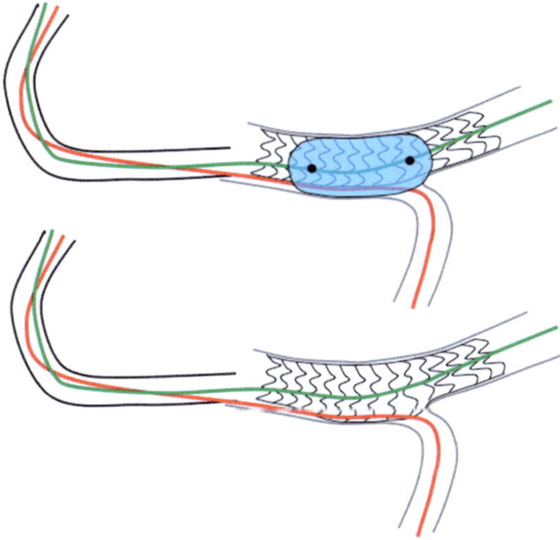

Fig. 8.5 Optimal balloon positioning for POT. This needs an optimal view of the bifurcation, with maximal separation between LAD and LCx. A balloon (semi or non-compliant) with two markers should be used in order to identify clearly the distal shoulder of the balloon. Upper panel: the distal shoulder is placed just proximal to the carina. Lower panel: after POT, good distal apposition and enlargement of stent struts, facilitating access to a distal strut, close to the carina. Note that proximal apposition at the level of the proximal edge of the stent is also crucial. Stent enhancement is very useful in this setting

8.3 Provisional Side Branch Stenting

The provisional approach is the recommended strategy for the majority of cases. At its core is a two-wire, one-stent technique that completes the procedure or otherwise is the foundation of a two-stent technique when required. Thus, the provisional approach is fully adaptable to the anatomical needs in the LMS and the cornerstone of a T, T and protrusion (TAP), or culotte technique (Fig. 8.6).

Critical to the success of the provisional technique is choosing the appropriate stent. The stent should be appropriately sized to the distal MB diameter. Care must be taken not to choose too large a stent as this can cause carina shift toward the SB and is one of the most common causes of acute SB loss. As previously discussed, the stent must then be adapted to the proximal MB using the POT. This should be performed immediately after MB stenting to correct proximal stent under expansion and mal apposition. Additionally, the POT facilitates SB access and rewiring as well as reducing the risk of accidental abluminal rewiring. POT is particularly important in LMS bifurcations where the larger SB magnifies the discrepancy between proximal and distal MV diameters. While clinical data in support of POT in LM PCI is limited, important benefits were demonstrated in an unpublished sub-study of the COBIS II registry. At 3 years follow-up MACE was significantly lower in a POT versus no POT cohort.

Particular care must be taken when positioning the balloon and performing the POT. It is critical to find an angiographic projection where the bifurcation is clearly seen in order to position the balloon marker at the level of the carina (Fig. 8.5). A POT performed too distally in the MB risks occlusion of the SB and if performed

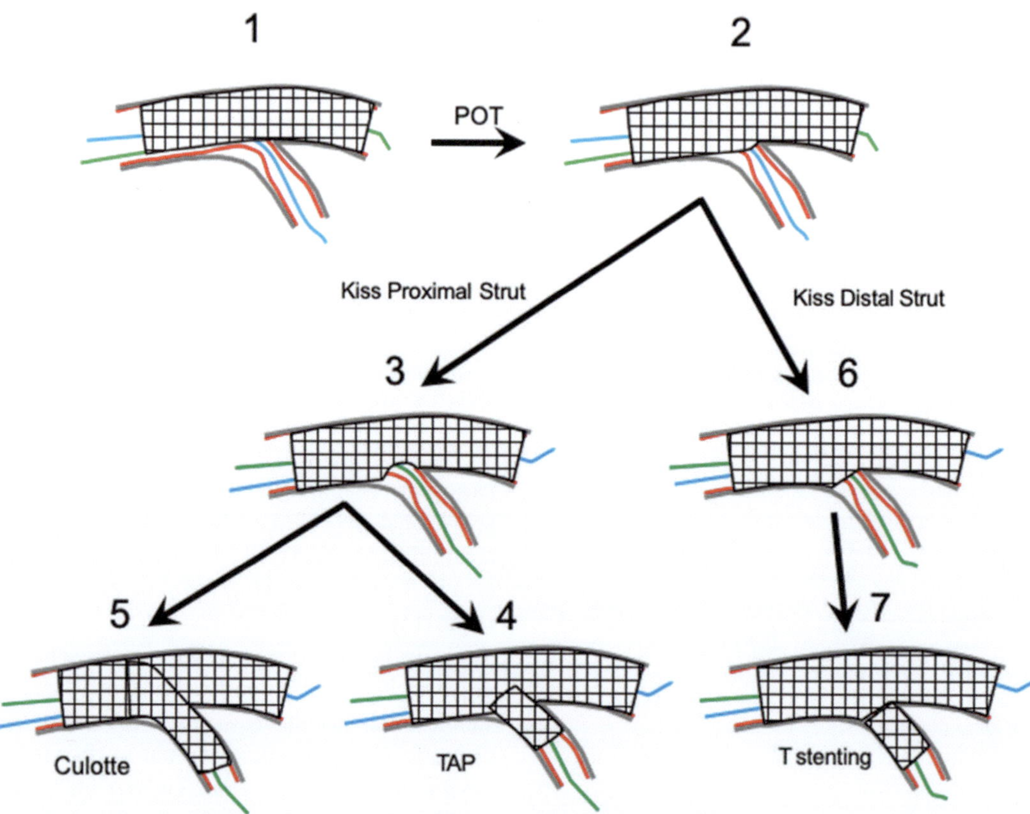

Fig. 8.6 Provisional SB stenting approach for LMS. (1) After wiring both branches, a stent sized to the distal reference is deployed. (2) POT is performed from the carina to the proximal edge of the stent. According to operator preference, the procedure can be stopped at this level. (3) After opening the strut toward the SB, careful evaluation of the angiogram shows that there is no protrusion of metal from the MB stent at the SB ostium (proximal strut) and there is a need for SB stenting. TAP (4) or culotte (5) is the best option. (6) There is a good projection of metal toward the SB ostium (distal strut). If SB stenting is needed, T stenting can be performed

too proximally does not adequately enlarge the stent cells at the level of the SB origin. The latter is the rationale for a re-POT in the case of SB compromise or difficult rewiring.

Following MB stenting and POT, the SB wire and the SB ostium are "jailed" by MB struts. The jailed wire increases procedural safety by helping to maintain SB patency and facilitate SB access by favorably modifying bifurcation angle. Care should be taken not to jail the wire on the radio-opaque segment as this part is more vulnerable to structural damage and fracture. In case of significant SB compromise and occlusion it serves as a useful ostial marker, and offers a bail-out strategy in case of loss in which a small (≤1.5 mm) balloon is passed along the jailed wire to restore flow (Fig. 8.7).

The aim of SB ballooning is to clear the SB of struts and facilitate further access to the SB. Struts across the ostium may act as a bridge for neo-endothelialization (Fig. 8.8) and impact target lesion revascularization (TLR). Given the importance of the SB in the LMS intervention, kissing balloon inflation is advocated although the data supporting this strategy is contradictory.

Before any intervention is undertaken in the SB however, the stent struts must be re-crossed. Several in vitro models have shown better SB scaffolding and less strut protrusion into the SB ostium when wire crossing is at the level of the most distal SB strut. For LMS interventions we advocate introduction of a third wire for strut re-crossing in order to maintain the MB wire position throughout the procedure.

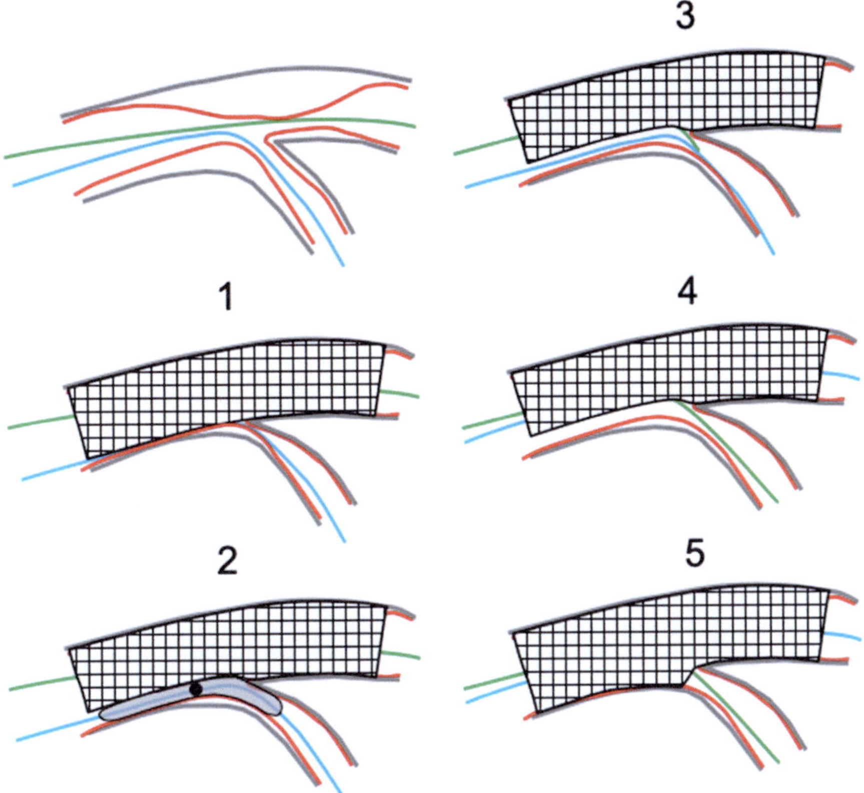

Fig. 8.7 Bail-out technique for SB reopening after stenting. (1) SB occlusion due to carina shifting (stent not sized according to distal reference). (2) After failure to rewire the lesion, a small balloon can be used on the jailed wire in order to restore the flow. Successful SB wiring through the MB stent is obtained in the majority of cases (3 and 4). Good result can be obtained after POT and kissing balloon inflation. If needed, provisional SB stenting (T, TAP, or culotte), can be performed

Because of a T shape angulation between the MB and the SB and because the MB is very large, care should be taken particularly in shaping the wire tip with enough angulation and a tip length at least equivalent to the distal MB diameter to facilitate access. Where possible the new wire should cross the stent in a loop to avoid passing outside the scaffold. The wire should be advanced beyond the SB. Using the right hand to orientate the tip toward the SB and the left hand to fix the position the wire is slowly withdrawn until seen to "fall" toward the SB ostium. The jailed SB wire is a useful guide to the position of wire crossing. If the new SB wire is distal to the jailed wire this is a good indicator that crossing was at the level of the distal strut. It can be also very useful to leave the radio-opaque part of wire at the level of the bifurcation and make a contrast injection to check that this wire is very close to the carina (Fig. 8.9) before removing the jailed wire.

Particular care must be taken to control the guide catheter when removing the jailed wire. The wire should be removed under continuous fluoroscopy, carefully observing guide position in relation to the proximal MB stent. As continuous traction is put on the jailed wire, the left hand must carefully control the guide position and avoid deep intubation.

Kissing balloon inflation (KBI) should be performed with NC balloons, especially for the SB in order to limit the risk of SB dissection. Our experience is that KBI is particularly useful for optimizing the stent deployment in the MB. For

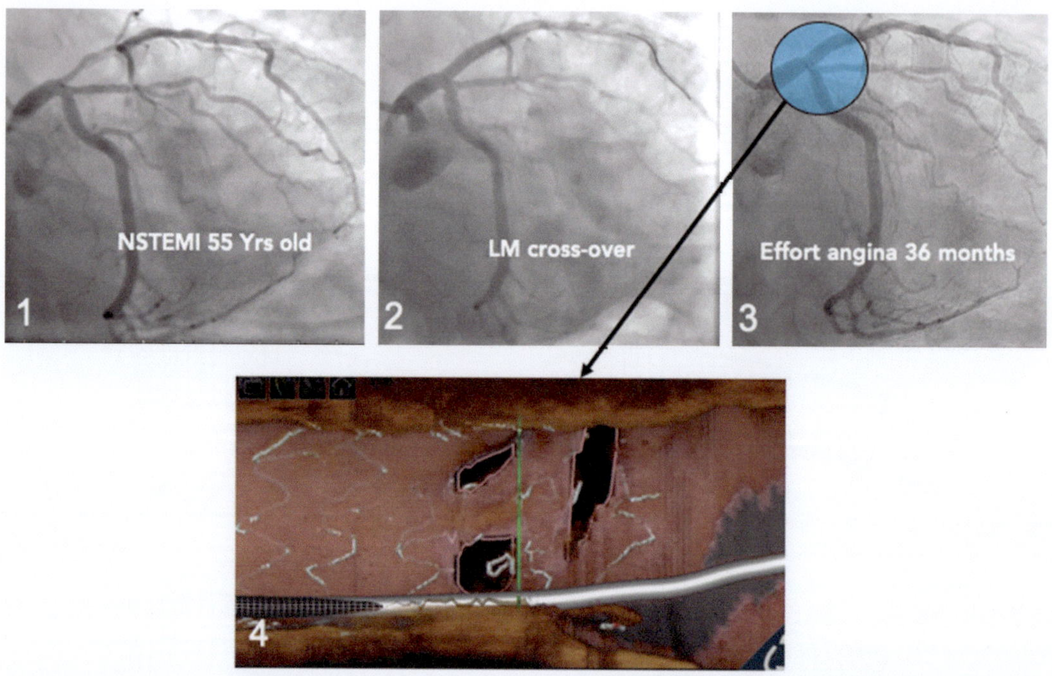

Fig. 8.8 Drawback of the simple cross-over stenting technique. Case example of a patient with a medina 0, 1, 0 lesion (1), treated with LM cross-over technique (2). Reoccurrence of angina 3 years related to ostial LCx stenosis (FFR 0.72) (3). OCT showing endothelial colonization of unopened stent struts (4)

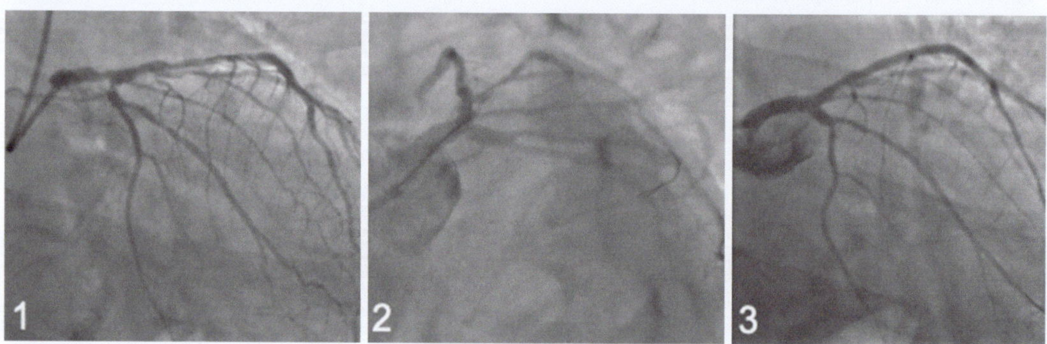

Fig. 8.9 Case example of 1, 0, 1 lesion treated with inverted provisional SB stenting approach. A 3.5 stent was deployed from LCx to LMS (1). POT was performed and the LCx wire was pulled-back in order to enter the distal strut toward the proximal LAD. Angiogram (2), confirm the position of the wire in a distal strut close to the carina. Final results after kissing balloon inflation (3)

large bifurcations requiring >3.5 mm NC balloons 7Fr guide catheters (GC) should be used. We recommend positioning the SB balloon first as manipulations in the GC are easier with a single balloon. Short balloons, appropriately sized to the distal MB and SB with minimal protrusion to the proximal MB, are recommended. While many sequences of inflation have been proposed the most important concepts are prolonged inflation (minimum 15 s) and simultaneous deflation in order to conserve the SB opening and strut clearance.

Provisional Side Branch Stenting

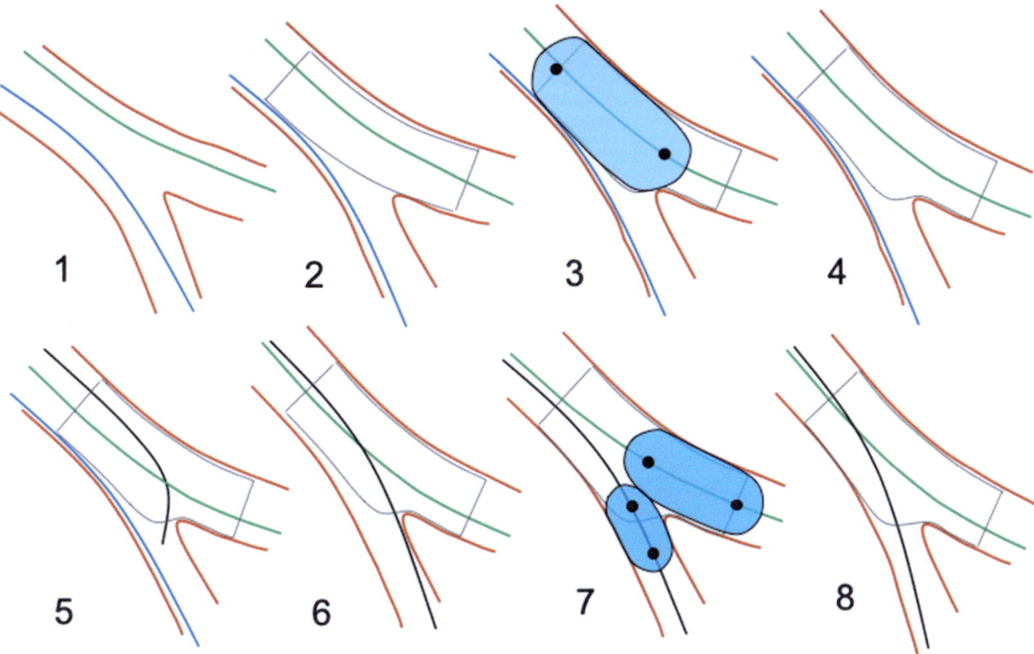

Fig. 8.10 Provisional SB stenting approach. (1) Wire both branches. (2) Stent the MB using a stent sized to the distal reference. (3) Do a POT (from the carina to the proximal edge of the stent). (5) Use a third wire and access the SB using a pull-back technique from the MB (optimal position can be checked by OCT or OFDI). (7) Do a kiss using two short balloons (ideally in the polygone of confluence). Prefer NC balloon for the SB. POT/Side/POT can be an alternative to kissing. (8) Optimal assessment of the result in both branches and decide to stent the SB or not

Schematic drawing of essential steps of provisional and inverted provisional approaches are represented in Figs. 8.10 and 8.11. In all cases a second stent can be used for performing a T, TAP or Culotte stenting according to the anatomy and the experience of the operator. The use of internal crush proposed many years ago as an alternative SB stenting after stenting the MB is not recommended and should be used only in a bail-out situation.

8.4　Systematic Two-Stent Approach

Although most LMS bifurcations can be treated with a provisional SB stenting approach, two-stent techniques are more frequently chosen for the LMS than other bifurcation lesions. The benefit of a two-stent strategy however relies on the technique applied to the specific anatomy. Given the angulation frequently encountered strategies such as T or TAP that avoid acute crossover into the MB are theoretically more attractive.

When and why a two-stent strategy is required depends on the evaluation and interpretation of the angiogram by the operator. The technique used is also heavily influenced by operator experience. Several anatomical complexities are taken into account including:

- Severity and extent (>5 mm from ostium) of SB disease
- SB angulation
- Presence of significant calcification
- Size discrepancy between the LM, LAD and circumflex

It must be remembered that a provisional strategy can be used in almost all of these

Inverted Provisional Side Branch Stenting

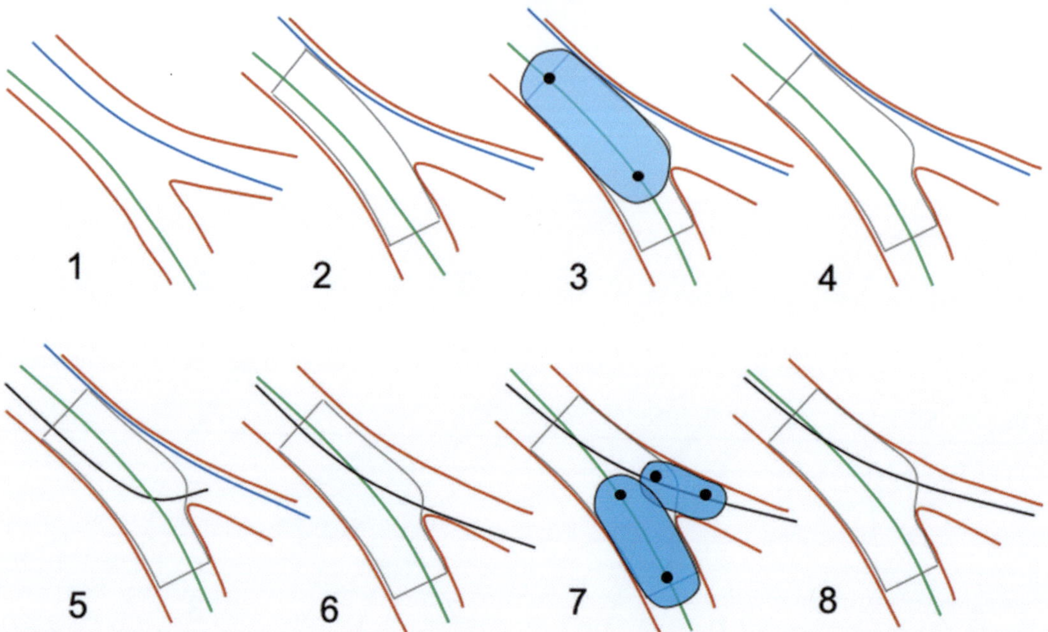

Fig. 8.11 Inverted provisional SB stenting approach. (1) Wire both branches. (2) Stent the SB using a stent sized to the distal reference. (3) Do a POT (from the carina to the proximal edge of the stent). (5) Use a third wire and access the MB using a pull-back technique from the SB (optimal position can be checked by OCT or OFDI). (7) Do a kiss using two short balloons (ideally in the polygone of confluence). Prefer NC balloon for the SB. POT/Side/POT can be an alternative to kissing. (8) Optimal assessment of the result in both branches and decide to stent the MB or not

circumstances where the operator wishes to secure the SB first by adopting an inverted provisional approach. In this technique, following SB stenting, POT, and SB rewiring, a decision to complete using a two-stent strategy can be made.

(i) A culotte technique (Fig. 8.12) when the LAD and Cx are similarly sized and the bifurcation angle is narrow.
(ii) A T or TAP technique (Fig. 8.6), limiting stent overlap in the proximal MB if the bifurcation angle is wide.

Favorable outcomes of a systematic two-stent strategy compared to a provisional approach have been reported in the DKCRUSH-V trial. The double kissing (DK) crush (Fig. 8.13) technique is technically more demanding and in experienced hands has shown lower rates of TLF and stent thrombosis. The technique, which is a progression of the original crush technique, employs triple POT, double kissing, and proximal cell recrossing (Fig. 8.13). It should however be noted that the operators were committed DKCRUSH specialists and the mean LCx lesion length was 17 mm which means that nearly all patients in the provisional SB stenting group should have been treated with two stents [8].

For two-stent strategies based on non-randomized studies and expert consensus, final high-pressure KBI is advocated [9]. More recent non-randomized insights from the Excel trial suggest that final KBI does not impact clinical outcomes. Similar outcomes were demonstrated with or without KBI for both one- and two-stent techniques. These data suggest that KBI may not be required if an angiographically acceptable result is achieved [10].

Culotte

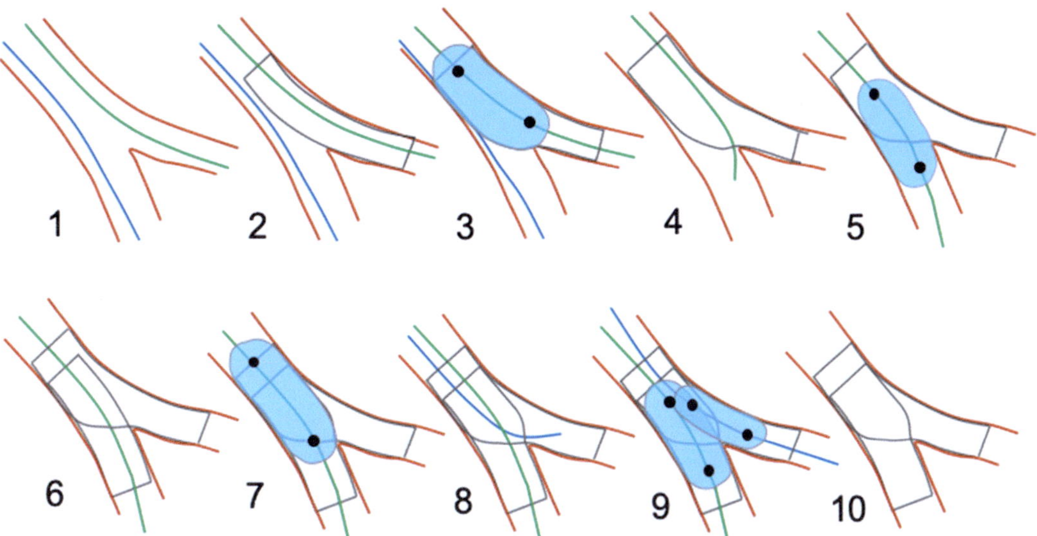

Fig. 8.12 Culotte technique (or inverted culotte). (1) Wire both branches. (2) Stent the MB using a stent sized to the distal reference. (3) Do a POT (from the carina to the proximal edge of the stent). (4) Use the pull-back technique from the MB to access the SB in a. distal strut (optimal position can be checked by OCT or OFDI). (5) Open the struts toward the SB. (6) Stent across LM and SB. (7) Do a POT (from the carina to the proximal edge of the stent kiss using two short balloons (ideally in the polygone of confluence). (8) Use a second wire to access the MB by using a pull-back technique from the SB (optimal position can be checked by OCT or OFDI). (9) Do a kiss using short balloons. A final POT is optional but recommended if long balloons are used

8.5   Difficult Wire Access

MB or SB access can be challenging before or after stenting. There are three main principals that should be applied to LM bifurcation lesion wiring:

1. Wire all important branches—i.e., branches that you do not want to lose.
2. Wire the most difficult branch first.
3. After MB stenting do not remove the jailed SB wire even if you have difficulties to access the SB through the MB stent.

It is important, when possible, to wire the most difficult branch first. Subsequent wires are then inserted by limiting the rotation to avoid wire wrap. Using a Torquer helps by allowing fine and more precise wire manipulations. Keeping the wires separated and identified on the table helps also prevent wire wrap during the procedure. A simple way of quickly identifying the wires is to arrange them in the same configuration as the working view (i.e., in an RAO caudal working view on the table the LAD wire on top and circumflex wire on bottom) using wet gauze to keep in position.

In case of difficult access we recommend a step-wise approach. The first step is to modify the workhorse wire tip shape (usually longer and more angulated) and try to enter the difficult branch using a pullback technique from the more accessible branch. Next try a very flexible or soft wire (such as fielder FC, Sion Blue). In case of failure it is better to continue the technical escalation as shown in Fig. 8.14, rather than performing a predilatation of the accessible vessel. The long U-shaped wire reverse technique can be also a very elegant solution (Fig. 8.15).

DK Crush

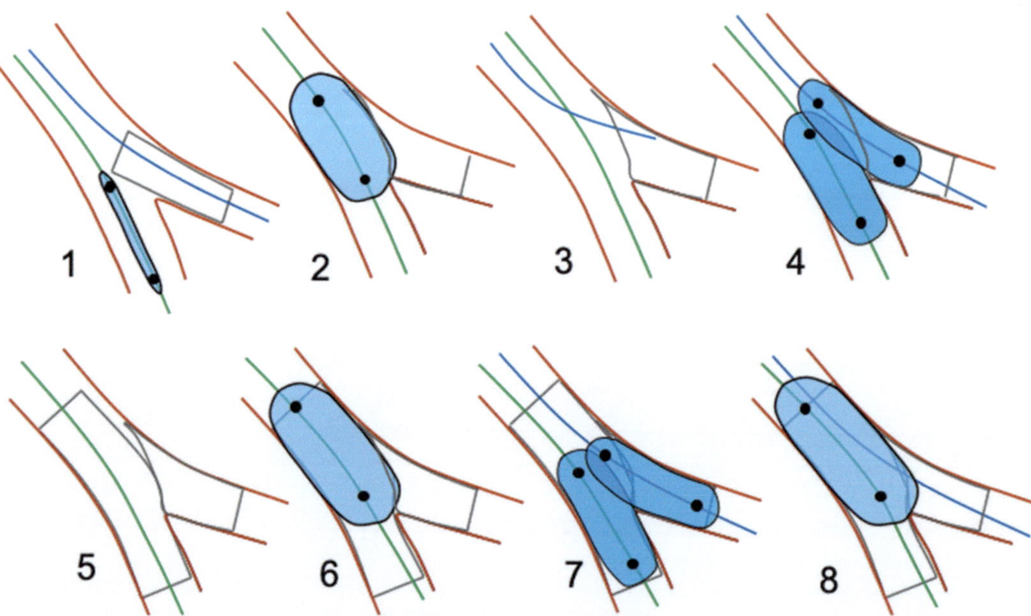

Fig. 8.13 DK Crush Technique. (1) Wire both branches, park a balloon for POT in the MB and stent the SB with the stent protruding in the LMS by 2 or 3 mm. (2) Remove the SB wire and pull-back the MB balloon and crush the LMS part of the SB stent by doing a POT. (3) Wire the SB through the proximal part of the SB stent. (4) Kissing balloon inflation. (5) Remove the SB wire and stent the main vessel using a stent sized to the distal reference. (6) POT (from the carina to the proximal edge of the stent). (7) Use a second wire to access the SB through a proximal or mid MB strut (optimal position can be checked by OCT or OFDI) and do a final kiss. (8) Final POT

Fig. 8.14 Wiring escalation for difficult MB or SB access before stenting

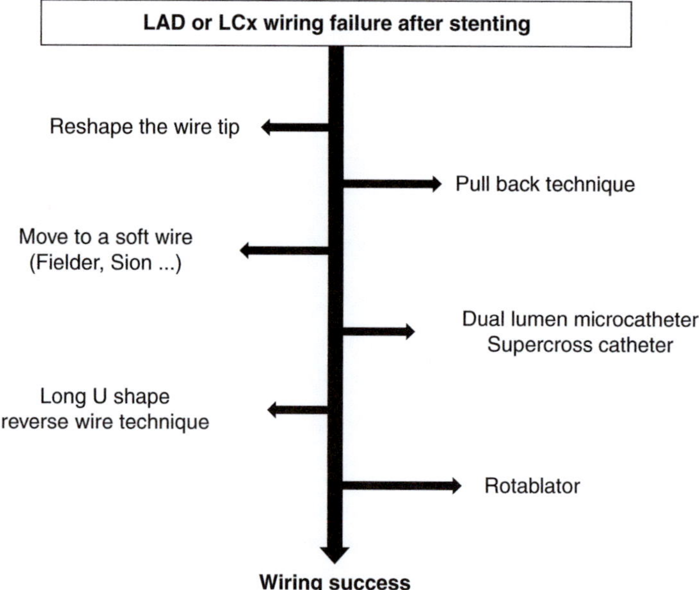

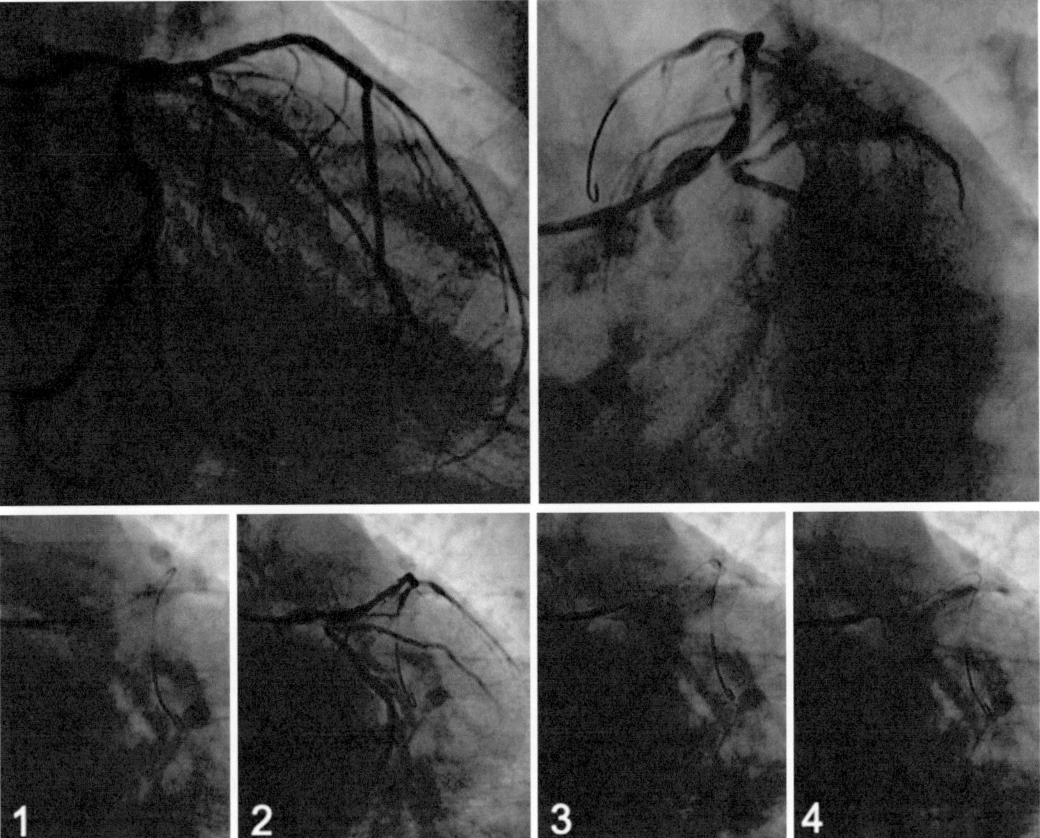

Fig. 8.15 Case example of a Medina 1, 0, 1 LMS lesion with difficult LCx access. Upper right panel (spider view) shows clearly the difficulty: eccentric lesion of the distal LMS pushing the wire away from the LCx and a severe angle >90° between LAD and LCx. After failure with a conventional approach, the long U shape reverse wire technique was used (same wire). The wire was pushed in the LAD and pulled-back slowly maintaining orientation toward the LCx (1). Continuing to pull-back, the wire entered the LCx (2), and progress into the LCx (3 and 4)

We recommend having at least one angled microcatheter available—i.e., Supercross 120° (Teleflex). This is extremely useful in challenging anatomy. The very soft tip should be first orientated toward the ostium and then a regular workhorse or soft wire used to access the branch. It is worth noting that removing the supercross can be challenging in a 6Fr GC. A standard balloon cannot be used to block the wire position in the guide and remove the device. Specific chronic total occlusion kit such as a Trapper (Boston Scientific) balloon or a wire extension may be required. As previously discussed rotablation can be an excellent approach to facilitate SB access when a calcified plaque protrudes in the lumen and deflects the wire.

Similar techniques may be employed to overcome difficulties in re-crossing the SB after MB stenting as illustrated in Fig. 8.16.

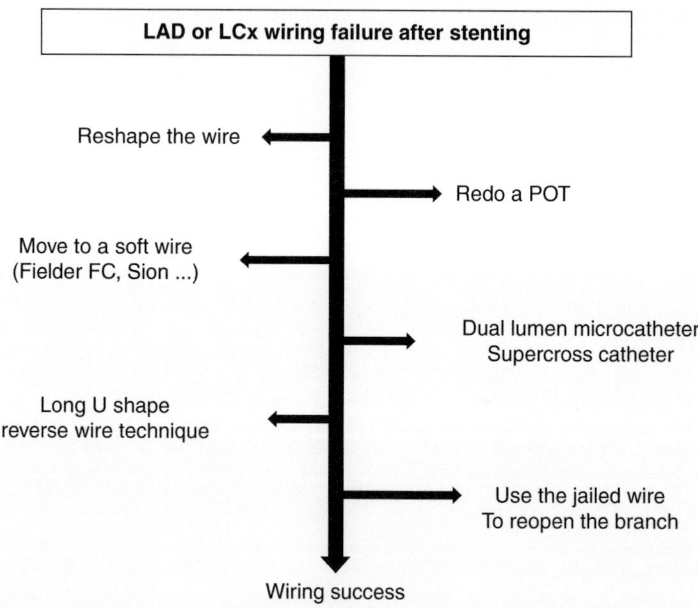

Fig. 8.16 Wiring escalation for difficult MB or SB access after stenting

8.6 Role of Intracoronary Imaging

Intracoronary imaging with intravascular ultrasound (IVUS) or optical coherence tomography (OCT) provides crucial insights in planning and optimizing bifurcation treatment. IC imaging has a role in all steps of the procedure from planning to final evaluation. Our experience is that intracoronary imaging is particularly important in the learning phase of LMS interventions and is extremely important in "calibrating" our eyes to the three diameters in the LMS bifurcation.

Angiographic ambiguity, particularly in relation to the circumflex ostium, is quite frequent and the use of adjunctive imaging tools can be valuable in characterizing plaque volume and distribution. Imaging provides far more insight into the degree, depth, and circumferential distribution of calcification in the bifurcation. With this understanding upfront debulking strategies can be employed in order to achieve better stent expansion. IC imaging allows for a detailed assessment of lesion length and vessel diameters in the bifurcation. This information informs stent choice and diameter in terms of anticipated over-expansion capacity in the proximal MB, and stent length.

Imaging also provides valuable information during the procedure for both one and two-stent strategies. IC is an excellent resource for evaluating the POT and the position of SB rewiring in relation to the distal strut. In complex anatomy requiring two-stent techniques or in the case of ambiguity imaging should be utilized to identify unintentional abluminal rewiring, assess the outcome of KBI and the result in the SB ostium. In the case of two-stent techniques, it is recommended to assess the result in both the SB and MB.

IVUS and OCT have different strengths depending on the clinical situation. IVUS is particularly useful in assessing ostial LMS when manual pullback is used and in cases with significant renal insufficiency where contrast. In contrast OCT offers better resolution and may be easier to interpret, and in particular 3-D modeling helps identify areas of under expansion and precisely localizes SB wire recrossing.

8.7 Role of Stent Enhancement

Stent enhancement is a very useful tool to check optimal deployment of the stent proximal and distal to the carina, eliminate stent distortion (Fig. 8.17), control the position of the balloon close to the carina

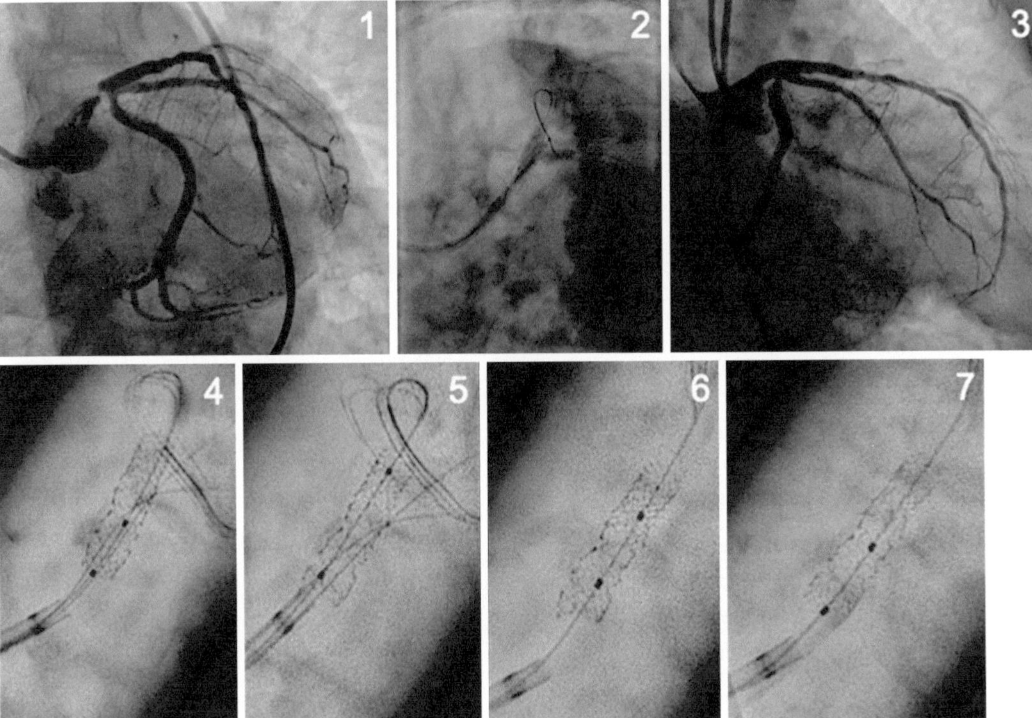

Fig. 8.17 Case example of a Medina 1, 0, 0, 0 LMS trifurcation lesion (1) treaded with provisional SB stenting approach using three wires and seven French guide. A stent was implanted from LM to LAD, followed by POT, wire exchange and trissing balloon inflation (2) with no need for SB stenting (3). Lower panel is a good illustration of the role of stent enhancement: positioning of the balloon for POT at the proximal edge of the stent (4), control of stent deformation after trissing balloon inflation, detection of a minor longitudinal compression during catheter manipulation (5). Correction of the stent deformation after final POT (6). Final result (7)

when doing POT and control the position of the stent when T or TAP stenting is performed.

8.8 Role of Mentorship

LMS bifurcations are complex angioplasties and require a certain level of experience and expertise. An analysis of 1900 LM interventions reinforced the impact of operator experience on clinical outcomes in LMS interventions [11]. Experienced operators (>15 interventions/year for 3 consecutive years) had significantly lower short- and long-term cardiovascular mortality than low volume operators, despite treating more complex disease. This makes a strong case for reserving complex angioplasties, such as LMS interventions to a small number of experienced operators and stresses the importance of sharing knowledge and experience through mentorship of less experienced interventionalists.

8.9 Tips and Tricks

- Think provisional.
- Discuss the case with experienced colleagues and have a plan A, B, C….
- Select your stent and balloons before the procedure respecting the fractal laws.
- Carefully position the POT at the level of the carina.
- Take the time to find the optimal working views (carina, access through a distal strut, LM ostium).
- Good GC support (Extra back-up except for severe ostial stenosis).
- If you think about rotablator, use it.
- If you think about hemodynamic risk, use IABP.
- Two (or three) wires and management of the wires (avoid wire criss-cross inside the patient, the catheter, and on the table).

- Know how to solve difficult MB or SB access before stenting and after stenting.
- Master at least one two-stent technique.
- Distal strut for provisional.
- Left-hand control to avoid longitudinal compression.
- Intracoronary imaging during the learning phase or when in doubt.
- Stent enhancement is very useful.

8.10 Conclusion

LMS disease is heterogeneous and complex and such complexity informs our management. The indication for PCI in the LMS has expanded over the last two decades and PCI is a viable alternative to CABG in selected cases. The majority of cases can be managed with a provisional approach that leaves the final strategy open to a two-stent technique if required.

Shared operator experience in LMS interventions, careful assessment of the baseline angiogram, and meticulous pre-procedural planning are critical for procedural success.

References

1. Stone GW, Sabik JF, Serruys PW, Simonton CA, Genereux P, Puskas J, et al. Everolimus-eluting stents or bypass surgery for left main coronary artery disease. N Engl J Med. 2016;375(23):2223–35.
2. Maehara A, Mintz GS, Castagna MT, Pichard AD, Satler LF, Waksman R, et al. Intravascular ultrasound assessment of the stenoses location and morphology in the left main coronary artery in relation to anatomic left main length. Am J Cardiol. 2001;88(1):1–4.
3. Naganuma T, Chieffo A, Meliga E, Capodanno D, Park SJ, Onuma Y, et al. Long-term clinical outcomes after percutaneous coronary intervention versus coronary artery bypass grafting for ostial/midshaft lesions in unprotected left main coronary artery from the DELTA registry: a multicenter registry evaluating percutaneous coronary intervention versus coronary artery bypass grafting for left main treatment. JACC Cardiovasc Interv. 2014;7(4):354–61.
4. Oviedo C, Maehara A, Mintz GS, Araki H, Choi SY, Tsujita K, et al. Intravascular ultrasound classification of plaque distribution in left main coronary artery bifurcations: where is the plaque really located? Circ Cardiovasc Interv. 2010;3(2):105–12.
5. Ng J, Foin N, Ang HY, Fam JM, Sen S, Nijjer S, et al. Over-expansion capacity and stent design model: an update with contemporary DES platforms. Int J Cardiol. 2016;221:171–9.
6. Watson T, Webster MWI, Ormiston JA, Ruygrok PN, Stewart JT. Long and short of optimal stent design. Open Heart. 2017;4(2):e000680.
7. Foin N, Sen S, Allegria E, Petraco R, Nijjer S, Francis DP, et al. Maximal expansion capacity with current DES platforms: a critical factor for stent selection in the treatment of left main bifurcations? EuroIntervention. 2013;8(11):1315–25.
8. Chen X, Li X, Zhang JJ, Han Y, Kan J, Chen L, et al. 3-year outcomes of the DKCRUSH-V trial comparing DK crush with provisional stenting for left main bifurcation lesions. JACC Cardiovasc Interv. 2019;12(19):1927–37.
9. Burzotta F, Lassen JF, Banning AP, Lefevre T, Hildick-Smith D, Chieffo A, et al. Percutaneous coronary intervention in left main coronary artery disease: the 13th consensus document from the European Bifurcation Club. EuroIntervention. 2018;14(1):112–20.
10. Kini AS, Dangas GD, Baber U, Vengrenyuk Y, Kandzari DE, Leon MB, et al. Influence of final kissing balloon inflation on long-term outcomes after PCI of distal left main bifurcation lesions: analysis from the EXCEL trial. EuroIntervention. 2019;16(3):218–24.
11. Xu B, Redfors B, Yang Y, Qiao S, Wu Y, Chen J, et al. Impact of operator experience and volume on outcomes after left main coronary artery percutaneous coronary intervention. JACC Cardiovasc Interv. 2016;9(20):2086–93.

Which Surgical Technique for Left Main Coronary Artery Bypass? A Mini-Invasive Approach

Bleri Çelmeta, Antonio Miceli, and Mattia Glauber

9.1 Introduction and History

The left main coronary artery is responsible for the vascularization of a large territory of the anterior and lateral myocardium. Consequently, a significant stenosis poses the patient in a life-threatening condition.

From the 1960s, the traditional full sternotomy CABG by the auxiliary of the CPB became the gold standard for treating the coronary artery disease (CAD) because of its safety, feasibility, and reproducibility. As the experience grew, it rapidly became evident that the CPB was associated with several postoperative adverse events (neurological, renal, infectious, hemorrhagic, etc.). On the other hand, full sternotomy could alter the respiratory mechanics of the rib cage and the physiologic pulmonary ventilation, leading to respiratory and infectious postoperative adverse events.

In this situation, MIDCAB was developed as a surgical strategy for the LAD revascularization which avoids the complications related to the CPB and to the full sternotomy. In the meanwhile, this approach offers all the benefits of the LIMA bypass graft which remains the gold standard for revascularization of the LAD and has stood the test of time [1].

This strategy has become particularly attractive for surgical high-risk patients with a counterindication for percutaneous revascularization: it is the case of anatomically complex coronary arteries, patients with diabetes or a contraindication for double antiplatelet therapy [2].

In cases of patients which present a left main coronary artery stenoses, MIDCAB and PCI can be performed together in the setting of a hybrid coronary revascularization (HCR) (surgical and percutaneous) in order to achieve a complete revascularization of the myocardial territory.

Interestingly, the first attempt of surgical coronary revascularization was performed through a left thoracotomy approach, by directly implanting LIMA into the myocardium of a beating heart [3]. In 1967, Kolesov performed for the first time directly sutured anastomoses between IMAs and coronary arteries through a left thoracotomy on a beating heart [4].

Subsequently, with the standardization of the CPB by a full sternotomy approach and the improvement of the cardioplegic solutions, CABG grew increasingly popular to become the gold standard for the surgical treatment of CAD.

In the early 1990s, Benetti proposed a mini-invasive approach for CABG through a right mini-thoracotomy which didn't involve CPB [5]. In the same years, a growing number of cardiac surgeons in different hospitals [6–8] reported on LIMA grafting to the LAD through a similar mini-invasive approach. Since then, the technique

B. Çelmeta · A. Miceli · M. Glauber (✉)
IRCCS Galeazzi-Sant'Ambrogio, Rho, Milano, Italy
e-mail: mattia.glauber@grupposandonato.it

© Springer Nature Switzerland AG 2022
B. Cortese (ed.), *Left Main Coronary Revascularization*,
https://doi.org/10.1007/978-3-031-05265-1_9

has gained popularity and is now performed in some of the best cardiac surgery hospitals in the world [9].

9.2 Indications

- MIDCAB is recommended to patients with an isolated proximal LAD and/or diagonal lesion whenever the percutaneous revascularization is not possible due to anatomical factors or due to a contraindication for the double anti-platelet therapy.
- Patients with a left main coronary artery disease could benefit from a MIDCAB associated with the percutaneous treatment of the non-LAD coronaries, the so-called hybrid approach. Moreover, this group of patients could receive a MICS-CABG by means of a totally arterial surgical revascularization. For this purpose, both internal thoracic mammary arteries and/or the radial artery can be used to achieve a mini-invasive surgical complete revascularization.
- Patients with restenosis of a previously stented LAD lesion could benefit from a MIDCAB. Similarly, patients with a failure of a saphenous bypass graft to LAD needing a single CABG could avoid higher risk redo surgery in favor of a minimally invasive MIDCABG.
- Patients with a surgical high risk and severe preoperative comorbidities (lung diseases, severe renal insufficiency, obesity, uncontrolled insulin-dependent diabetes mellitus, previous cerebrovascular disease or severe cerebral or peripherical vascular diseases, hematological disorders, advanced age, calcified ascending aorta) could benefit from an off-pump surgery by a sternal sparing approach. In these settings, the MIDCAB could offer the best solution in terms of in-hospital death, neurological events, and perioperative myocardial infarction [8].

There are a series of anatomical and patient-related factors which could favor and make MIDCAB more feasible and easier to perform. A slim patient, with a thin and vertically positioned heart, offers an optimal access from the right anterior mini-thoracotomy. On the other hand, a non-calcified good caliber LAD (diameter > 1.75 mm) with a mid-distal presentation (2–4 cm distal to the second diagonal branch) facilitates the conducting of the surgery [1].

9.3 Contraindications

- The presence of a hemodynamically instable patient with an acute myocardial infarction due to a left main coronary artery stenosis is considered an absolute contraindication, as MIDCAB and MICS-CABG in general don't offer the fastest surgical solution in the context of the need of an emergency revascularization. This is due to longer time needed to harvest the IMAs when compared to the great saphenous vein on one side and to the easier and faster approach by means of a full traditional median sternotomy.
- The presence of an occluded left subclavian artery is also an absolute contraindication for MIDCAB as the LIMA wouldn't guarantee the blood support needed to the LAD.

Some patient-related and coronary artery-related conditions could render more difficult and technically demanding the performance of a MIDCAB surgery. In the first case, severe obesity, pectus excavatum, severe scoliosis, small width of intercostal spaces, and previous thoracotomy with important adhesions of the left hemithorax are all patient-related relative contraindications for MIDCAB. In the second case, the LAD-related unfavorable characteristics could be: a relatively short non "apex-forming" LAD, a deep intra-myocardial course, or a small-sized LAD with a heavily calcified arterial wall.

9.4 Surgical Procedure

The patient is placed in a supine position with an insufflated pressure bag under the left scapula to help the widening of the intercostal spaces and the exposition of the LIMA. The left groin and the sternum are always available for an eventual change of strategy (sternotomy, CPB) if necessary or in cases of emergency. The perfusionist and the CPB machine are always ready in stand-by in the operative room. An oro-tracheal intubation with a Carlens tube is used to easily achieve a single lung selective ventilation. The hemodynamic parameters are monitored by the insertion of a radial and a jugular catheter. The catheterization of the bladder is performed to quantify the diuresis and to monitor the body temperature. In cases of a preoperative pulmonary hypertension or low left ventricular ejection fraction (LVEF), a Swan-Ganz catheter is placed for a correct estimation of pressures in the right heart chambers, the pulmonary artery, and the pulmonary capillaries (wedge pressure). As in all mini-invasive procedures, external defibrillator pads are positioned before the incision. The heart rhythm is monitored by a five-channel electrocardiogram. The probe for the transesophageal echocardiography is positioned in all patients before the incision. A warming blanket is always used to maintain physiological body temperature.

An incision of circa 5 cm for anterolateral mini-thoracotomy is made in the fourth intercostal space, 4–5 cm from the lateral border of the sternum. The subcutaneous and muscular tissue is dissected and cauterized with caution, avoiding the injury of the intercostal and/or mammary pedicle. It is important to divide the muscles over a length larger than the cutaneous incision to facilitate retraction and to decrease tension or fraction of the ribs. After the single lung selective ventilation is activated, the intercostal space is entered.

A particular rib retractor, designed specifically for IMA harvesting, is used. The rib retraction should always be gradual and careful in order to avoid rib fracture or excessive tension to the soft tissue, which may lead to tissue necrosis. The LIMA is harvested under direct vision in a pediculized or skeletonized fashion. Harvesting should be as proximal as possible, ideally involving all the vessel's length. However, as Calafiore and colleagues have previously shown, a length of 9 cm or less is suffi-

cient to perform the LAD revascularization in some 77% of cases [7]. In all cases, it is of outmost importance that the vessel leans without tension on the medial mediastinum.

Subsequently, 100–150 IU/kg of intravenous heparin is delivered in order to maintain the activated clotting time (ACT) at a level superior to 300 s. A small rib retractor is inserted and progressively retracted. A redundant pericardial fat is prepared to cover and protect the future anastomosis site. The pericardium is then opened in a longitudinal fashion. The LAD is identified, and a suction cardiac tissue stabilizer is used to immobilize the anastomosis site (Fig. 9.1). The vessel is occluded proximally by means of a pledgeted 4-0 polypropylene suture to achieve a bloodless operative field. If hemodynamic instability or electrocardiographic changes of the ST segment are noted, an intravascular shunt is placed through the anastomosis site to assure intracoronaric blood flow throughout the execution of the surgical anastomosis. The anastomosis is performed by a 8-0 polypropylene suture, afterward protamine is administered for the reversion of the heparinization (Fig. 9.2). The pericardium is closed, the fatty extrapericardial tissue is approximated above the distal part of the LIMA for further protection, and a chest drain is positioned.

It is of note that in case of a left main critical stenosis, the diagonal or the obtuse marginal coronary arteries can be also revascularized in the

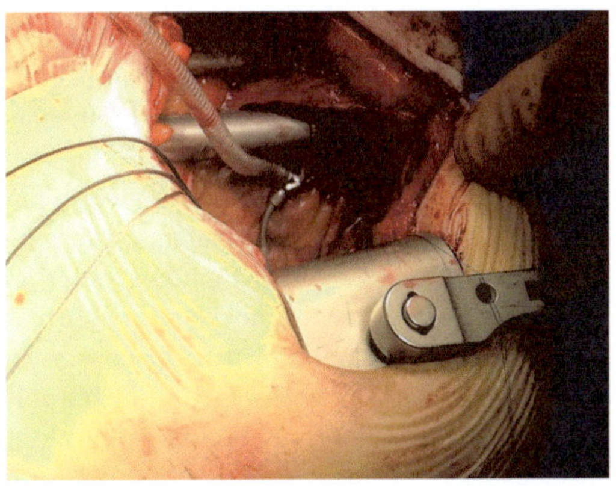

Fig. 9.1 Mini-thoracotomic approcah for CABG LIMA/LAD (MIDCAB)

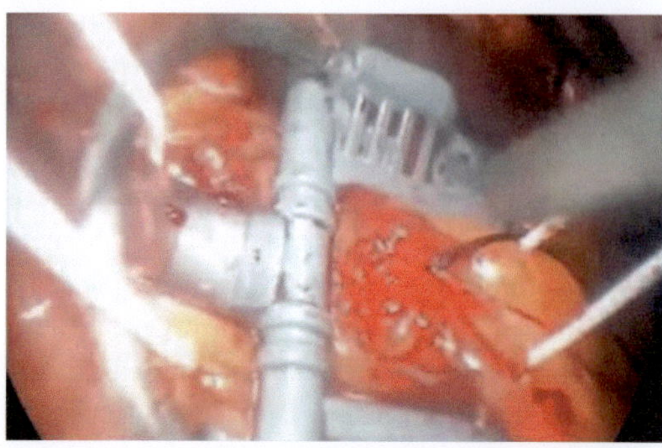

Fig. 9.2 Final anastomosis after MIDCAB procedure

contest of a MICS-CABG surgery by means of a radial artery or a great saphenous vein, previously anastomosed termino-laterally in Y graft to the LIMA. In all cases, aorta is not manipulated surgically.

After finishing the surgical anastomoses, the anesthesiologist gently reinsuflates the left lung: it is of outmost importance to assure that the LIMA sits freely above the heart and medial to the lung with no angulation and with no risk of avulsion, as these adverse events are frequently associated to fatal outcomes.

The ribs are subsequently reapproximated and the thoracotomy is closed in layers.

9.5 Outcomes and Comparison to Other Revascularization Strategies

The current 2018 European Society of Cardiology and European Association for Cardio-Thoracic Surgery guidelines for myocardial revascularization recommend CABG or PCI as first-line management for left main coronary disease in cases of low anatomical complexity expressed by a low SYNTAX score. In all cases, patient comorbidities and preferences are also a guiding factor for the decision of the therapeutical strategy [10].

Since the introduction of percutaneous myocardial revascularization through PCI, first and second generation of drug eluting stents, the treatment of the ischemic cardiopathy has changed forever. In Germany, Ohlmeier et al. have reported a relative increase in the overall PCI and PCI-DES rate of 38% and 548%, respectively from 2004 to 2011 [11]. Similar results published from many other Hospitals demonstrate a similar trend worldwide.

In the meanwhile, the surgical treatment has evolved as well, mostly with the advent of mini-invasive cardiac surgery. This type of surgery offers a reduced blood products transfusion, Intensive Care Unit (ICU) length of stay, and reduced hospitalization times when compared to traditional cardiac surgery, especially in the hands of experienced mini-invasive surgeons in high-volume surgery hospitals [12, 13]. Specifically for MIDCAB in patients who had a LIMA-LAD anastomosis, by avoiding the full sternotomy, Hu et al. reported that these patients had lower intensive care unit time, intubation time, and hospital stay when compared to full sternotomy off-pump coronary artery bypass (OPCAB) grafting patients [14].

The quality of life in the months following the intervention is higher when compared to that of the patients who received a sternotomy: Al-Ruzzeh et al. have found that patient who received MIDCAB had an excellent general health perception (assessed by the Short Form health survey SF-36 and the Hospital Anxiety and Depression Scale HADS) when compared to the traditional CABG group [15–17]. Often, physical recovery from sternotomy takes about 3–6 months. Especially in older patients, this time frame could make up an important proportion of the remaining life and therefore can significantly reduce the perception of the postoperative quality of life.

The first systematic review of the postoperative outcomes in MIDCAB was published by Kettering and colleagues in 2004 [18]. Postoperative mortality in the MIDCAB varies from 0 to 4.9%. Recently, a large meta-analysis including 37 studies with 31,728 patients was published by Indja and colleagues [19], comparing early and late postoperative outcomes between percutaneous coronary intervention with first- and second-generation drug-eluting stents (DESs), OPCAB and MIDCAB in patients with involvement of left main or left anterior descending disease. Early and late mortality was found to be similar between the groups. Another large study demonstrated similar early mortality between MIDCAB and full sternotomy CABG for isolated proximal LAD stenosis (2.0 vs. 2.5%) [20].

In the MIDCAB surgery, the aortic manipulation is avoided: the aorta is not clamped, no CPB is needed and no proximal anastomosis for the bypass graft is performed. This may extend the LIMA to LAD surgery benefits even in patients with a heavily calcified aorta. More importantly, this aspect may contribute to the reduction of peri-operative stroke. In fact, stroke rate varies from 0.6 to 4% after standard CABG [21, 22] and from 0.4 to 0.6% after MIDCAB [23, 24]. On the other hand, when compared to percutaneous revascularization performed for proximal LAD coronary artery disease, MIDCAB had similar periprocedural stroke rates, as shown from previous major RCTs and meta-analyses [19, 25–28].

This favorable outcome could also be partly explained by a lower rate of postoperative atrial fibrillation (AF) in off-pump cardiac surgery [29]. AF is a well-known independent predictor for perioperative stroke [30]. Its role has been re-evaluated in the recent times, as new-onset AF following coronary bypass surgery was found to be associated with significantly higher risk of mortality in short- and long-term follow-up. This difference in the survival rate remains important and valid up to the following 15 years after the surgery [31]. However, it remains unclear whether the role of the AF over the outcomes is direct, or if it acts as a surrogate of more compromised preoperative conditions.

Early myocardial infarction and early repeated revascularization are rare events in the MIDCAB, with no significant difference compared to patients receiving a percutaneous revascularization with DES implantation or to patients receiving an OPCAB [19].

However, patients receiving MIDCAB have shown significantly less late myocardial infarction, recurrent angina, and target vessel revascularization (TVR) when compared to patients receiving DESs. MIDCAB is associated with a significant reduction in late TVR of 82% com-pared to first-generation DES (OR 0.18, 95% CI 0.09–0.32) and 67% compared to second-generation DES (OR 0.33, 95% CI 0.13–0.75) [19]. Goy and colleagues demonstrated that compared to the MIDCAB, the patients with isolated proximal LAD stenosis undergoing PCI suffered from a higher rate of recurrent angina at median follow-up of 2.5 years [32]. Similarly, other studies confronting the long-term results between MIDCAB and PCI with bare metal stents (BMS) demonstrated that the first group had a significantly lower rate of recurrent angina and TVR [32–36].

Effectively, these late benefits of the surgical versus the percutaneous treatment could be explained in two different planes.

On one side, the long-term benefits of the LIMA as the ultimate conduit for the coronary revascularization are well-known. IMA has a minor susceptibility for atherosclerosis, a good resistance to endothelial damage due to surgical harvesting and may go through a remarkable arterial remodeling over time which leads to an increase in blood flow to the coronary artery. The patency rates at 10 years were reported to be from 90 to 95% [37–39]. Its usage to treat CAD is directly associated with prolonged survival in the long-term period.

On the other side, performing a coronary artery bypass creates a "surgical collateraliza-tion" of the coronary tree. The development of anatomic collateral coronary arteries offers a fundamental protection from myocardial infarction in cases of significant coronary stenoses; in some cases, even total coronary occlusions may not provoke anginous symptoms nor myocardial tissue damage. In a similar fashion, performing a coronary artery bypass creates a "surgical" collateral network. This offers a protection from late myocardial infarction, related not only to already existing "flow-limiting" CAD but also to future coronary stenoses in case of progression of the disease (i.e., plaque rupture of a "non-flow limiting" CAD resulting in vessel occlusion). Percutaneous coronary revascularization on the other side can only offer a treatment of the existing "flow-limiting" stenoses but does not address an eventual progression of the CAD disease [40].

An important potential drawback for performing MIDCAB is related to its learning curve, not only for the surgeon but also for the entire medical (anesthesiologists or cardiologists) and nursing team. Technical errors (stenotic or occluded anastomosis, dissected or twisted LITA graft), associated with increased intra-hospital morbidity and mortality, are inversely related to the surgical load, to the frequency of performing the operation, and the level of experience [41, 42]. This steep learning curve, associated with the highly selected target group of patients may have influenced the fact that after all these years of experience and excellent results reported for MIDCAB, the technique makes up only a small part of surgical myocardial revascularization worldwide.

9.6 Hybrid Coronary Revascularization

HCR is the performance in the same patient of a LIMA to LAD bypass in the setting of a mini-invasive surgery (off-pump non-sternotomy or robotic surgery) associated with percutaneous myocardial revascularization. This approach assures all the well-known long-term survival benefits of a LIMA to LAD bypass graft by maintaining in the meanwhile a low morbidity in the immediate postoperative time, combining the benefits of both procedures.

HCR may offer an optimal solution for patients with a left main critical stenosis. It is true that total arterial myocardial surgical revascularization has demonstrated to be superior in terms of survival and outcomes [44], but nonetheless saphenous vein graft (SVG) remains the most used bypass graft for non-LAD coronary arteries [45]. Venous bypass grafts have a limited durability in long-term follow-up: 20% of all SVGs occludes in the first year, and up to 70% are occluded 15 years after performing the CABG [46]. Bearing in mind that last generation DESs have shown a good durability in time, percutaneous revascularization for the circumflex, obtuse marginal or diagonal coronary arteries may offer a feasible and reasonable solution for patients with left main stenosis.

9.6.1 Timing of the HCR

HCR may be performed as a one- or two-step procedure.

In the one-step procedure, the surgical and percutaneous stages are developed in sequence in a hybrid operative room during the same operative time. It offers the advantage that the surgical anastomosis is immediately assessed by an intra-operative coronarography while the percutaneous step is made with the surgical team at the bedside for any possible complication or unsuccessful PCI [47]. On the other hand, the hybrid operative room is not present in all cardiac surgery hospitals. Moreover, the need of DAPT immediately after a surgical procedure may increase the risk of postoperative bleeding.

The two-step procedure for HCR is performed in the majority of cases by a MIDCAB first, followed by the PCI and/or DES implantation in the next days to the next months, depending on the medical team's preference and experience. In this case, all eventual anastomotic stenoses can be addressed during the percutaneous step, while DAPT is initiated later after the surgery without the risk of mediastinal bleeding. On the other hand, non-treated non-LAD stenotic coronary arteries (i.e., circumflex, obtuse marginal, or diagonal in case of a left main stenosis) may cause anginous symptoms or even a myocardial infarction, imposing a precocious non-planned percutaneous treatment.

In rare cases, a so-called reverse HCR is necessary (PCI before MIDCAB): it is the case of acute coronary syndromes in which the culprit lesion is located in a non-LAD vessel (or occasionally in stable CAD when the severity of the non-LAD stenoses are significantly greater than that of the LAD) [43]. However, as surgical procedures are followed by a systemic inflammatory response and platelets activation, the risk of stent thrombosis increases, especially after early interruption of DAPT. To avoid this scenario, the surgical step is usually performed at least 30 days after the percutaneous one [43, 48].

9.6.2 HCR Outcomes

Many studies have shown encouraging and promising results after HCR. Shen et al. [49] reported a comparison of propensity-matched patients who had one-step HCR versus isolated CABG via sternotomy versus multivessel PCI. At 3-year follow-up, the cumulative MACCE rate of the hybrid group (6.4%) was significantly lower than that of the PCI group (22.7%; $p < 0.001$), but was nonsignificantly different from that of the CABG group (13.5%; $p = 0.14$). The POL-MIDES (Safety and Efficacy Study of Hybrid Revascularization in Multivessel Coronary Artery Disease) trial, a randomized prospective trial of 200 patients with multivessel CAD presented by Gasior and colleagues, demonstrated that there was no statistically significant difference between HCR and CAGB in terms of mortality, myocardial infarction, repeat revascularization and major bleeding at a follow-up of 1 year [50]. Similar results were presented by Tajstra and colleagues at a 5-year follow-up after HCR or CABG [51].

Specifically for left main coronary artery stenosis, Halkos et al. demonstrated that HCR patients had reduced blood transfusions and mechanical ventilation time when compared to OPCAB, while maintaining a similar MACCE rate [52].

The large-scale National Heart, Lung, and Blood Institute-sponsored, randomized Hybrid Trial (Hybrid Coronary Revascularization Trial) was introduced and developed to compare short- and long-term results between HCR and fully percutaneous myocardial revascularization. The results of the 2-year follow-up of 200 patients will become available in the near future [43].

9.7 Conclusions

With an always more patient-friendly therapeutical solution for CAD, the future of surgical myocardial revascularization will involve less and less frequently a full sternotomy with a CPB. The mini-invasive approach, offered as an all surgical or hybrid strategy for patients with left main stenosis, could constitute a valid therapeutical alternative. Although being a more challenging approach with a steep learning curve, its short- and long-term outcomes are excellent and encouraging when performed in high-volume cardiac centers by experienced surgeons.

References

1. Garg S, Raja SG. Minimally invasive direct coronary artery bypass (MIDCAB) grafting. AME Med J. 2020;5:19.
2. Serruys PW, Morice MC, Kappetein AP, Colombo A, Holmes DR, Mack MJ, et al. Percutaneous coronary intervention versus coronary-artery bypass grafting for severe coronary artery disease. N Engl J Med. 2009;360:961–72.
3. Vineberg AM. Development of an anastomosis between the coronary vessels and a transplanted internal mammary artery. Can Med Assoc J. 1946;55(2):117–9.
4. Kolesov VI. [Initial experience in the treatment of stenocardia by the formation of coronary-systemic vascular anastomoses]. Kardiologiia 1967;7:20–5. Russian.
5. Benetti FJ, Ballester C, Sani G, et al. Video assisted coronary bypass surgery. J Card Surg. 1995;10:620–5.
6. Benetti FJ, Naselli G, Wood M, Geffner L. Direct myocardial revascularization without extracorporeal circulation. Experience in 700 patients. Chest. 1991;100:312–6.
7. Calafiore AM, Di Gammarco G, Teodori G, et al. Left anterior descending coronary artery grafting via left anterior small thoracotomy without cardiopulmonary bypass. Ann Thorac Surg. 1996;61:1658–65.
8. Jacobs S, Holzhey D, Falk V, et al. High-risk patients with multivessel disease--is there a role for incomplete myocardial revascularization via minimally invasive direct coronary artery bypass grafting? Heart Surg Forum. 2007;10:E459–62.
9. Melly L, Torregrossa G, Lee T, et al. Fifty years of coronary artery bypass grafting. J Thorac Dis. 2018;10:1960–7.
10. Sousa-Uva M, Neumann FJ, Ahlsson A, Alfonso F, Banning AP, Benedetto U, et al. 2018 ESC/EACTS guidelines on myocardial revascularization. Eur J Cardiothorac Surg. 2019;55:4–90.
11. Ohlmeier C, Czwikla J, Enders D, et al. Perkutane koronare Interventionen: Einsatz zwischen 2004 und 2012 in Deutschland [percutaneous coronary interventions: use between 2004 and 2012 in Germany]. Bundesgesundheitsblatt Gesundheitsforschung Gesundheitsschutz. 2016;59(6):783–8.
12. Marin Cuartas M, Javadikasgari H, Pfannmueller B, et al. Mitral valve repair: robotic and other minimally invasive approaches. Prog Cardiovasc Dis. 2017;60(3):394–404.

13. Vicol C, Nollert G, Mair H, et al. Midterm results of beating heart surgery in 1-vessel disease: minimally invasive direct coronary artery bypass versus off-pump coronary artery bypass with full sternotomy. Heart Surg Forum. 2003;6:341–4.

14. Hu FB, Cui LQ. Short-term clinical outcomes after hybrid coronary revascularization versus off-pump coronary artery bypass for the treatment of multivessel or left main coronary artery disease: a meta-analysis. Coron Artery Dis. 2015;26:526–34.

15. Al-Ruzzeh S, Mazrani W, Wray J, et al. The clinical outcome and quality of life following minimally invasive direct coronary artery bypass surgery. J Card Surg. 2004;19(1):12–6.

16. Simchen E, Galai N, Braun D, et al. Sociodemographic and clinical factors associated with low quality of life one year after coronary bypass operations: the Israeli coronary artery bypass study (ISCAB). J Thorac Cardiovasc Surg. 2001;121:909–19.

17. Zigmond A, Snaith R. The hospital anxiety and depression scale. Acta Psychiatr Scand. 1983;67:361–70.

18. Kettering K, Dapunt O, Baer FM. Minimally invasive direct coronary artery bypass grafting: a systematic review. J Cardiovasc Surg. 2004;45:255–64.

19. Indja B, Woldendorp K, Black D, Bannon PG, Wilson MK, Vallely MP. Minimally invasive surgical approaches to left main and left anterior descending coronary artery revascularization are superior compared to first- and second-generation drug-eluting stents: a network meta-analysis. Eur J Cardiothorac Surg. 2020;57:18–27.

20. Raja SG, Garg S, Rochon M, et al. Short-term clinical outcomes and long-term survival of minimally invasive direct coronary artery bypass grafting. Ann Cardiothorac Surg. 2018;7:621–7.

21. Lamy A, Devereaux PJ, Prabhakaran D, et al. Off-pump or on-pump coronary-artery bypass grafting at 30 days. N Engl J Med. 2012;366(16):1489–97.

22. Mack MJ, Head SJ, Holmes DR Jr, et al. Analysis of stroke occurring in the SYNTAX trial comparing coronary artery bypass surgery and percutaneous coronary intervention in the treatment of complex coronary artery disease. JACC Cardiovasc Interv. 2013;6(4):344–54.

23. McGinn JT Jr, Usman S, Lapierre H, Pothula VR, Mesana TG, Ruel M. Minimally invasive coronary artery bypass grafting: dual-center experience in 450 consecutive patients. Circulation. 2009;120(11 Suppl):S78–84.

24. Rabindranauth P, Burns JG, Vessey TT, Mathiason MA, Kallies KJ, Paramesh V. Minimally invasive coronary artery bypass grafting is associated with improved clinical outcomes. Innovations. 2014;9(6):421–6.

25. Blazek S, Rossbach C, Borger MA, Fuernau G, Desch S, Eitel I, et al. Comparison of sirolimus-eluting stenting with minimally invasive bypass surgery for stenosis of the left anterior descending coronary artery: 7- year follow-up of a randomized trial. JACC Cardiovasc Interv. 2015;8:30–8.

26. Blazek S, Holzhey D, Jungert C, Borger MA, Fuernau G, Desch S, et al. Comparison of bare-metal stenting with minimally invasive bypass surgery for stenosis of the left anterior descending coronary artery: 10- year follow-up of a randomized trial. JACC Cardiovasc Interv. 2013;6:20–6.

27. Deppe AC, Liakopoulos OJ, Kuhn EW, Slottosch I, Scherner M, Choi YH, et al. Minimally invasive direct coronary bypass grafting versus percutaneous coronary intervention for single-vessel disease: a meta-analysis of 2885 patients. Eur J Cardiothorac Surg. 2015;47:397–406.

28. Wang XW, Qu C, Huang C, Xiang XY, Lu ZQ. Minimally invasive direct coronary bypass compared with percutaneous coronary intervention for left anterior descending artery disease: a meta-analysis. J Cardiothorac Surg. 2016;11:125.

29. Jakubová M, Mitro P, Stančák B, et al. The occurrence of postoperative atrial fibrillation according to different surgical settings in cardiac surgery patients. Interact Cardiovasc Thorac Surg. 2012;15(6):1007–12.

30. Kosmidou I, Chen S, Kappetein AP, et al. New-onset atrial fibrillation after PCI or CABG for left Main disease: the EXCEL trial. J Am Coll Cardiol. 2018;71(7):739–48.

31. Maimari M, Baikoussis NG, Gaitanakis S, et al. Does minimal invasive cardiac surgery reduce the incidence of post-operative atrial fibrillation? Ann Card Anaesth. 2020;23(1):7–13.

32. Goy JJ, Eeckhout E, Burnand B, et al. Coronary angioplasty versus left internal mammary artery grafting for isolated proximal left anterior descending artery stenosis. Lancet. 1994;343:1449–53.

33. Reeves BC, Angelini GD, Bryan AJ, et al. A multicenter randomised controlled trial of minimally invasive direct coronary bypass grafting versus percutaneous transluminal coronary angioplasty with stenting for proximal stenosis of the left anterior descending coronary artery. Health Technol Assess. 2004;8:1–43.

34. Shirai K, Lansky AJ, Mehran R, et al. Minimally invasive coronary artery bypass grafting versus stenting for patients with proximal left anterior descending coronary artery disease. Am J Cardiol. 2004;93:959–62.

35. Kim JW, Lim DS, Sun K, et al. Stenting or MIDCAB using ministernotomy for revascularization of proximal left anterior descending artery? Int J Cardiol. 2005;99:437–41.

36. Deo SV, Sharma V, Shah IK, et al. Minimally invasive direct coronary artery bypass graft surgery or percutaneous coronary intervention for proximal left anterior descending artery stenosis: a meta-analysis. Ann Thorac Surg. 2014;97:2056–65.

37. Sabik JF 3rd, Lytle BW, Blackstone EH, Houghtaling PL, Cosgrove DM. Comparison of saphenous vein and internal thoracic artery graft patency by coronary system. Ann Thorac Surg. 2005;79(2):544–51.

38. Waheed A, Klosterman E, Lee J, et al. Assessing the long-term patency and clinical outcomes of venous and arterial grafts used in coronary artery bypass grafting: a meta-analysis. Cureus. 2019;11(9):e5670. https://doi.org/10.7759/cureus.5670.
39. Zhu YY, Hayward PA, Hare DL, Reid C, Stewart AG, Buxton BF. Effect of lipid exposure on graft patency and clinical outcomes: arteries and veins are different. Eur J Cardiothorac Surg. 2014;45(2):323–8.
40. Doenst T, Haverich A, Serruys P, Bonow RO, Kappetein P, Falk V, et al. PCI and CABG for treating stable coronary artery disease: JACC review topic of the week. J Am Coll Cardiol. 2019;73:964–76.
41. Davierwala PM, Verevkin A, Bergien L, et al. Twenty-year outcomes of minimally invasive direct coronary artery bypass surgery: the Leipzig experience [published online ahead of print, 2021 Feb 17]. J Thorac Cardiovasc Surg. 2021;S0022–5223(21)00343-3.
42. Holzhey DM, Jacobs S, Walther T, Mochalski M, Mohr FW, Falk V. Cumulative sum failure analysis for eight surgeons performing minimally invasive direct coronary artery bypass. J Thorac Cardiovasc Surg. 2007;134:663–9.
43. Moreno PR, Stone GW, Gonzalez-Lengua CA, Puskas JD. The hybrid coronary approach for optimal revascularization: JACC review topic of the week. J Am Coll Cardiol. 2020;76(3):321–33.
44. Rocha RV, Tam DY, Karkhanis R, et al. Long-term outcomes associated with total arterial revascularization vs non-total arterial revascularization. JAMA Cardiol. 2020;5(5):507–14.
45. Head SJ, Milojevic M, Taggart DP, Puskas JD. Current practice of state-of-the-art surgical coronary revascularization. Circulation. 2017;136(14):1331–45.
46. Parang P, Arora R. Coronary vein graft disease: pathogenesis and prevention. Can J Cardiol. 2009;25(2):e57–62.
47. Bachinsky WB, Abdelsalam M, Boga G, Kiljanek L, Mumtaz M, McCarty C. Comparative study of same sitting hybrid coronary artery revascularization versus off-pump coronary artery bypass in multivessel coronary artery disease. J Interv Cardiol. 2012;25(5):460–8.
48. Panoulas VF, Colombo A, Margonato A, Maisano F. Hybrid coronary revascularization: promising, but yet to take off. J Am Coll Cardiol. 2015;65(1):85–97.
49. Shen L, Hu S, Wang H, et al. One-stop hybrid coronary revascularization versus coronary artery bypass grafting and percutaneous coronary intervention for the treatment of multivessel coronary artery disease: 3-year follow-up results from a single institution. J Am Coll Cardiol. 2013;61(25):2525–33.
50. Gąsior M, Zembala MO, Tajstra M, et al. Hybrid revascularization for multivessel coronary artery disease. JACC Cardiovasc Interv. 2014;7(11):1277–83.
51. Tajstra M, Hrapkowicz T, Hawranek M, et al. Hybrid coronary revascularization in selected patients with multivessel disease: 5-year clinical outcomes of the prospective randomized pilot study. JACC Cardiovasc Interv. 2018;11(9):847–52.
52. Halkos ME, Vassiliades TA, Douglas JS, et al. Hybrid coronary revascularization versus off-pump coronary artery bypass grafting for the treatment of multivessel coronary artery disease. Ann Thorac Surg. 2011;92(5):1695–702.

Preoperative IVUS Assessment of the Left Main

Gianluca Caiazzo, Maria Scalamogna,
Luigi Di Serafino, Luca Golino,
Vincenzo Manganiello, Mario De Michele,
Giovanni Esposito, Adrian Banning,
and Luciano Fattore

10.1 Introduction

Atherosclerotic disease of the left main coronary artery (LMCA) is particularly relevant in the context of coronary lesions for the vast amount of myocardium subtended to this coronary segment. For this reason, acute complications occurring during LMCA intervention may have a rapid progression toward hemodynamic instability. Moreover, LMCA treatment usually requires technically challenging procedures, since atherosclerosis within this segment is often diffuse, with frequent involvement of the coronary bifurcation and/or of the ostium. Recent trials have highlighted the role of coronary stenting in the LMCA setting, particularly in patients with less complex LMCA disease and patients unsuitable for surgery [1, 2]. All coronary stenoses of 50% or more located at the LMCA level, as well as stenoses of the proximal left anterior descending artery (LAD), are currently considered to be treated according to the European Society of Cardiology guidelines on myocardial revascularization which indicate PCI of the LMCA as safe and effective as surgical revascularization (Class I, level of evidence A) in case of a low SYNTAX score (0–22) (Fig. 10.1) [3]. Although guidelines' recommendations are largely extrapolated from studies based on angiographic images, it is diffusely recognized that angiography presents several limitations in assessing the severity of stenotic plaques, especially in case of LMCA disease [4]. The main issue is represented by diffuse atherosclerotic involvement and the absence of a normal reference segment, especially when the LMCA is short. Stenosis diameter is then difficult to calculate and is often underestimated. Since intracoronary imaging techniques like intravascular ultrasound (IVUS) and optical coherence tomography (OCT) have been introduced in the clinical scenario, interventional cardiologists experimented the opportunity to overcome this issue. OCT technology allows a better visualization of the vessel wall, with a tenfold higher axial resolution (14 μm) compared to IVUS. Thus, OCT represents a precious imaging modality to identify stent failures (i.e., stent malapposition, dissection, tissue protrusion, and thrombus). Unfortunately, OCT is not able to measure the plaque burden due

G. Caiazzo · L. Golino · V. Manganiello
M. De Michele · L. Fattore
Cardiology Unit, "San Giuseppe Moscati" Hospital,
Aversa (CE), Italy

M. Scalamogna · L. Di Serafino · G. Esposito
Department of Advanced Biomedical Sciences,
University of Naples Federico II, Naples, Italy

A. Banning (✉)
Cardiology Unit, "San Giuseppe Moscati" Hospital,
Aversa (CE), Italy

Department of Advanced Biomedical Sciences,
University of Naples Federico II, Naples, Italy
e-mail: Adrian.Banning@ouh.nhs.uk

© Springer Nature Switzerland AG 2022
B. Cortese (ed.), *Left Main Coronary Revascularization*,
https://doi.org/10.1007/978-3-031-05265-1_10

	CAGB		PCI	
	Class	Level	Class	Level
Left Main disease with low SYNTAX score (0–22).	I	A	I	A
Left Main disease with intermediate SYNTAX score (23–32).	I	A	IIa	A
Left Main disease with high SYNTAX score (>33).	I	A	III	B

Fig. 10.1 Recommendation for the type of revascularization in patients with stable coronary artery disease with suitable coronary anatomy for both procedures and low predicted surgical mortality. (2018 ESC/EACTS Guidelines on myocardial revascularization)

to its shallow penetration depth (1–2 mm) [5]. For this reason, and given the wide availability of IVUS-guided PCI clinical data and the presence of standardized criteria for optimizing stent implantation, IVUS still represents the reference for intracoronary imaging trials [6], especially in the LMCA setting. In particular, in the last two decades several large studies have been published showing the importance of IVUS in order to recognize the morphological characteristics of plaques, quantify their severity, achieve optimal stent expansion, lower stent malapposition rates, and, consequently, better clinical outcomes, especially in complex PCIs as multivessel disease and/or left main coronary artery stenting [7–12].

10.2 Intravascular Ultrasound (IVUS) Technology

The size of current IVUS catheters are ranging from 2.6 to 3.5 French (0.87–1.17 mm) and are inserted into the coronary arteries through 6-French guiding catheters. The principle of IVUS imaging is based on the oscillatory movement (expansion and contraction) of a piezoelectric transducer (crystal) in order to produce sound waves when electrically excited. There are two major different transducer designs [13]: (1) the mechanical single element rotating device and (2) the electronic phased array. The mechanical rotating element device uses a single piezoelectric transducer that rotates with 1800 rotations per minute, while the electronic phased array device uses multiple stationary placed piezoelectric transducers which are sequentially activated. The generated sound waves by the transducers propagate through the different tissues and are reflected according to the acoustic properties of the tissue it travels through [14].

Gray-scale-based plaque classification is limited due to its low spatial resolution and for the usual IVUS transducers (20 and 40 MHz) for which the axial resolution is 200 μm and the lateral 200–250 μm. Based on their visual estimation at gray-scale IVUS, atheromas have been classified into four categories [15] (Fig. 10.2):

1. Soft plaque (lesion echogenicity less than the surrounding adventitia)
2. Fibrous plaque (intermediate echogenicity between soft (echolucent) atheromas and highly echogenic calcified plaques)
3. Calcified plaque (echogenicity higher than the adventitia with acoustic shadowing)
4. Mixed plaques (no single acoustical subtype represents >80% of the plaques)

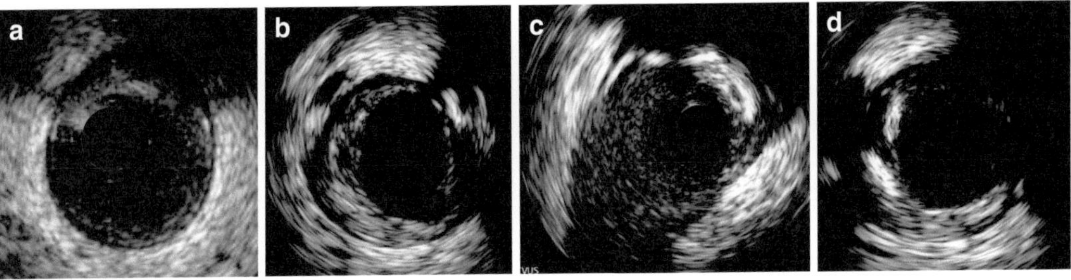

Fig. 10.2 Atheromas classified into four categories according to visual estimation at gray-scale IVUS: soft plaque (**a**); fibrous plaque (**b**); calcified plaque (**c**); mixed plaque (**d**)

Recent technological improvements in the field allowed the introduction of IVUS catheters with 60 MHz wideband transducer which increases lateral and axial resolution (6 mm penetration depth) to visualize all three vessel layers, plaque morphology, and improves stent strut visibility. To overcome the limitations of qualitative visual interpretation of the IVUS images and to describe the coronary plaque morphology, several post-processing methods for computer-assisted quantification have been developed during the recent years. There are two basic different approaches: (1) Signal-based analysis (the so-called raw radiofrequency analysis or RF analysis) and (2) Image-based analysis. The first RF-signal-based tissue composition analysis tool was the so-called virtual histology (VH-IVUS, Volcano Therapeutics) software. It uses in-depth analysis of the backscattered RF signal in order to provide a more detailed description of the atheromatous plaque composition. The main principle of this technique is that it uses not only the envelope amplitude of the reflected RF signals (as gray-scale IVUS does), but uses also the underlying frequency content to analyze the tissue components present in coronary plaques. This combined information is processed and identifies four basic plaque tissue components: (1) Fibrous tissue (dark green), (2) Fibrofatty tissue (light green), (3) Necrotic core (red), and (4) dense calcium (white) [16]. However, the use of VH-IVUS is currently limited due to the lack of clinical evidence of its value.

10.3 The Role of IVUS in Pre-operative LMCA Assessment

Due to all these technical characteristics, IVUS imaging is currently considered the gold standard tool for LMCA stenosis evaluation. Multiple reasons have to be taken into account. In contrast to coronary angiography, as said, IVUS is accurate in assessing both the coronary lumen and wall characteristics and, it has a higher tissue penetration compared to OCT which uses infrared light. Moreover, IVUS represents a unique imaging tool for ostial lesions assessment: as a matter of fact, OCT requires complete blood removal with contrast medium to obtain good-quality images which is almost impossible at the ostium level where the guiding catheter needs to be selectively positioned. The reasons IVUS is helpful and has been increasingly used in such procedures can be resumed into four main points:

1. To assess the nature of the lesion; the detection by IVUS of highly calcified plaques gives important information for treatment strategy.
2. To measure the minimum lumen area (MLA) in the LMCA in order to assess the severity of the stenosis. In other words, LMCA is the only coronary segment where IVUS allows to establish the indication for revascularization.
3. To check the presence of disease at ostial LAD and/or left circumflex (LCX) for procedural planning (two-stents technique vs. provisional stenting).
4. To size the main vessel and the side branches for subsequent stent selection.

10.3.1 Plaque Morphology at IVUS

When IVUS is used in a normal vessel, it is not easy to differentiate the lumen border from the vessel border. The lumen border is drawn inside the intima or plaque and the intimal layer is normally not seen unless it has begun to thicken. The media is the dark band between the adventitia and the intima (Fig. 10.3). The gray-scale-based imaging modality identifies different types of plaques, but it has some limitations for the identification of its tissue composition [17]. Soft (echolucent) plaques have been related either to high lipid content or presence of smooth muscle cells [18]. While fibrous plaques usually have an intermediate echogenicity, sometimes very dense fibrous plaques can also appear as calcified lesions. Traditionally, acoustic shadowing has been considered as a sign of calcification, but necrotic tissue can also cause shadowing [19]. Calcium is indicated by very bright areas with acoustic shadowing that blocks out the image behind. This shadowing occurs because the high density of calcium dampens the ultrasound echo. IVUS detects only the leading edge of calcium and therefore cannot determine its thickness. Calcification on IVUS is usually described by its circumferential angle (arc), longitudinal length, and depth. Importantly, IVUS is the only intracoronary imaging tool able to detect deep calcium plaques, which can have important procedural implications (see Fig. 10.2).

Our current understanding of plaque biology suggests that ~60% of clinically evident plaque rupture originates within an inflamed thin-capped fibroatheroma (TCFA) [20].

The definition of an IVUS-derived TCFA has been proposed as a lesion fulfilling the following criteria in at least three frames: (1) plaque burden ≥40%; (2) *confluent* necrotic core ≥10% in direct contact with the lumen (i.e., no visible overlying tissue) [21]. The first small-size study aimed at systematically characterizing plaque ruptures in the LMCA found that ruptured plaques that involve the LMCA present with an acute coronary syndrome and have an angiographically complex appearance. Interestingly, this study

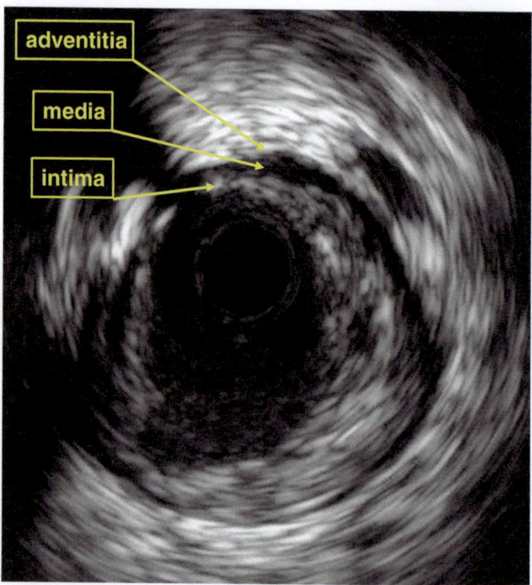

Fig. 10.3 IVUS image showing three layers (intima, media, and adventitia) within the context of a diseased (eccentric plaque) LMCA

also showed that ruptured plaques rarely compromise the lumen and almost exclusively involve the LMCA bifurcation opposite the distal flow divider [22]. Such findings have been confirmed by other groups; lesions involving the bifurcation LAD-LCX have been found to be predominantly located in the outer wall of the carina, and such locations were often associated with a larger necrotic core content [23].

Ruptured plaques may have a variable appearance on IVUS. Most commonly, IVUS may reveal ulceration depicted as an echo-lucent cavity beginning at the luminal-intimal border (Fig. 10.4). These features should be distinguished from dissections which appear as longitudinal tears of the intima and media (Fig. 10.5).

The pathophysiologic natural consequence of a ruptured plaque is thrombus which also represent the ultimate pathological feature leading to ACS. Thrombus is usually recognized as an echolucent intraluminal mass, often with a layered or pedunculated appearance by IVUS [15]. Fresh or acute thrombus may appear also as an echo-dense intraluminal tissue, which does not follow the circular appearance of the vessel wall, while older, more organized thrombus has a darker ultrasound appearance.

An in-depth analysis on IVUS-derived plaque types and on their relationship with adverse coronary events was performed in an international prospective study, the Providing Regional Observations to Study Predictors of Events in the Coronary Tree study (PROSPECT study) [24]. The aim of this natural-history study was to provide prospective in vivo confirmation of the hypothesis that acute coronary syndromes arise from atheromas with specific histopathological characteristics, not necessarily dependent on the angiographic severity of the stenosis. Notably, most of the lesions responsible for major adverse cardiovascular events during follow-up were angiographically mild, whereas intravascular ultrasonography showed that most had a small luminal area and/or a large plaque burden. In particular, a baseline plaque burden of at least 70% and a minimal luminal area of 4.0 mm^2 or less were independent predictors of non-culprit-lesion–related MACE. Moreover, thanks to VH-IVUS, it was possible to demonstrate that events related to non-culprit lesions typically occurred at sites that were classified as thin-cap fibroatheromas, a finding that is consistent with the established concept of vulnerable plaque [24].

Further important information provided by IVUS analysis on LMCA in the pre-assessment phase is represented by the geometric disposition of plaques and by their distributions along coronary branches. Concentric plaques are distributed circumferentially in the vessel and tend to occur in areas of negative remodeling. Conversely, eccentric plaques are distributed non-circumferentially in the vessel and this makes the assessment of disease by angiography prone to

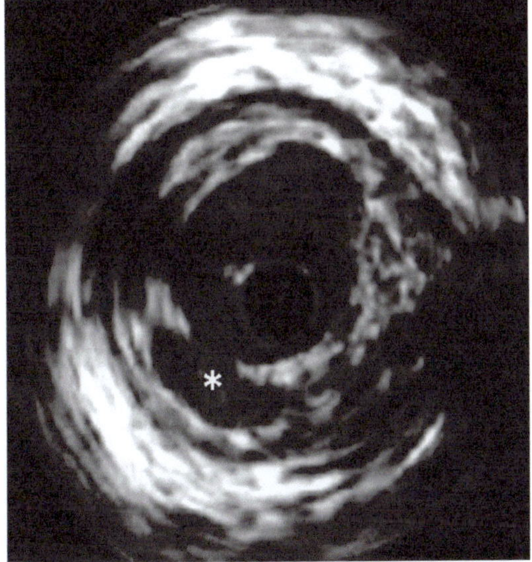

Fig. 10.4 Echo-lucent cavity (see asterisk) beginning at the luminal-intimal border of a fibrous plaque indicating an ulcerated/ruptured plaque

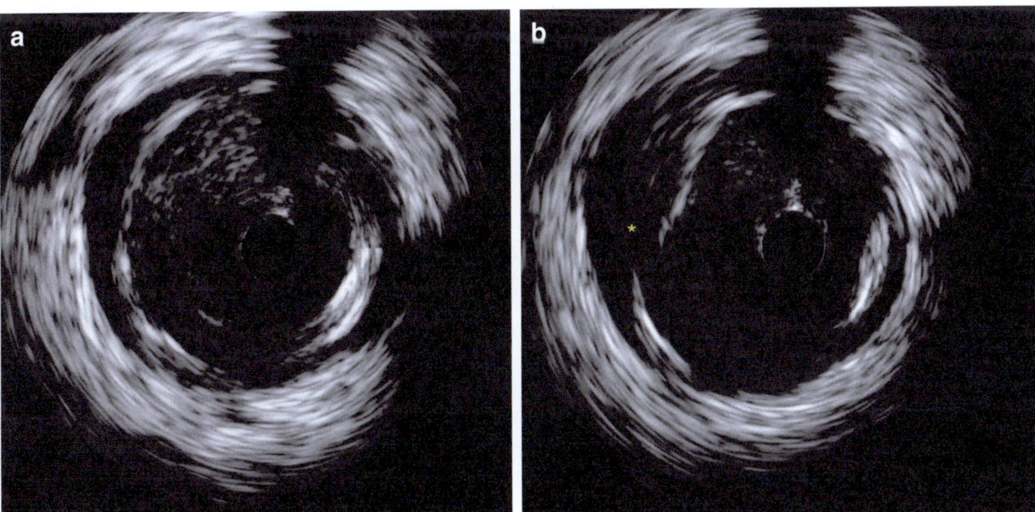

Fig. 10.5 Type D-E (NHLBI) circumferential LMCA dissection. (**b**) The asterisk indicates intimal flap dynamic fluctuation toward the vessel lumen

underestimation or overestimation depending on the angle of view (Fig. 10.6). As said, lesions involving the distal LMCA bifurcation into LAD and LCX branches are predominantly located in the outer wall of the carina; such plaque distribution recognition by IVUS can have important technical implications in order to select the best two-stent technique strategy for PCI (see Sect. 10.3.1). Moreover, several IVUS studies have shown different lesion characteristics between ostial and distal left main lesions. Maehara et al. reported that non-ostial plaques were more calcific than ostial lesions [25] (Fig. 10.7). Tyczynski et al. reported that all left main ruptured plaques occurred in the distal half of the left main artery [22]. In a study by Sano et al., distal lesions were

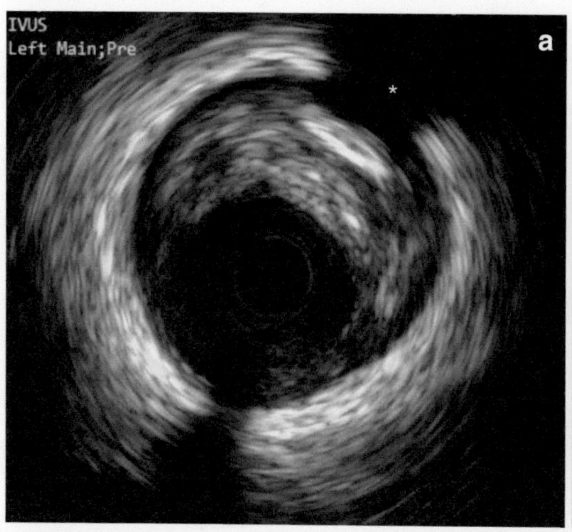

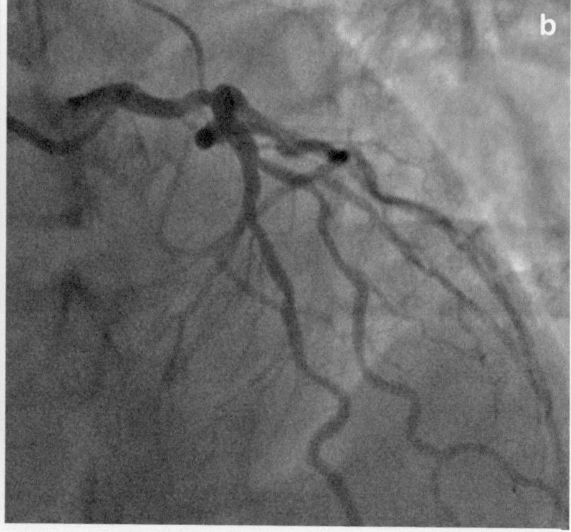

Fig. 10.6 Severe distal LMCA stenosis caused by a large fibrocalcific eccentric plaque (**a**); eccentric plaques are distributed non-circumferentially in the vessel and this makes the assessment of disease by angiography prone to underestimation or overestimation depending on the angle of view as shown in panel (**b**) where the angiographic view seems not to underline evident stenosis of the distal LMCA; the asterisk shows a spot deep calcification within the context of the fibrous plaque (**a**)

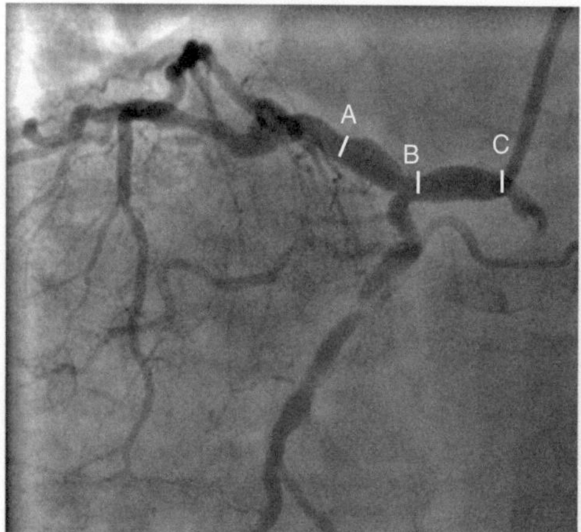

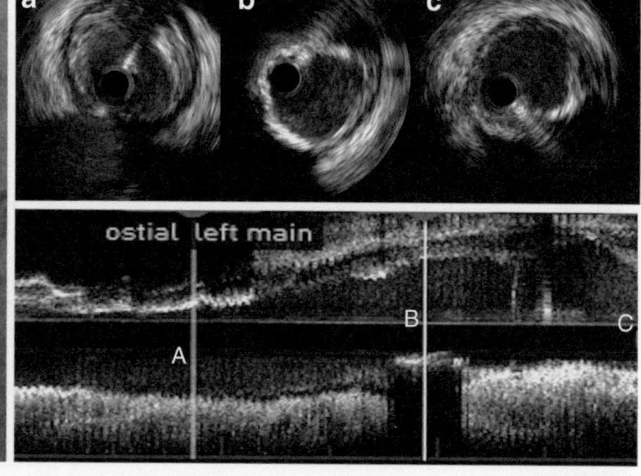

Fig. 10.7 Non-ostial LMCA plaques are generally more calcific than ostial lesions; the angiographic view on the left shows a diseased LMCA where calcific stenoses are not clearly evident as compared to IVUS images on the right. The IVUS cross-sections show typical LMCA plaque characteristics with accentuated calcification concentrated in the distal segment (**b**) as compared to the ostium (**c**) and proximal LAD (**a**)

more calcified and had the largest plaque burdens; on the other hand, ostial lesions were more fibrotic and had the smallest plaque burdens. These findings suggested a different etiology between ostial and distal left main lesions, ostial lesions being more often of non-atherosclerotic nature [26].

10.3.2 IVUS-Based Indication for Treatment and Relationship with Functional Evaluation

Precise angiographic assessment of the severity of left main coronary artery (LMCA) lesions is difficult and in some cases, impossible. The misclassification of an intermediate LM stenosis, solely based on the angiography, might occur in up to 50% of the cases. Factors such as the absence of a proximal reference point, vessel tortuosity and overlap, or eccentric or bifurcating plaque distribution all increase the challenge. Further, angiography provides no detail regarding the vessel wall characteristics. Also, it is well documented that interobserver grading of angiographic stenoses is inconsistent, and these findings are even more pronounced in the assessment of LMCA [27]. For these reasons, as said, IVUS has been selected as gold standard imaging tool for evaluation and treatment guidance of LMCA lesions that are angiographically indeterminate. The use of IVUS-based MLA measurement as parameter for decision making is well established whereas one other approach would be to use the degree of area stenosis, as we usually do with the degree of diameter stenosis used in angiography, which is obtained by dividing the lumen area at the lesion site by the lumen area at a normal reference site. A 50% diameter stenosis, which is the angiographic criterion for defining significant lesions, would be equivalent to a 75% area stenosis. However, when angiography is compared with the functional evaluation, this threshold might underestimate the LM stenosis, being the optimal cut-off values for predicting "hemodynamically significant" LM stenosis close to 40% [28]. Furthermore, as said, the LMCA is generally a short vessel and may be

diffusely diseased, leaving little chance for a normal reference segment [27]. Moreover, LMCA atherosclerosis assessment can be complicated by arterial remodeling, which can be either "negative" or "positive", and may affect the whole LMCA [29]. Hence, absolute measurements such as MLA or MLD may be more representative of flow impairment and of long-term outcome than lumen area stenosis and plaque burden [30]. Several small-sample size studies have been performed through the last two decades aiming to find an MLA cut-off which could correlate with clinical events. Among the first studies investigating IVUS MLA cut-offs, Fassa et al. conducted IVUS studies on 214 patients with angiographically indeterminate LMCA lesions, and deferral of revascularization was recommended when the MLA was larger than the predetermined value of 7.5 mm^2. Long-term follow-up (mean 3.3 ± 2.0 years) showed no significant difference in MACE (target vessel revascularization, acute myocardial infarction, and death) between patients with an MLA < 7.5 mm^2 who underwent revascularization and those with an MLA $\geq$7.5 mm^2 deferred for revascularization ($p = 0.28$) [31]. Subsequently, De la Torre et al. published a prospective non-randomized study providing such information, the LITRO study, including 358 patients undergoing IVUS examination of intermediate LMCA lesions. This study supports the safety of using the IVUS-derived cutoff value of 6 mm^2 of MLA for the decision-making in intermediate LMCA lesions [32]. From the introduction in the clinical practice of functional evaluation of coronary stenoses by fractional flow reserve (FFR), several studies have been conducted aiming to correlate IVUS-derived cut-offs to functional measurements (Fig. 10.8). Although the FFR does not provide any anatomical information, it allows the interventionalists to better understand the functional significance of intermediate LM stenosis, thereby suggesting whether or not to perform a percutaneous or surgical revascularization. The FFR represents the ratio of the simultaneously recorded mean arterial pressure distal to the stenosis (Pd) and the mean aortic pressure measured at the tip of the guiding catheter (Pa) during a stable steady state adenosine-

Angiography   Functional evaluation   Imaging

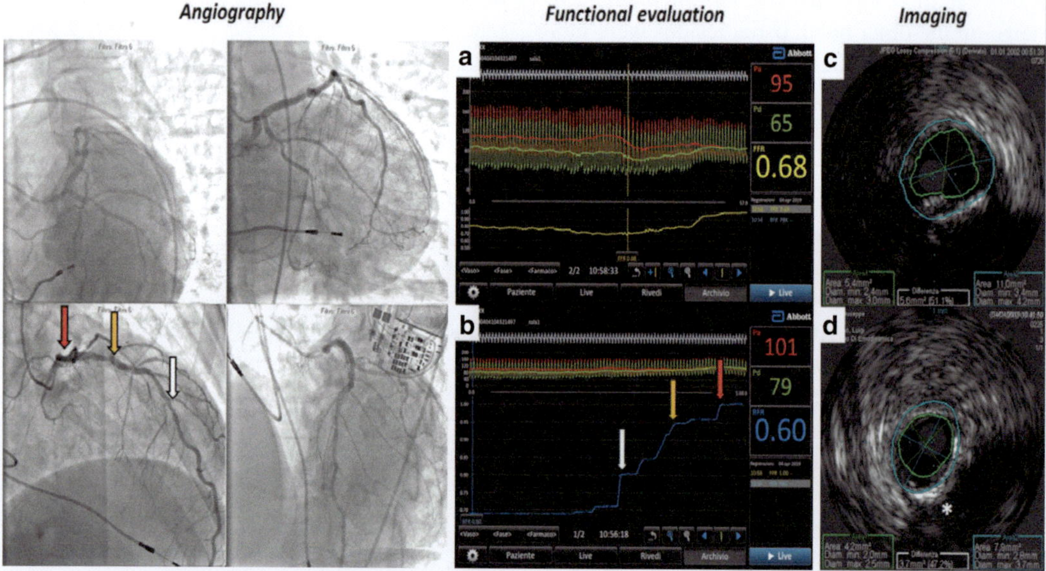

Fig. 10.8 The angiography shows an intermediate stenosis of the LMCA (red arrow) and two stenosis of the LAD located at the proximal (orange arrow) and the middle (white arrow) segment. At functional evaluation, the combination of all the stenoses was responsible for myocardial ischemia being the FFR value of 0.68 (panel **a**). FFR evaluation was performed by intracoronary administration of adenosine (200 mg), thereby it was not possible to discriminate the lesion with the highest ischemic value. The Resting Full Cycle Ratio (RFR) analysis (panel **b**), without adenosine administration, demonstrates the highest functional value of the proximal stenosis of the LAD (orange arrow). However, since the cross-talk of the lesions might have potentially led to the underestimation of the LMCA stenosis (red arrow), IVUS has been performed before deciding the treatment strategy. IVUS allowed to better evaluate the stenosis of the LMCA which is severe (MLA < 6 mm^2) (**c**). In addition, it was also possible to evaluate the morphology of the mid-LAD stenosis, with mild calcification (asterisk) and a reduced MLA (**d**)

induced maximal hyperemia. This functional evaluation requires some care in the manipulation of both the guiding catheter and the pressure wire: (1) it is important, indeed, to disengage the guiding catheter during the FFR measurement, in order to prevent pressure dampening, due to the interaction between the guiding catheter and the stenosis, especially when the ostium is involved; (2) maximal hyperemia should be maintained for all the time needed for the pullback [33]. As it normally occurs for other segments of the coronary three, also during the assessment of an intermediate LM stenosis an FFR value ≤0.80 identifies a functional significant stenosis associated with the presence of inducible myocardial ischemia. However, some limitations of this tool in this setting should be disclosed: there is a lack of randomized data confirming the long-term safety of this approach; an FFR assessment across the LM is influenced by the presence of one or multiple stenoses within the distal coronary segments. Thus, the presence of a significant stenosis within the LAD or LCX may lead to an overestimation of the FFR value across the LM. Thereby, after PCI of the distal stenosis, LM stenosis might result significantly at the FFR evaluation. For these reasons, and in this particular setting, the functional evaluation should be supported by an additional imaging modality, such as IVUS, which might be helpful not only for deciding on the need for revascularization, but also to guide the best treatment strategy. As said, an IVUS minimal lumen area (MLA) of 6 mm^2 is conventionally considered an indication for revascularization in the European population according to the EBC recommendations. This value was obtained from Murray's law and has been supported by several studies [32, 34]. However, the LM-MLA 6 mm^2

cut-off value seems to be population-dependent. In 112 Asian patients, Park et al. showed an IVUS MLA of <4.5 mm^2 was an independent predictor of an FFR value <0.80 [35]. Yet, the adjustments of MLA for the body mass index, body surface area, and left ventricular (LV) mass assessed by echocardiography did not improve the diagnostic accuracy. However, the sensitivity (77%) and negative predictive value (75%) for a 4.5 mm^2 cut-off were suboptimal. Notably, among the 54 lesions with LM-MLA > 4.5 mm^2, 13 (24.1%) had an FFR of <0.80. The proposal of 4.5 mm^2 as a LM-MLA optimal cut-off value should be taken very cautiously until further clinical data supports its prognostic validity [36, 37]. In general, the correlation between IVUS MLA and FFR is higher for LMCA stenosis as compared with non-LM stenosis. This was previously attributed to the simplicity of the morphologic characteristics of isolated ostial and shaft LMCA stenosis, including the uniformly large vessel size, short lesion length and lack of side branches, and other anatomical factors that could potentially affect the FFR. Finally, the available clinical evidence supports the use of IVUS with an MLA > 6 mm^2 for safe deferral. The finding of an MLA 5–6 mm^2 might require further evaluation with FFR, while a MLA < 5 mm^2 indicates the need for revascularization. Additional evaluation through the use of both IVUS and FFR measurements is therefore strongly recommended, especially when the functional significance of the LM disease is equivocal and in the context of complex clinical scenario. Notably, in the Fractional Flow Reserve and Intravascular Ultrasound Relationship Study (FIRST study), Waksman et al. confirmed the concept that the optimal cut-off for an MLA to FFR < 0.8 is vessel-dependent [38]. The FIRST study was a multicenter, prospective registry of patients with intermediate coronary lesions, defined as 40–80% stenosis by angiography. In total, 350 patients (367 lesions) were enrolled at 10 U.S. and European sites. Also of interest, this study found that an MLA < 3.6 mm^2 (AUC = 0.68) was best for reference vessel diameters > 3.5 mm while FFR correlated with plaque burden ($r = -0.220$, $p < 0.001$) but not with other plaque morphology [38]. The usefulness of FFR use for

LMCA lesions assessment still represents a developing field of research. Recently, Mallidi et al. performed a meta-analysis of six prospective cohort studies involving 525 patients looking at the long-term outcomes of FFR-guided revascularization of ambiguous left main coronary artery (LMCA) lesions; patients underwent revascularization (revascularization group) or medical therapy (deferred group) based on FFR. There was no statistically significant difference between the groups in the rates of primary endpoint ($p = 0.15$), all-cause mortality ($p = 0.06$) or nonfatal myocardial infarctions ($p = 0.76$). However, there was a significant increase in the rate of subsequent revascularizations in the deferred patients ($p = 0.002$) [39].

10.3.3 IVUS-Guided LMCA Assessment: Impact on Therapeutic Strategies

IVUS offers consistent measures when assessing LMCA bifurcation and is currently widely used in the pre-PCI phase. As said, atherosclerotic plaques have a peculiar distribution in the LMCA context and IVUS have represented a useful tool to clarify such characteristics. Of note, short LMCAs are usually diseased at the ostium while longer LMCAs tend to develop atherosclerosis at the distal bifurcation site [25]. It has been noted in a small population of patients that, irrespective of angiographic Medina classification, the carina and both sides of the flow divider were almost always free of significant atherosclerotic plaques (Fig. 10.9). Other IVUS-based studies have shown that certain plaque distribution patterns are more frequent than others. On this topic, in a series by Oviedo et al., continuous plaque from the LMCA into the proximal LAD was seen in 90% and from the LMCA into the LCX in 66%, with disease from the LMCA into both the LAD and LCX in 62% [40]. For better plaque distribution evaluation during pre-PCI LMCA assessment, it has been suggested that IVUS should be performed from both the left LAD and LCX to define the MLA within the LMCA and to assess accurately the extension of the disease at the

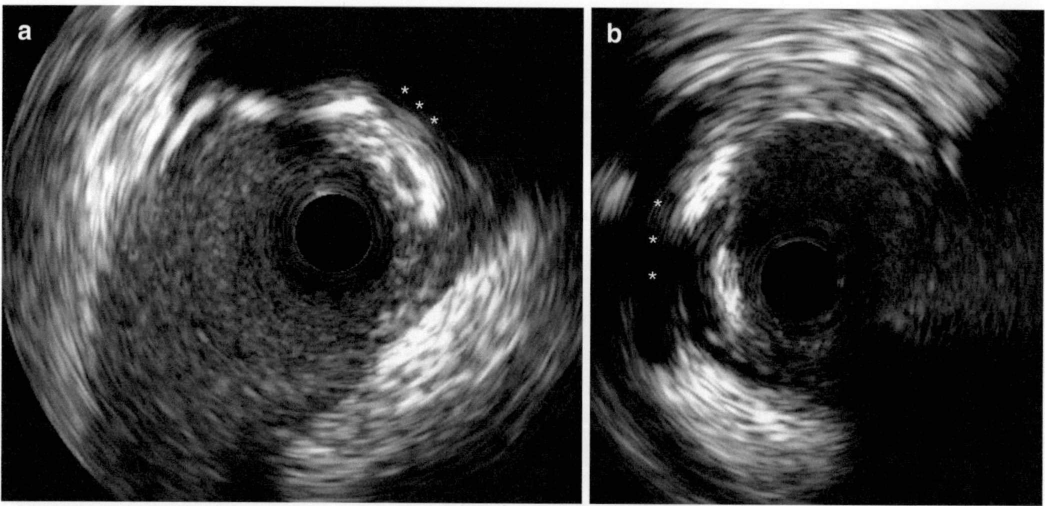

Fig. 10.9 IVUS cross-sections show typical plaque disposition within two different LMCA; yellow asterisks show eccentric fibrocalcific plaques opposite to the side-branch (LCX) origin

LAD and LCX ostia. It has been shown that an MLA > 4.0 mm^2 and a plaque burden < 50% at the LCX ostium are rarely associated with an FFR < 0.8 after single stent crossover [41]. All these pre-PCI evaluations can have important consequences on procedural planning. When the bifurcation is involved, the segment to be stented should go from the LMCA toward the vessel presenting the largest size and the tightest stenosis. Moreover, the carina angle evaluation with IVUS could help during the bifurcation stenting technique selection. As a matter of fact, patients who have a "vulnerable" carina or significant calcium identified by IVUS longitudinal reconstruction are at particular risk of adverse carina shift towards the SB. Accurate vessel sizing represents the first issue to be overcome when facing LMCA PCIs. In fact, it has been demonstrated that incorrect stent sizing is associated with stent under-expansion which is a powerful predictor of early stent thrombosis and restenosis after DES implantation according to numerous IVUS studies [42–45]. Of note, fractal geometry also represents a useful method in order to size LMCA including its bifurcation into the LAD and LCX by using Murray's law. However, IVUS has an important role during this phase, given the serious limitations that angiography has and that we

have previously described. Moreover, IVUS can be used not only to select stent diameter, but also to identify optimal proximal and distal stent edge landing zones and select stent length using motorized transducer pullback to measure the distance between the proximal and distal landing zones. The ability of IVUS to visualize true vessel size permits upsizing a stent to maximize final stent dimensions; true vessel size is larger than lumen dimensions because of accumulated plaque and positive remodeling. Optimal landing zones are the largest lumens with the smallest plaque burden in the same coronary artery segment, ideally a plaque burden < 50%. Similarly, the aorto-ostial junction should be covered if the plaque burden is >50%. Conversely, an aggressive stent sizing strategy should be avoided in lesions with IVUS-detected negative remodeling because of the risk of perforation [46]. Other important IVUS-based information which can significantly impact on PCI strategy is represented by plaque characteristics. In example, severe calcification has several implications for procedural planning and is often not clearly visible at angiography [46] (Fig. 10.10). There is general agreement that a total calcium arc > 180° and increased calcium thickness > 0.5 mm are associated with greater risk of stent under-expansion whereas evidence

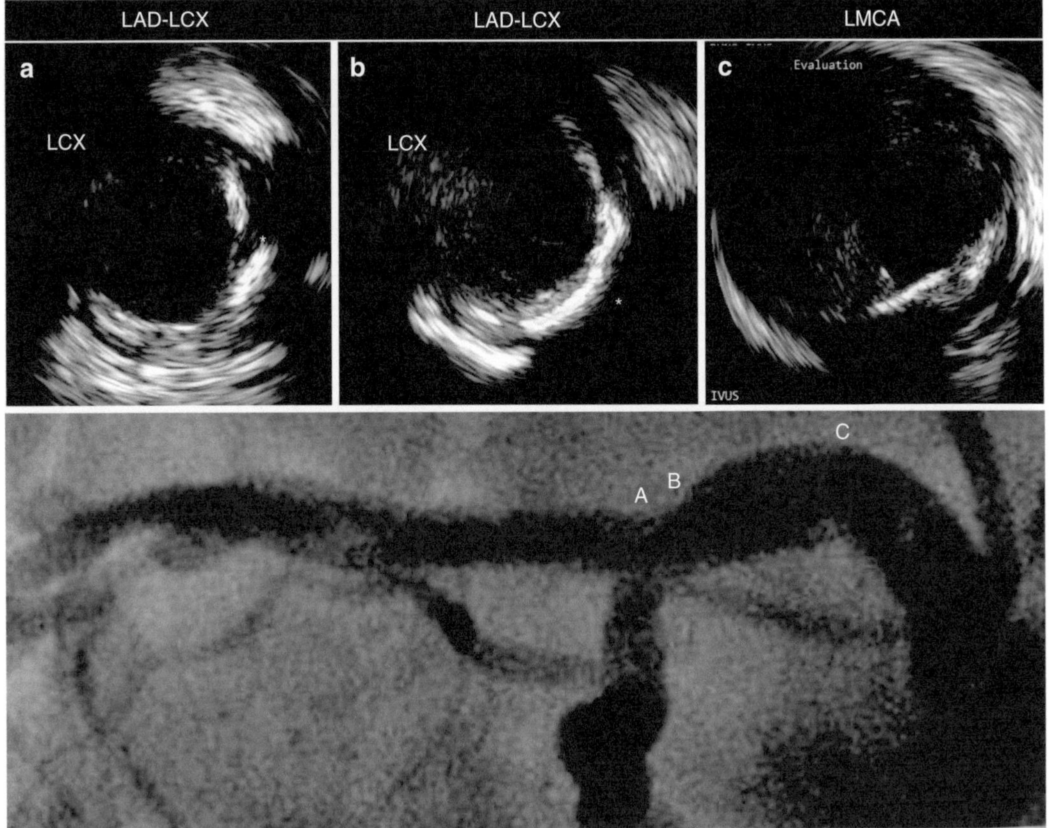

Fig. 10.10 The upper panel shows IVUS cross-sections of distal LMCA. (**a** and **b**) An eccentric calcific plaque opposite to the LCX origin; asterisks show superficial calcium less represented into the LMCA (**c**). In the lower panel, the angiographic view shows the LMCA bifurcation with the absence of clearly visible calcifications

of calcium fractures following lesion preparation is associated with improved stent expansion. In case of large (>180°) calcium pools and absence of calcium fracture following the initial lesion preparation, a more aggressive lesion preparation should be considered [47]. Moreover, IVUS studies have shown that localized calcium deposits or the transition from calcified to non-calcified plaques (or to normal vessel wall) are associated with PCI-related dissections. As a practical consideration, it is generally accepted that deep calcifications are better treated by means of scoring balloons whereas atherectomy-based techniques are suitable for calcific plaques closer to the vessel lumen. Nevertheless, it is easier to prevent stent under-expansion than it is to struggle to correct it.

10.4 IVUS-Guided LMCA PCI: Clinical Evidences

In the last two decades, several evidences have been accumulated on the impact on clinical outcomes of IVUS utilization during PCI with DES in patients with unprotected LMCA disease. Among the first studies, Agostoni et al. evaluated the differential impact of IVUS guidance on the short- and mid-term clinical events in a small population of patients (n = 58) referred for LMCA percutaneous revascularization with DES. In that study, no significant clinical benefit occurred in the IVUS sub-group [48]. The first study to demonstrate the possible benefit of IVUS guidance in reducing long-term mortality undergoing PCI for unprotected LMCA disease is represented by a sub-study of the MAIN-COPMPARE registry [10]. In this analysis, patients who underwent elective stenting of the unprotected LMCA were divided into those undergoing stent implantation under IVUS guidance (756, 77.5%) and those undergoing stent placement under conventional angiography guidance (291, 22.5%). After propensity score matching, a total of 201 matched pairs of patients were created and the risk of 3-year mortality for IVUS guidance was 60% lower than that for angiography guidance in the matched population. Three-year clinical outcomes were also assessed in a patient-level pooled analysis of four registries of patients with LM disease treated with DES in Spain [49]. In this analysis, a total of 1670 patients were included, and 505 patients (30.2%) underwent DES implantation under IVUS guidance (IVUS group). After matching, 505 patients without the use of IVUS during revascularization were selected (no-IVUS group). Survival free of cardiac death, myocardial infarction, and target lesion revascularization was 88.7% in the IVUS group and 83.6% in the no-IVUS group ($p = 0.04$) for the overall population whereas the incidence of definite and probable thrombosis was significantly lower in the IVUS group (0.6 vs. 2.2%; $p = 0.04$). Also, IVUS-guided revascularization was identified as an independent predictor for major adverse events. In a nationwide population-based study, Andell et al. included 2468 patients, where IVUS guidance was used in 621 (25.2%) cases. Authors found that, after adjustment for confounders, the primary endpoint of mortality, restenosis, or definite ST occurred significantly less in the IVUS group (HR, 0.65; 95% confidence interval [CI], 0.50–0.84; $p = 0.001$). In that study, the authors conclude that potential mediators of the benefit found include larger and more appropriately sized stents, perhaps translating into lower risk of subsequent ST [50]. The two most recent randomized clinical trials testing revascularization strategies for unprotected left main disease, EXCEL and NOBLE, yielded conflicting results [1, 2]. In the EXCEL study, investigators randomized 948 patients with left main coronary artery disease to PCI with an everolimus-eluting stent and 957 patients to CABG. The pri-

mary endpoint (a composite that included all-cause mortality, stroke, or MI at 3 years) occurred in 15.4% of patients treated with PCI and 14.7% of patients treated with CABG ($p = 0.02$ for non-inferiority) [47]. In NOBLE, PCI with primarily a biolimus-eluting stent was associated with a higher rate of major adverse cardiac and cerebrovascular events at 5 years. However, there was no difference in all-cause mortality between the two treatment groups, but the rate of non-procedural MI was significantly higher among PCI-treated patients (6.9 vs. 1.9%; HR 2.88; 95% CI 1.40–5.90). Similarly, repeat revascularizations were significantly higher with PCI compared with surgery (16.2 vs. 10.4%; HR 1.50; 95% CI 1.04–2.17) [48]. Interestingly, in the subgroup analysis of the EXCEL trial, LMCA stenting was aided by the use of IVUS in 77% of cases (and MSA < 8.7 mm^2 was associated with worse MACE outcomes) whereas less than half of PCI-treated patients had a pre-PCI IVUS assessment in the NOBLE trial.

10.5 Conclusions

In conclusion, the use of IVUS within the LMCA has a strong evidence base but there is still limited practical guidance about how to use it. Its usefulness has been described at each step of LMCA pre-assessment: to decide whether or not revascularize, to decide whether a one-stent technique might be sufficient, and to size the stent and select the optimum landing zones. Finally, IVUS has reported good relationship with FFR as a diagnostic tool with the advantage of unique morphological and plaque characteristics insights which can be crucial during percutaneous revascularization procedures.

References

1. Stone GW, Sabik JF, Serruys PW, Simonton CA, Généreux P, Puskas J, Kandzari DE, Morice MC, Lembo N, Brown WM 3rd, Taggart DP, Banning A, Merkely B, Horkay F, Boonstra PW, van Boven AJ, Ungi I, Bogáts G, Mansour S, Noiseux N, Sabaté M, Pomar J, Hickey M, Gershlick A, Buszman P,

Bochenek A, Schampaert E, Pagé P, Dressler O, Kosmidou I, Mehran R, Pocock SJ, Kappetein AP, Trial EXCEL, Investigators. Everolimus eluting stents or bypass surgery for left main coronary artery disease. N Engl J Med. 2016;375(23):2223–35.

2. Mäkikallio T, Holm NR, Lindsay M, Spence MS, Erglis A, Menown IB, Trovik T, Eskola M, Romppanen H, Kellerth T, Ravkilde J, Jensen LO, Kalinauskas G, Linder RB, Pentikainen M, Hervold A, Banning A, Zaman A, Cotton J, Eriksen E, Margus S, Sørensen HT, Nielsen PH, Niemelä M, Kervinen K, Lassen JF, Maeng M, Oldroyd K, Berg G, Walsh SJ, Hanratty CG, Kumsars I, Stradins P, Steigen TK, Fröbert O, Graham AN, Endresen PC, Corbascio M, Kajander O, Trivedi U, Hartikainen J, Anttila V, Hildick-Smith D, Thuesen L, Christiansen EH, Noble Study Investigators. Percutaneous coronary angioplasty versus coronary artery bypass grafting in treatment of unprotected left main stenosis (NOBLE): a prospective, randomised, open-label, non-inferiority trial. Lancet. 2016;388(10061):2743–52.

3. Neumann FJ, Sousa-Uva M, Ahlsson A, Alfonso F, Banning AP, Benedetto U, Byrne RA, Collet JP, Falk V, Head SJ, Jüni P, Kastrati A, Koller A, Kristensen SD, Niebauer J, Richter DJ, Seferovic PM, Sibbing D, Stefanini GG, Windecker S, Yadav R, Zembala MO, ESC Scientific Document Group. 2018 ESC/EACTS guidelines on myocardial revascularization. Eur Heart J. 2019;40(2):87–165.

4. Chakrabarti AK, Grau-Sepulveda MV, O'Brien S, Abueg C, Ponirakis A, Delong E, Peterson E, Klein LW, Garratt KN, Weintraub WS, Gibson CM. Angiographic validation of the American College of Cardiology Foundation—the Society of Thoracic Surgeons Collaboration on the Comparative Effectiveness of Revascularization Strategies Study. Circ Cardiovasc Interv. 2014;7:11–8.

5. Gomez-Lara J, Diletti R, Brugaletta S, Onuma Y, Farooq V, Thuesen L, McClean D, Koolen J, Ormiston JA, Windecker S, Whitbourn R, Dudek D, Dorange C, Veldhof S, Rapoza R, Regar E, Garcia-Garcia HM, Serruys PW. Angiographic maximal luminal diameter and appropriate deployment of the everolimus-eluting bioresorbable vascular scaffold as assessed by optical coherence tomography: an ABSORB cohort B trial sub-study. EuroIntervention. 2012;8(2):214–24.

6. Waksman R, Kitabata H, Prati F, Albertucci M, Mintz GS. Intravascular ultrasound versus optical coherence tomography guidance. J Am Coll Cardiol. 2013;62(17 Suppl):S32–40. https://doi.org/10.1016/j.jacc.2013.08.709.

7. Chieffo A, Latib A, Caussin C, Presbitero P, Galli S, Menozzi A, Varbella F, Mauri F, Valgimigli M, Arampatzis C, Sabate M, Erglis A, Reimers B, Airoldi F, Laine M, Palop RL, Mikhail G, Maccarthy P, Romeo F, Colombo A. A prospective, randomized trial of intravascular-ultrasound guided compared to angiography guided stent implantation in complex coronary lesions: the AVIO trial. Am Heart J. 2013;165(1):65–72.

8. Roy P, Steinberg DH, Sushinsky SJ, Okabe T, Pinto Slottow TL, Kaneshige K, Xue Z, Satler LF, Kent KM, Suddath WO, Pichard AD, Weissman NJ, Lindsay J, Waksman R. The potential clinical utility of intravascular ultrasound guidance in patients undergoing percutaneous coronary intervention with drug-eluting stents. Eur Heart J. 2008;29(15):1851–7.

9. Claessen BE, Mehran R, Mintz GS, Weisz G, Leon MB, Dogan O, de Ribamar Costa J Jr, Stone GW, Apostolidou I, Morales A, Chantziara V, Syros G, Sanidas E, Xu K, Tijssen JG, Henriques JP, Piek JJ, Moses JW, Maehara A, Dangas GD. Impact of intravascular ultrasound imaging on early and late clinical outcomes following percutaneous coronary intervention with drug-eluting stents. JACC Cardiovasc Interv. 2011;4(9):974–81. Erratum in: JACC Cardiovasc Interv. 2011 Nov;4(11):1255

10. Park SJ, Kim YH, Park DW, Lee SW, Kim WJ, Suh J, Yun SC, Lee CW, Hong MK, Lee JH, Park SW, Main-Compare Investigators. Impact of intravascular ultrasound guidance on long-term mortality in stenting for unprotected left main coronary artery stenosis. Circ Cardiovasc Interv. 2009;2(3):167–77.

11. Mudra H, di Mario C, de Jaegere P, Figulla HR, Macaya C, Zahn R, Wennerblom B, Rutsch W, Voudris V, Regar E, Henneke KH, Schächinger V, Zeiher A, OPTICUS (Optimization with ICUS to Reduce Stent Restenosis) Study Investigators. Randomized comparison of coronary stent implantation under ultrasound or angiographic guidance to reduce stent restenosis (OPTICUS Study). Circulation. 2001;104(12):1343–9.

12. Oemrawsingh PV, Mintz GS, Schalij MJ, Zwinderman AH, Jukema JW, Van der Wall EE, TULIP Study. Thrombocyte activity evaluation and effects of ultrasound guidance in long intracoronary stent placement. Intravascular ultrasound guidance improves angiographic and clinical outcome of stent implantation for long coronary artery stenoses: final results of a randomized comparison with angiographic guidance (TULIP Study). Circulation. 2003;107(1):62–7.

13. Garcìa-Garcìa HM, Gogas BD, Serruys PW, Bruining N. IVUS-based imaging modalities for tissue characterization: similarities and differences. Int J Cardiovasc Imaging. 2011;27(2):215–24.

14. Bartorelli AL, Potkin BN, Almagor Y, Keren G, Roberts WC, Leon MB. Plaque characterization of atherosclerotic coronary arteries by intravascular ultrasound. Echocardiography. 1990;7(4):389–95.

15. Mintz GS, Nissen SE, Anderson WD, Bailey SR, Erbel R, Fitzgerald PJ, Pinto FJ, Rosenfield K, Siegel RJ, Tuzcu EM, Yock PG. American College of Cardiology clinical expert consensus document on standards for acquisition, measurement and reporting of intravascular ultrasound studies (IVUS). A report of the American College of Cardiology Task Force on clinical expert consensus documents. J Am Coll Cardiol. 2001;37(5):1478–92.

16. Nair A, Kuban BD, Tuzcu EM, Schoenhagen P, Nissen SE, Vince DG. Coronary plaque classification

with intravascular ultrasound radiofrequency data analysis. Circulation. 2002;106(17):2200–6.

17. Di Mario C, Görge G, Peters R, Kearney P, Pinto F, Hausmann D, von Birgelen C, Colombo A, Mudra H, Roelandt J, Erbel R. Clinical application and image interpretation in intracoronary ultrasound. Study Group on Intracoronary Imaging of the Working Group of Coronary Circulation and of the Subgroup on Intravascular Ultrasound of the Working Group of Echocardiography of the European Society of Cardiology. Eur Heart J. 1998;19(2):207–29.

18. Prati F, Arbustini E, Labellarte A, Dal Bello B, Sommariva L, Mallus MT, Pagano A, Boccanelli A. Correlation between high frequency intravascular ultrasound and histomorphology in human coronary arteries. Heart. 2001;85(5):567–70.

19. De Maria AN, Narula J, Mahmud E, Tsimikas S. Imaging vulnerable plaque by ultrasound. J Am Coll Cardiol. 2006;47(8 Suppl):C32–9.

20. Virmani R, Burke AP, Farb A, Kolodgie FD. Pathology of the vulnerable plaque. J Am Coll Cardiol. 2006;47(8 Suppl):C13–8.

21. García-García HM, Goedhart D, Schuurbiers JC, Kukreja N, Tanimoto S, Daemen J, Morel MA, Bressers M, van Es GA, Wentzel JJ, Gijsen F, van der Steen AF, Serruys PW. Virtual histology and remodelling index allow in vivo identification of allegedly high-risk coronary plaques in patients with acute coronary syndromes: a three vessel intravascular ultrasound radiofrequency data analysis. EuroIntervention. 2006;2(3):338–44.

22. Tyczynski P, Pregowski J, Mintz GS, Witkowski A, Kim SW, Waksman R, Satler L, Pichard A, Kalinczuk L, Maehara A, Weissman NJ. Intravascular ultrasound assessment of ruptured atherosclerotic plaques in left main coronary arteries. Am J Cardiol. 2005;96(6):794–8.

23. Rodriguez-Granillo GA, García-García HM, Wentzel J, Valgimigli M, Tsuchida K, van der Giessen W, de Jaegere P, Regar E, de Feyter PJ, Serruys PW. Plaque composition and its relationship with acknowledged shear stress patterns in coronary arteries. J Am Coll Cardiol. 2006;47(4):884–5.

24. Stone GW, Maehara A, Lansky AJ, de Bruyne B, Cristea E, Mintz GS, Mehran R, McPherson J, Farhat N, Marso SP, Parise H, Templin B, White R, Zhang Z, Serruys PW, Prospect Investigators. A prospective natural-history study of coronary atherosclerosis. N Engl J Med. 2011;364(3):226–35.

25. Maehara A, Mintz GS, Castagna MT, Pichard AD, Satler LF, Waksman R, Laird JR Jr, Suddath WO, Kent KM, Weissman NJ. Intravascular ultrasound assessment of the stenoses location and morphology in the left main coronary artery in relation to anatomic left main length. Am J Cardiol. 2001;88:1–4.

26. Sano K, Mintz GS, Carlier SG, de Ribamar Costa J Jr, Qian J, Missel E, Shan S, Franklin-Bond T, Boland P, Weisz G, Moussa I, Dangas GD, Mehran R, Lansky AJ, Kreps EM, Collins MB, Stone GW, Leon MB, Moses JW. Assessing intermediate left main coronary lesions using intravascular ultrasound. Am Heart J. 2007 Nov;154(5):983–8.

27. Fisher LD, Judkins MP, Lesperance J, Cameron A, Swaye P, Ryan T, Maynard C, Bourassa M, Kennedy JW, Gosselin A, Kemp H, Faxon D, Wexler L, Davis KB. Reproducibility of coronary arteriographic reading in the coronary artery surgery study (CASS). Catheter Cardiovasc Diagn. 1982;8(6):565–75.

28. Toth G, Hamilos M, Pyxaras S, Mangiacapra F, Nelis O, De Vroey F, Di Serafino L, Muller O, Van Mieghem C, Wyffels E, Heyndrickx GR, Bartunek J, Vanderheyden M, Barbato E, Wijns W, De Bruyne B. Evolving concepts of angiogram: fractional flow reserve discordances in 4000 coronary stenoses. Eur Heart J. 2014;35:2831–8.

29. Glagov S, Weisenberg E, Zarins CK, Stankunavicius R, Kolettis GJ. Compensatory enlargement of human atherosclerotic coronary arteries. N Engl J Med. 1987;316:1371–5.

30. Ricciardi MJ, Meyers S, Choi K, Pang JL, Goodreau L, Davidson CJ. Angiographically silent left main disease detected by intravascular ultrasound: a marker for future adverse cardiac events. Am Heart J. 2003;146:507–12.

31. Fassa AA, Wagatsuma K, Higano ST, Mathew V, Barsness GW, Lennon RJ, Holmes DR Jr, Lerman A. Intravascular ultrasound-guided treatment for angiographically indeterminate left main coronary artery disease: a long-term follow-up study. J Am Coll Cardiol. 2005;45(2):204–11.

32. de la Torre Hernandez JM, Hernandez Hernandez F, Alfonso F, Rumoroso JR, Lopez-Palop R, Sadaba M, Carrillo P, Rondan J, Lozano I, Ruiz Nodar JM, Baz JA, Fernandez Nofrerias E, Pajin F, Garcia Camarero T, Gutierrez H, LITRO Study Group. Prospective application of pre-defined intravascular ultrasound criteria for assessment of intermediate left main coronary artery lesions results from the multicenter LITRO study. J Am Coll Cardiol. 2011;58:351–8.

33. Puri R, Kapadia SR, Nicholls SJ, Harvey JE, Kataoka Y, Tuzcu EM. Optimizing outcomes during left main percutaneous coronary intervention with intravascular ultrasound and fractional flow reserve: the current state of evidence. JACC Cardiovasc Interv. 2012;5:697–707.

34. Jasti V, Ivan E, Yalamanchili V, Wongpraparut N, Leesar MA. Correlations between fractional flow reserve and intravascular ultrasound in patients with an ambiguous left main coronary artery stenosis. Circulation. 2004;110:2831–6.

35. Park SJ, Ahn JM, Kang SJ, Yoon SH, Koo BK, Lee JY, Kim WJ, Park DW, Lee SW, Kim YH, Lee CW, Park SW. Intravascular ultrasound-derived minimal lumen area criteria for functionally significant left main coronary artery stenosis. JACC Cardiovasc Interv. 2014;7:868–74.

36. Park SJ, Kang SJ, Ahn JM. Reply: the optimal cut-off value for left main minimal lumen area of 4.5 mm(2): a word of caution. JACC Cardiovasc Interv. 2015;8:123–4.

37. de la Torre Hernandez JM, Hernandez F, Alfonso F. The optimal cutoff value for left main minimal lumen area of 4.5 mm(2): a word of caution. JACC Cardiovasc Interv. 2015;8:122–3.

38. Waksman R, Legutko J, Singh J, Orlando Q, Marso S, Schloss T, Tugaoen J, DeVries J, Palmer N, Haude M, Swymelar S, Torguson R. FIRST: fractional flow reserve and intravascular ultrasound relationship study. J Am Coll Cardiol. 2013;61:917–23.

39. Mallidi J, Atreya AR, Cook J, Garb J, Jeremias A, Klein LW, Lotfi A. Long-term outcomes following fractional flow reserve-guided treatment of angiographically ambiguous left main coronary artery disease: a meta-analysis of prospective cohort studies. Catheter Cardiovasc Interv. 2015;86:12–8.

40. Oviedo C, Maehara A, Mintz GS, Araki H, Choi SY, Tsujita K, Kubo T, Doi H, Templin B, Lansky AJ, Dangas G, Leon MB, Mehran R, Tahk SJ, Stone GW, Ochiai M, Moses JW. Intravascular ultrasound classification of plaque distribution in left main coronary artery bifurcations: where is the plaque really located? Circ Cardiovasc Interv. 2010;3:105–12.

41. Kang SJ, Ahn JM, Kim WJ, Lee JY, Park DW, Lee SW, Kim YH, Lee CW, Park SW, Park SJ. Functional and morphological assessment of side branch after left main coronary artery bifurcation stenting with cross-over technique. Catheter Cardiovasc Interv. 2014;83:545–52.

42. ChoiS-Y WB, Maehara A, Lansky AJ, Guagliumi G, Brodie B, Kellett MA, Dressler O, Parise H, Mehran R, Dangas GD, Mintz GS, Stone GW. Intravascular ultrasound findings of early stent thrombosis after primary percutaneous intervention in acute myocardial infarction: a harmonizing outcomes with revascularization and stents in acute myocardial infarction (HORIZONS-AMI) sub-study. Circ Cardiovasc Interv. 2011;4:239–47.

43. Kang S-J, Ahn J-M, Song H, Kim W-J, Lee J-Y, Park D-W, Yun S-C, Lee S-W, Kim Y-H, Lee CW, Mintz GS, Park S-W, Park S-J. Comprehensive intravascular ultrasound assessment of stent area and its impact on restenosis and adverse cardiac events in 403 patients with unprotected left main disease. Circ Cardiovasc Interv. 2011;4:562–9.

44. Sonoda S, Morino Y, Ako J, Terashima M, Hassan AHM, Bonneau HN, Leon MB, Moses JW, Yock PG, Honda Y, Kuntz RE, Fitzgerald PJ. Impact of final stent dimensions on long-term results following sirolimus-eluting stent implantation: serial intravascular ultrasound analysis from the Sirius Trial. J Am Coll Cardiol. 2004;43:1959–63.

45. Song H-G, Kang S-J, Ahn J-M, Kim W-J, Lee J-Y, Park D-W, Lee S-W, Kim Y-H, Lee CW, Park S-W, Park S-J. Intravascular ultra- sound assessment of optimal stent area to prevent in-stent restenosis after zotarolimus-, everolimus-, and sirolimus-eluting stent implantation. Catheter Cardiovasc Interv. 2014;83:873–8.

46. Mintz GS. Intravascular imaging of coronary calcification and its clinical implications. JACC Cardiovasc Imaging. 2015;8:461–71.

47. Räber L, Mintz GS, Koskinas KC, Johnson TW, Holm NR, Onuma Y, Radu MD, Joner M, Yu B, Jia H, Meneveau N, de la Torre Hernandez JM, Escaned J, Hill J, Prati F, Colombo A, Di Mario C, Regar E, Capodanno D, Wijns W, Byrne RA, Guagliumi G. Clinical use of intracoronary imaging. Part 1: guidance and optimization of coronary interventions. An expert consensus document of the European Association of Percutaneous Cardiovascular Interventions. EuroIntervention. 2018;14(6):656–77.

48. Agostoni P, Valgimigli M, Van Mieghem CA, Rodriguez-Granillo GA, Aoki J, Ong AT, Tsuchida K, McFadden EP, Ligthart JM, Smits PC, de Jaegere P, Sianos G, Van der Giessen WJ, De Feyter P, Serruys PW. Comparison of early outcome of percutaneous coronary intervention for unprotected left main coronary artery disease in the drug-eluting stent era with versus without intravascular ultrasonic guidance. Am J Cardiol. 2005;95(5):644–7.

49. De la Torre Hernandez JM, Baz Alonso JA, Gómez Hospital JA, Alfonso Manterola F, Garcia Camarero T, Gimeno de Carlos F, et al. Clinical impact of intravascular ultrasound guidance in drug-eluting stent implantation for unprotected left main coronary disease: pooled analysis at the patient- level of 4 registries. JACC Cardiovasc Interv. 2014;7:244–54.

50. Andell P, Karlsson S, Mohammad MA, Götberg M, James S, Jensen J, Fröbert O, Angerås O, Nilsson J, Omerovic E, Lagerqvist B, Persson J, Koul S, Erlinge D. Intravascular ultrasound guidance is associated with better outcomes in patients undergoing unprotected left main coronary artery stenting compared with angiography guidance alone. Circ Cardiovasc Interv. 2017;10:e004813.

Preoperative Functional Assessment of the Left Main and Postoperative Side Branch Evaluation

11

Luigi Di Serafino and Emanuele Barbato

11.1 Left Main Anatomy and Atherosclerotic Process

The LM represents the proximal segment of the left coronary artery that usually arises from the left aortic sinus and bifurcates into the left anterior descending (LAD) and left circumflex (LCX) arteries [1, 2]. In a right dominant system, it supplies the left ventricle with more than four-fifth of the blood flow [3, 4]. The atherosclerotic involvement of the LMS bifurcation is usually accelerated in the lateral walls, being these latter areas of low shear stress, conversely, the bifurcation carina is frequently free of disease. However, bifurcation disease is rarely focal and plaque extension from the LM into the proximal LAD is common [5].

11.2 Limitations of the Angiography for LMS Evaluation

Equivocal left main stenosis is not an infrequent angiographic finding. Despite the widespread adoption of a 50% angiographic diameter stenosis as a cut-off value to consider a lesion signifi-

cant and to indicate revascularization, underestimation of the true severity of the disease is frequent given a considerable intra- and interobserver variability in the angiographic assessment [6]. This is mainly due to the following technical limitations:

- Catheter-related issues:
  - Catheter-induced spasm
  - Catheter overlap with the LM ostium might induce contrast medium spill-over and incomplete mixing of blood and contrast medium in the proximal part of the LM
  - Reflux of contrast in aortic sinus might mask ostial stenosis
- LM anatomy-related issues:
  - An angulated LM makes difficult the interpretation of the stenosis severity
  - Reverse tapering phenomenon: despite the absence of any atherosclerotic disease, the LM ostium may be smaller in caliber as compared with the distal segment
  - In case of diffuse disease or ostial stenosis, a reference segment might be missing
- Foreshortening issues with overlapping of the bifurcation branches

As a result of the angiography-based evaluation of a LM stenosis, a misclassification might occur in up to 50% of the cases. In addition, in comparison with fractional flow reserve (FFR), the optimal angiographic cut-off value for

L. Di Serafino · E. Barbato (✉)
Department of Advanced Biomedical Sciences, University of Naples Federico II, Naples, Italy
e-mail: luigi.diserafino@unina.it;
emanuele.barbato@unina.it

© Springer Nature Switzerland AG 2022
B. Cortese (ed.), *Left Main Coronary Revascularization*,
https://doi.org/10.1007/978-3-031-05265-1_11

predicting "hemodynamically significant" stenosis is close to 40% [7]. In a study including 213 patients with an angiographically intermediate left main stenosis undergoing FFR evaluation, only 35% of patients underwent revascularization with a bypass graft. Of note, up to 23% of patients presented with a LM stenosis <50%, but with an FFR <0.80. In addition, at 5-year follow-up the clinical outcome was similar between patients with functionally non-significant stenosis and patients treated with bypass graft [8].

Similarly, an instantaneous wave-free ratio (iFR)-deferral strategy of LM stenosis in 314 patients was associated with no significant difference in the primary composite endpoint of all-cause death, non-fatal myocardial infarction, and ischemia-driven target lesion revascularization as compared with patients in whom LM was revascularized (9.2 vs. 14.6%, $p = 0.26$) at a median follow-up of 30 months [9].

Nevertheless, most of the currently available clinical evidence about the management of LM stenosis is actually mainly based on the angiographic estimation [10, 11]. In both the EXCEL and NOBEL trial, the inclusion criteria were LM stenosis >70% (EXCEL) or >50% (NOBLE) at visual estimation, or the presence of hemodynamically significant LM stenosis determined by the means of non-invasive or invasive assessment.

11.3 FFR and iFR: Principles

The FFR is the ratio between the maximal hyperemic blood flow through an epicardial stenosis and the maximal hyperemic blood flow in the hypothetical absence of the stenosis; it reflects both the severity of the stenosis and the amount of myocardium subtended. It is normally calculated by measuring the distal mean coronary artery pressure with a specific 0.014″ pressure-sensor guidewire during maximal hyperemia, while the contemporary measured aortic pressure represents the pressure in the theoretical absence of the stenosis [12–14]. After the publication of FAME and FAME II trials which respectively showed the superiority of the FFR-based

treatment as compared with the angiographic guidance and, the superiority of PCI for functionally significant stenosis with medical treatment as compared with medical treatment alone, improving the clinical outcomes in patients with coronary artery disease, the use of FFR has been implemented into the current coronary revascularization guidelines for patients with equivocal coronary artery disease [15–19].

The instantaneous wave-free ratio (iFR) has been introduced as an alternative to the FFR; it does not require hyperemic drugs since it samples intracoronary pressure during the "diastolic wave-free" period, where microvascular resistance is supposed to be lower and stable [20]. Recently, two large-scale randomized trials showed the iFR to be clinically non-inferior to the FFR, thereby they are equally recommended by the European guidelines for the assessment of the ischemic potential of equivocal coronary artery stenoses [21–24].

11.4 Tips and Tricks for LM Functional Assessment

The assessment of the equivocal stenosis of the LM using the FFR or iFR is more challenging in comparison with non-LM stenosis. In case of ostial stenosis, some issues may arise since the beginning of the invasive functional assessment, namely at the time of the "equalization" or "normalization" of the two pressures. In fact, after the guiding catheter is flushed with saline, in order to remove any residual contrast used, the pressure-wire should be positioned with its sensor at 1 or 2 mm distal to the tip of the guiding catheter. At that location, the two pressures should be equal. In case of ostial disease of the LM, the "equalization" can be performed with the guiding catheter disengaged and the sensor of the pressure-wire positioned in the aorta at the tip of the guiding catheter (Fig. 11.1) [25].

The presence of the ostial stenosis could make difficult the intracoronary administration of the hyperemic agent, such as the adenosine. In this case, intravenous administration of adenosine (140 mg/kg of body weight/min) or regadenosone

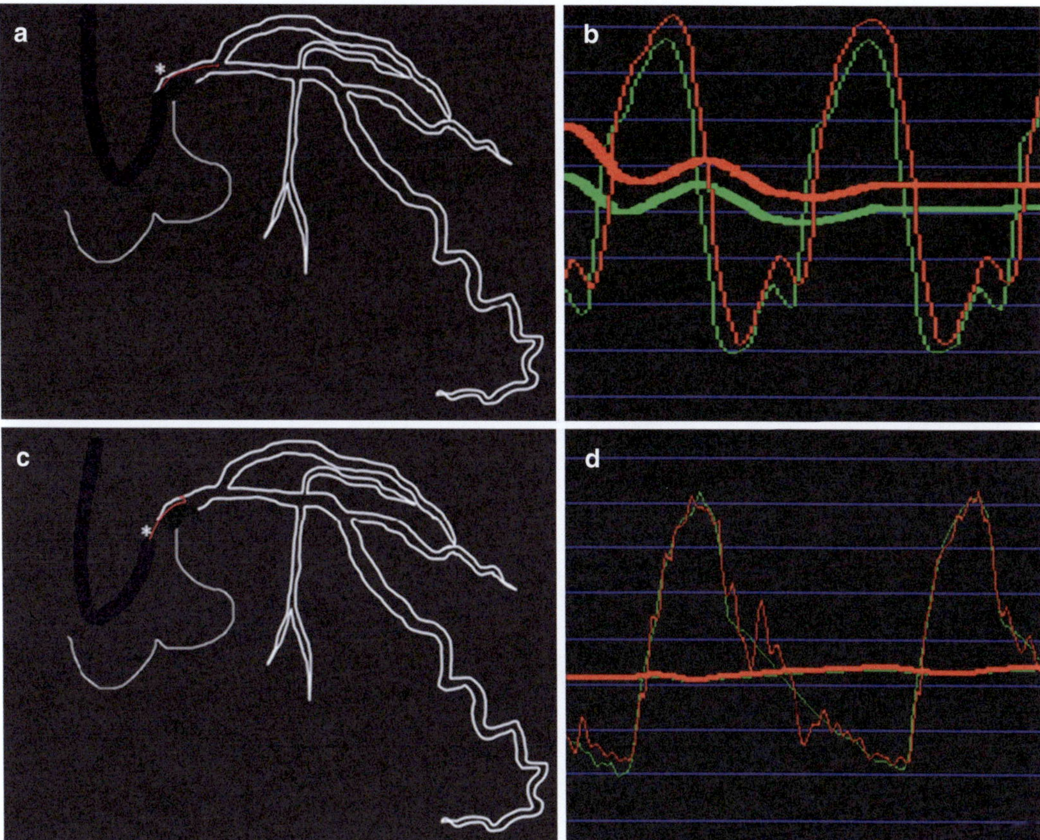

Fig. 11.1 Ostial LM stenosis assessment. In case of an ostial stenosis of the LM, the equalization should be performed avoiding any interaction between the guiding catheter and the coronary ostium (Panel **a**), thereby avoiding the "ventricularization" of the aortic pressure (Panel **b**). As soon the pressure-wire has crossed the stenosis, the catheter should be dislodged from the ostium (Panel **c**) together with the wire sensor (*), allowing for a correct pressure tracing (Panel **d**) before the equalization

(400 mg i.v. bolus) should be preferred (Table 11.1) [25]. However, intracoronary bolus of adenosine is still possible with some skill and care: performed the equalization and with the pressure-wire positioned in the distal vessel, the guiding catheter (without side-holes) should be advanced into the ostium and, after the intracoronary bolus of adenosine is given, rapidly disengaged in order to correctly measure the proximal (aortic) pressure.

Another issue is represented by the position of the pressure-wire. In general, for the assessment of stenosis involving the LM only, the pressure-wire should be positioned distally in the left anterior descending artery, which represents the largest myocardial territory subtended by the stenosis. The sensor should be placed in the same position where ideally the surgeon would place the anastomosis, in case the patient would be referred to CABG [25]. At the variance, for the assessment of equivocal stenosis of the LM involving the bifurcation and the proximal segment of both the LAD and the LCX, the FFR measurement should be performed both with the wire positioned in the LAD and through the LCX (Fig. 11.2).

The assessment of the LM stenosis with the pressure-wire might even be more challenging in case the LAD is also diseased and presenting with an equivocal stenosis at the proximal

Table 11.1 Hyperemic agents for functional assessment of the LM

Drug	Administration	Dosage	Duration	Plateau	Indications
Adenosine	I.C. bolus	200 µg	20″	No	
	I.V. infusion	140 µg/kg/min	60″ since the end of the infusion	Yes	Recommended for serial and ostial stenosis
Regadenoson	I.V. bolus	0.4 mg	2–5′	yes	Recommended for serial and ostial stenosis
Papaverine	I.C. bolus	20 mg	Up to 60″	Yes	Recommended for serial stenosis

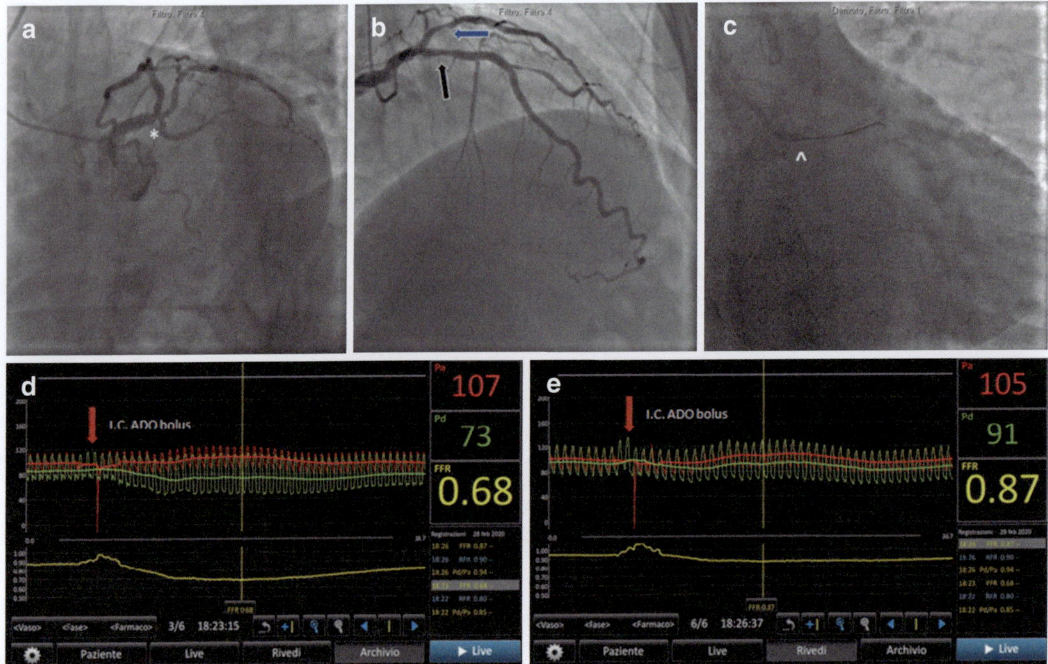

Fig. 11.2 Functional assessment of a distal LM stenosis. Functional evaluation of a distal LM stenosis involving a trifurcation (Panel **a**, *). The proximal LAD is also diseased (Panel **b**, black arrow) as well as the proximal ramus (Panel **b**, blue arrow). The pressure-wire equalization is performed with the wire positioned through the LAD and the sensor at the same location of the tip of the guiding catheter (Panel **c**, ^). With the pressure-wire in the distal LAD, an intra-coronary bolus of adenosine is rapidly given (200 µg—Panel **d**, red arrow) and the guiding catheter dislocated from the ostium and the lowest FFR value is considered (0.68). The same procedure is repeated with the pressure-wire through the ramus (Panel **e**) with the same adenosine administration

segment. In this case, indeed, the FFR measurement should be performed at the steady state of the maximal hyperemia, i.e., induced by systemic infusion of adenosine, in order to perform a gentle pull-back of the pressure-wire while looking for the largest step-up of the pressure gradient produced by the "functionally tightest" stenosis (Fig. 11.3) [13, 14]. However, the pos-

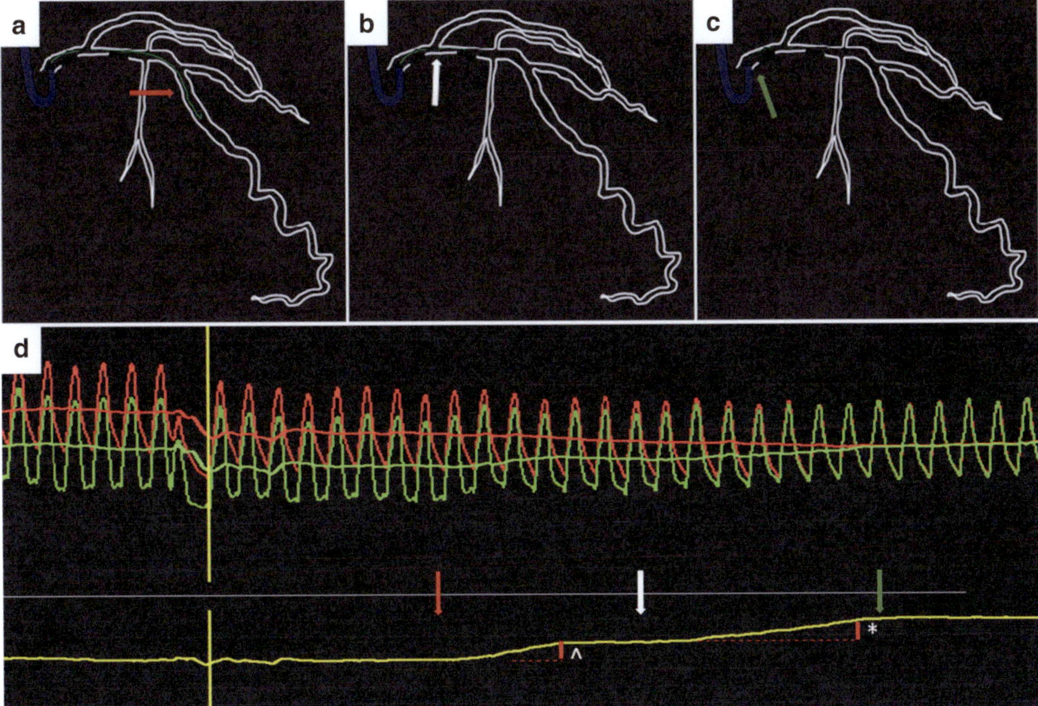

Fig. 11.3 Functional assessment of serial stenoses. With the pressure wire positioned in the distal LAD (Panel **a**), maximal hyperemia is induced with I.V. adenosine administration in order to obtain a stable hyperemic plateau. The lowest FFR value is registered (Panel **d**, red arrow) and the wire is slowly pulled-back and, as soon as the pressure sensor is in between the two stenosis (Panel **b**, white arrow) a clear step up (Panel **d**, ^) is recorded and a new FFR value is registered (Panel **d**, white arrow). Finally, the wire is pulled-back with the sensor proximal to the LM stenosis (Panel **c**, green arrow) obtaining a perfect overlapping of the pressure curves (Panel **d**, green arrow) and a second step up (Panel **d**, *) due to the presence of the LM stenosis

sible "cross-talk" between the stenosis might affect the functional assessment of the LM stenosis. In fact, the presence of a stenosis in the LAD might underestimate the FFR value of the LM stenosis when the pressure-wire is placed through the LAD; on the contrary, even if the pressure-wire is placed in the non-diseased LCX an overestimation of the FFR value might also occur (Fig. 11.4) [26]. However, this scenario might have clinical implications only when the downstream disease in the stenosed vessel is proximal and very severe [26].

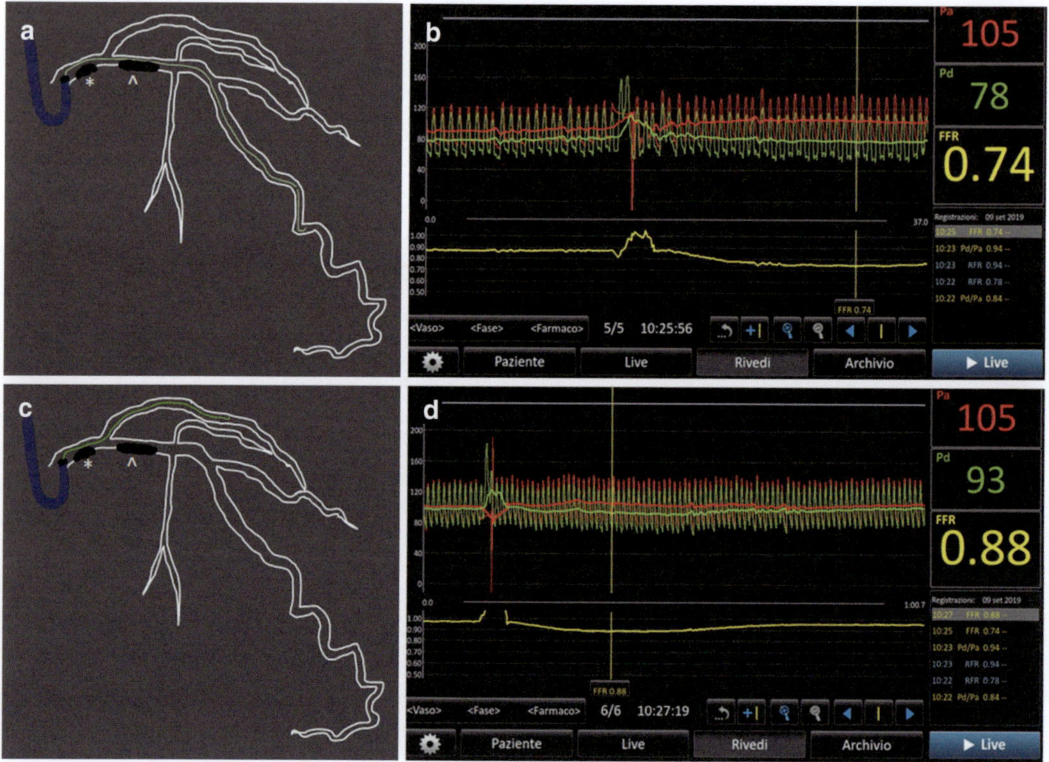

Fig. 11.4 LM stenosis assessment in the presence of a critical stenosis in the proximal LAD. In case of the presence of an equivocal stenosis of the LM (*) together with a critical stenosis in the very proximal segment of the LAD (^), the measurement of the FFR with the pressure-wire positioned in the distal LAD (Panel **a**) might lead to an underestimation of the FFR value and therefore a functional overestimation of the LM stenosis (Panel **b**). In contrast, positioning the pressure-wire in the distal LCX (Panel **c**) might lead to an overestimation of the FFR value which in turn means a functional underestimation of the LM (Panel **d**)

11.5   Assessment of the Distal LM Bifurcation Post PCI

In a bifurcation lesion, after stenting the main branch, the potential plaque shift determining a stenosis at the ostium of the side branch might represent a challenging diagnostic issue. In fact, unless flow limiting, the side branch lesion is often of limited functional significance [27]. Only a quarter of cases with an angiographically significant residual stenosis at the side branch ostium have been found to be also "functionally" significant [28]. This discrepancy also occurs in the context of the distal LM bifurcation and it has been hypothesized to be also associated with an optical phenomenon produced by angiography [29–32]. However, the main mechanism of the acute lumen loss at the LCX ostium, after cross-over LM-LAD stenting, has been shown to be associated with carina rather than plaque shift which is more frequent when the angle between the LAD and the LCX is particularly narrowed [32–36]. However, the "bigger the better" paradigm would suggest that a larger side-branch ostial area might be less susceptible to the risk of restenosis compared with a smaller one [37, 38]. In addition, struts over a side-branch ostium may act as a trigger for neointimal proliferation leading to potential impairment of the side-branch ostium [39]. Conversely, the presence of "floating struts" at the side branch has been reported to be associated with a reduced incidence of strut coverage which in turn increases the risk of stent thrombosis [40]. Thus, the aim of the final kissing balloon, after the treatment of a coronary bifurcation, especially of the LM, is to limit the presence of floating struts, even though the long-term clinical impact of this approach is yet to be determined [32, 41–45]. Nevertheless, after LM-LAD crossover stenting, the percentage diameter stenosis of the jailed LCX ostium rarely correlates with the FFR value, even though the angiographic appearance might suggest the presence of a critical stenosis. In a study including 83 patients who underwent LM-LAD crossover stenting, only 14 patients (17%) presented with a positive FFR value (<0.80) at the LCX ostium [46]. In addition, a positive FFR value was an independent predictor of the risk for a 5-year target lesion failure [46]. In this context, the FFR assessment of the side branch appears to be useful to guide revascularization strategy of the side branch, avoiding unnecessary complex procedures.

After crossover stenting, the FFR measurement of the jailed side-branch ostium with a pressure-wire might result more difficult as compared with any other regular wire. Although not designed to be jailed, some operators used the pressure wire to protect the side-branch when performing a PCI of a coronary bifurcation according to the provisional technique, avoiding side-branch rewiring and possible interventions, thereby reducing the procedural time. However, some difficulties could be encountered while removing the jailed pressure-wire and, in this case, rather than forcing, a low-profile over-the-wire balloon may facilitate the removal of the wire, in order to avoid pressure-wire fracture/damage/rupture [47, 48]. However, in the setting of the LM bifurcation, the pressure-wire jailing during provisional treatment of the bifurcation has never been tested. Of note, in case of crossover LM-LAD stenting, the jailed pressure-wire, as the other regular wires, can also be damaged by the guiding catheter when this latter is advanced into the stent, particularly if the LM ostium is also covered; in this case indeed, the deep intubation with the guiding catheter should be avoided if the jailed wire is still in place.

An alternative option to ease the side-branch functional assessment after stenting the main branch is the use of pressure-sensored microcatheters able to slide onto regular workhorse guidewires, therefore reducing the risk of vascular dissection or guidewire fracture.

11.6 Conclusions

A correct assessment of a left main stenosis might be challenging, in particular when it is based on angiography alone [49]. A functional evaluation with FFR and/or iFR might be useful to correctly identify those lesions which need to be treated rather than left to medical treatment, even though the association with other imaging modalities might be required in some cases. The knowledge of the common issues more often associated with the functional assessment of the LM stenosis, and the tips and tricks for overcoming the complex anatomies is mandatory, in order to better identify the correct treatment strategy even in more complex cases.

References

1. Reig J, Petit M. Main trunk of the left coronary artery: anatomic study of the parameters of clinical interest. Clin Anat. 2004;17(1):6–13.
2. Park SJ, Park DW. Percutaneous coronary intervention with stent implantation versus coronary artery bypass surgery for treatment of left main coronary artery disease: is it time to change guidelines? Circ Cardiovasc Interv. 2009;2(1):59–68.
3. Sianos G, Morel MA, Kappetein AP, Morice MC, Colombo A, Dawkins K, et al. The SYNTAX score: an angiographic tool grading the complexity of coronary artery disease. EuroIntervention. 2005;1(2):219–27.
4. Leaman DM, Brower RW, Meester GT, Serruys P, van den Brand M. Coronary artery atherosclerosis: severity of the disease, severity of angina pectoris and compromised left ventricular function. Circulation. 1981;63(2):285–99.
5. Oviedo C, Maehara A, Mintz GS, Araki H, Choi SY, Tsujita K, et al. Intravascular ultrasound classification of plaque distribution in left main coronary artery bifurcations: where is the plaque really located? Circ Cardiovasc Interv. 2010;3(2):105–12.
6. Kassimis G, de Maria GL, Patel N, Raina T, Scott P, Kharbanda RK, et al. Assessing the left main stem in the cardiac catheterization laboratory. What is "significant"? Function, imaging or both? Cardiovasc Revasc Med. 2018;19(1 Pt A):51–6.
7. Toth G, Hamilos M, Pyxaras S, Mangiacapra F, Nelis O, De Vroey F, et al. Evolving concepts of angiogram: fractional flow reserve discordances in 4000 coronary stenoses. Eur Heart J. 2014;35(40):2831–8.
8. Hamilos M, Muller O, Cuisset T, Ntalianis A, Chlouverakis G, Sarno G, et al. Long-term clinical outcome after fractional flow reserve-guided treatment in patients with angiographically equivo-

cal left main coronary artery stenosis. Circulation. 2009;120(15):1505–12.

9. Warisawa T, Cook CM, Rajkumar C, Howard JP, Seligman H, Ahmad Y, et al. Safety of revascularization deferral of left main stenosis based on instantaneous wave-free ratio evaluation. JACC Cardiovasc Interv. 2020;13(14):1655–64.

10. Stone GW, Sabik JF, Serruys PW, Simonton CA, Généreux P, Puskas J, et al. Everolimus-eluting stents or bypass surgery for left main coronary artery disease. N Engl J Med. 2016;375(23):2223–35.

11. Mäkikallio T, Holm NR, Lindsay M, Spence MS, Erglis A, Menown IB, et al. Percutaneous coronary angioplasty versus coronary artery bypass grafting in treatment of unprotected left main stenosis (NOBLE): a prospective, randomised, open-label, non-inferiority trial. Lancet. 2016;388(10061):2743–52.

12. Park SJ, Ahn JM, Kang SJ. Paradigm shift to functional angioplasty: new insights for fractional flow reserve- and intravascular ultrasound-guided percutaneous coronary intervention. Circulation. 2011;124(8):951–7.

13. Mangiacapra F, Di Serafino L, Barbato E. The role of fractional flow reserve to guide stent implantation. Minerva Cardioangiol. 2011;59(1):39–48.

14. Di Serafino L, Barbato E. [Invasive functional assessment of coronary artery stenosis using fractional flow reserve]. G Ital Cardiol (Rome) 2020;21(1):16–24.

15. Tonino PA, Fearon WF, De Bruyne B, Oldroyd KG, Leesar MA, Ver Lee PN, et al. Angiographic versus functional severity of coronary artery stenoses in the FAME study fractional flow reserve versus angiography in multivessel evaluation. J Am Coll Cardiol. 2010;55(25):2816–21.

16. Pijls NH, Fearon WF, Tonino PA, Siebert U, Ikeno F, Bornschein B, et al. Fractional flow reserve versus angiography for guiding percutaneous coronary intervention in patients with multivessel coronary artery disease: 2-year follow-up of the FAME (Fractional Flow Reserve Versus Angiography for Multivessel Evaluation) study. J Am Coll Cardiol. 2010;56(3):177–84.

17. Tonino PA, De Bruyne B, Pijls NH, Siebert U, Ikeno F, van't Veer M, et al. Fractional flow reserve versus angiography for guiding percutaneous coronary intervention. N Engl J Med. 2009;360(3):213–24.

18. De Bruyne B, Fearon WF, Pijls NH, Barbato E, Tonino P, Piroth Z, et al. Fractional flow reserve-guided PCI for stable coronary artery disease. N Engl J Med. 2014;371(13):1208–17.

19. Neumann FJ, Sousa-Uva M, Ahlsson A, Alfonso F, Banning AP, Benedetto U, et al. 2018 ESC/EACTS Guidelines on myocardial revascularization. Eur Heart J. 2019;40(2):87–165.

20. Sen S, Escaned J, Malik IS, Mikhail GW, Foale RA, Mila R, et al. Development and validation of a new adenosine-independent index of stenosis severity from coronary wave-intensity analysis: results of the ADVISE (ADenosine Vasodilator Independent Stenosis Evaluation) study. J Am Coll Cardiol. 2012;59(15):1392–402.

21. Davies JE, Sen S, Escaned J. Instantaneous wave-free ratio versus fractional flow reserve. N Engl J Med. 2017;377(16):1597–8.

22. Götberg M, Fröbert O. Instantaneous wave-free ratio versus fractional flow reserve. N Engl J Med. 2017;377(16):1596–7.

23. Knuuti J, Wijns W, Saraste A, Capodanno D, Barbato E, Funck-Brentano C, et al. 2019 ESC Guidelines for the diagnosis and management of chronic coronary syndromes. Eur Heart J. 2020;41(3):407–77.

24. Collet JP, Thiele H, Barbato E, Barthélémy O, Bauersachs J, Bhatt DL, et al. 2020 ESC Guidelines for the management of acute coronary syndromes in patients presenting without persistent ST-segment elevation. Eur Heart J. 2020;42(14): 1289–367.

25. Toth GG, Johnson NP, Jeremias A, Pellicano M, Vranckx P, Fearon WF, et al. Standardization of fractional flow reserve measurements. J Am Coll Cardiol. 2016;68(7):742–53.

26. Yong AS, Daniels D, De Bruyne B, Kim HS, Ikeno F, Lyons J, et al. Fractional flow reserve assessment of left main stenosis in the presence of downstream coronary stenoses. Circ Cardiovasc Interv. 2013;6(2):161–5.

27. Koh JS, Koo BK, Kim JH, Yang HM, Park KW, Kang HJ, et al. Relationship between fractional flow reserve and angiographic and intravascular ultrasound parameters in ostial lesions: major epicardial vessel versus side branch ostial lesions. JACC Cardiovasc Interv. 2012;5(4):409–15.

28. Koo BK, Kang HJ, Youn TJ, Chae IH, Choi DJ, Kim HS, et al. Physiologic assessment of jailed side branch lesions using fractional flow reserve. J Am Coll Cardiol. 2005;46(4):633–7.

29. Nam CW, Hur SH, Koo BK, Doh JH, Cho YK, Park HS, et al. Fractional flow reserve versus angiography in left circumflex ostial intervention after left main crossover stenting. Korean Circ J. 2011;41(6):304–7.

30. Farooq V, Heo JH, Raber L, Brugaletta S, Radu M, Gogas BD, et al. Tools & techniques: risk stratification and diagnostic tools in left main stem intervention. EuroIntervention. 2011;7(6):747–53.

31. Kang SJ, Mintz GS, Kim WJ, Lee JY, Oh JH, Park DW, et al. Changes in left main bifurcation geometry after a single-stent crossover technique: an intravascular ultrasound study using direct imaging of both the left anterior descending and the left circumflex coronary arteries before and after intervention. Circ Cardiovasc Interv. 2011;4(4):355–61.

32. Farooq V, Okamura T, Onuma Y, Gogas BD, Serruys PW. Unravelling the complexities of the coronary bifurcation: is this raising a few eyebrows? EuroIntervention. 2012;7(10):1133–41.

33. Vassilev D, Gil RJ. Relative dependence of diameters of branches in coronary bifurcations after stent

implantation in main vessel—importance of carina position. Kardiol Pol. 2008;66(4):371–8. discussion 9

34. Gil RJ, Vassilev D, Formuszewicz R, Rusicka-Piekarz T, Doganov A. The carina angle-new geometrical parameter associated with periprocedural side branch compromise and the long-term results in coronary bifurcation lesions with main vessel stenting only. J Interv Cardiol. 2009;22(6):E1–E10.

35. Suárez de Lezo J, Medina A, Martín P, Novoa J, Pan M, Caballero E, et al. Predictors of ostial side branch damage during provisional stenting of coronary bifurcation lesions not involving the side branch origin: an ultrasonographic study. EuroIntervention. 2012;7(10):1147–54.

36. Farooq V, Serruys PW, Heo JH, Gogas BD, Okamura T, Gomez-Lara J, et al. New insights into the coronary artery bifurcation hypothesis-generating concepts utilizing 3-dimensional optical frequency domain imaging. JACC Cardiovasc Interv. 2011;4(8):921–31.

37. Romagnoli E, Sangiorgi GM, Cosgrave J, Guillet E, Colombo A. Drug-eluting stenting: the case for post-dilation. JACC Cardiovasc Interv. 2008;1(1):22–31.

38. McDaniel MC, Douglas JS. Stent area by intravascular ultrasound and outcomes in left main intervention with drug-eluting stents: small stents, more events. Circ Cardiovasc Interv. 2011;4(6):542–4.

39. Foin N, Viceconte N, Chan PH, Lindsay AC, Krams R, Di Mario C. Jailed side branches: fate of unapposed struts studied with 3D frequency-domain optical coherence tomography. J Cardiovasc Med (Hagerstown). 2011;12(8):581–2.

40. Gutiérrez-Chico JL, Regar E, Nüesch E, Okamura T, Wykrzykowska J, di Mario C, et al. Delayed coverage in malapposed and side-branch struts with respect to well-apposed struts in drug-eluting stents: in vivo assessment with optical coherence tomography. Circulation. 2011;124(5):612–23.

41. Niemelä M, Kervinen K, Erglis A, Holm NR, Maeng M, Christiansen EH, et al. Randomized comparison of final kissing balloon dilatation versus no final kissing balloon dilatation in patients with coronary bifurcation lesions treated with main vessel stenting: the Nordic-Baltic Bifurcation Study III. Circulation. 2011;123(1):79–86.

42. Hoye A, Iakovou I, Ge L, van Mieghem CA, Ong AT, Cosgrave J, et al. Long-term outcomes after stenting of bifurcation lesions with the "crush" technique: predictors of an adverse outcome. J Am Coll Cardiol. 2006;47(10):1949–58.

43. Hildick-Smith D, Lassen JF, Albiero R, Lefevre T, Darremont O, Pan M, et al. Consensus from the 5th European Bifurcation Club meeting. EuroIntervention. 2010;6(1):34–8.

44. Stankovic G, Darremont O, Ferenc M, Hildick-Smith D, Louvard Y, Albiero R, et al. Percutaneous coronary intervention for bifurcation lesions: 2008 consensus document from the fourth meeting of the European Bifurcation Club. EuroIntervention. 2009;5(1):39–49.

45. Banning AP, Lassen JF, Burzotta F, Lefèvre T, Darremont O, Hildick-Smith D, et al. Percutaneous coronary intervention for obstructive bifurcation lesions: the 14th consensus document from the European Bifurcation Club. EuroIntervention. 2019;15(1):90–8.

46. Lee CH, Choi SW, Hwang J, Kim IC, Cho YK, Park HS, et al. 5-Year outcomes according to FFR of left circumflex coronary artery after left main crossover stenting. JACC Cardiovasc Interv. 2019;12(9):847–55.

47. Hidalgo F, Pan M, Ojeda S, Suárez de Lezo J, Lostalo A, Luque A, et al. Feasibility and efficacy of the jailed pressure wire technique for coronary bifurcation lesions. JACC Cardiovasc Interv. 2019;12(1):109–11.

48. Bilge M, Ali S, Alemdar R, Yasar AS, Erdogan M. First experience with the jailed pressure wire technique in the provisional side branch stenting of coronary bifurcation lesions. EuroIntervention. 2014;10(5):570–3.

49. Fisher LD, Judkins MP, Lesperance J, Cameron A, Swaye P, Ryan T, et al. Reproducibility of coronary arteriographic reading in the coronary artery surgery study (CASS). Catheter Cardiovasc Diagn. 1982;8(6):565–75.

Is There a Role for OCT for Left Main Assessment Before and After PCI?

Rocco Vergallo, Carlo Trani, Bernardo Cortese, and Francesco Burzotta

12.1 Introduction

The left main (LM) stem is the first segment of the left coronary artery, and it generally supplies more than 75% of the left ventricular myocardial territory in subjects with a right dominant circulation, making significant LM disease often associated with severe ischemia, arrhythmias, and other life-threatening sequelae [1, 2]. Substantial evidence from real-world registries, randomized trials, and meta-analyses suggest that percutaneous coronary intervention (PCI), when performed in experienced centers, represents a valuable option for myocardial revascularization in selected patients with unprotected LM disease [3, 4]. It thus appears clear the importance of an accurate assessment of the significance of LM stenosis as well as the detailed characterization of its atherosclerotic involvement, particularly when an angiographically moderate or indeterminate lesion is present. Coronary angiography is the initial invasive modality for LM evaluation [5]. According to the European guidelines, myocardial revascular-

ization is indicated for patients with LM angiographic diameter stenosis >50% and evidence of myocardial ischemia [6]. Yet, in clinical practice, evidence of myocardial ischemia may be equivocal, and an accurate assessment of the extent and characteristics of LM disease is often challenging due to the two-dimensional nature of angiography, particularly when an eccentric distribution of atherosclerotic disease and/or a complex anatomy with tortuous overlapping coronary segments are present. For this reason, adjunctive techniques (i.e., intravascular imaging/functional assessment) have been introduced to aid the evaluation of LM disease severity and to guide invasive treatment [7]. Several seminal intravascular ultrasound (IVUS) studies assessed LM disease severity using different parameters, and a minimal lumen area (MLA) cut-off value of 6 mm^2 has been traditionally considered as the most robust IVUS-derived threshold [8, 9]. Nevertheless, a number of studies from different groups investigated the possible relation between IVUS-derived MLA and fractional flow reserve (FFR) in LM stenosis, providing inconsistent results [8]. Data supporting the use of optical coherence tomography (OCT) as an alternative to IVUS for LM disease assessment are increasing [7, 10–13]. Thanks to its higher spatial resolution (10 times greater than IVUS), OCT allows an unprecedented characterization of the morphology of the LM wall structure and a precise definition of its lumen dimensions, particularly in the mid/distal LM seg-

R. Vergallo · C. Trani · F. Burzotta (✉)
Institute of Cardiology, Fondazione Policlinico Universitario A. Gemelli IRCCS, Università Cattolica del Sacro Cuore, Rome, Italy
e-mail: francesco.burzotta@unicatt.it

B. Cortese
Fondazione Ricerca e Innovazione Cardiovascolare, Milano, Italy

ments, while proximal/ostial LM disease assessment is often technically difficult [7, 10, 13, 14]. The present chapter will provide some practical tips and tricks on how to perform a correct assessment of LM disease by OCT, as well as a summary of available evidence on the potential use of OCT for the definition of left main disease, and for the guidance and optimization of LM PCI.

12.2 Left Main Stem Anatomy and Atherosclerotic Disease Distribution

The LM arises from the left sinus of Valsalva, although anomalous take-off from (or above) the right sinus of Valsalva represents a relatively common anatomic variant [1, 2]. The LM is a large diameter artery with a non-trivial variability across different subjects. A large IVUS study found that LM mean reference diameter is 5 mm, ranging between 3.5 and 6.5 mm [15]. Based on angiographic findings, LM anatomy (and disease) is typically divided into three segments: "ostial", "mid-shaft", and "distal" (Fig. 12.1). After an average length of 10.5 ± 5.3 mm, the LM divides into the left anterior descending artery (LAD) and the left circumflex artery (LCX), while a distal trifurcation is observed in one-fourth of cases due to the presence of an intermediate branch [16]. Of note, the size of the normal LM and of its branches can be predicted using fractal geometry and Finet's law. The prevalence of LM atherosclerotic disease in patients referred for coronary angiography is

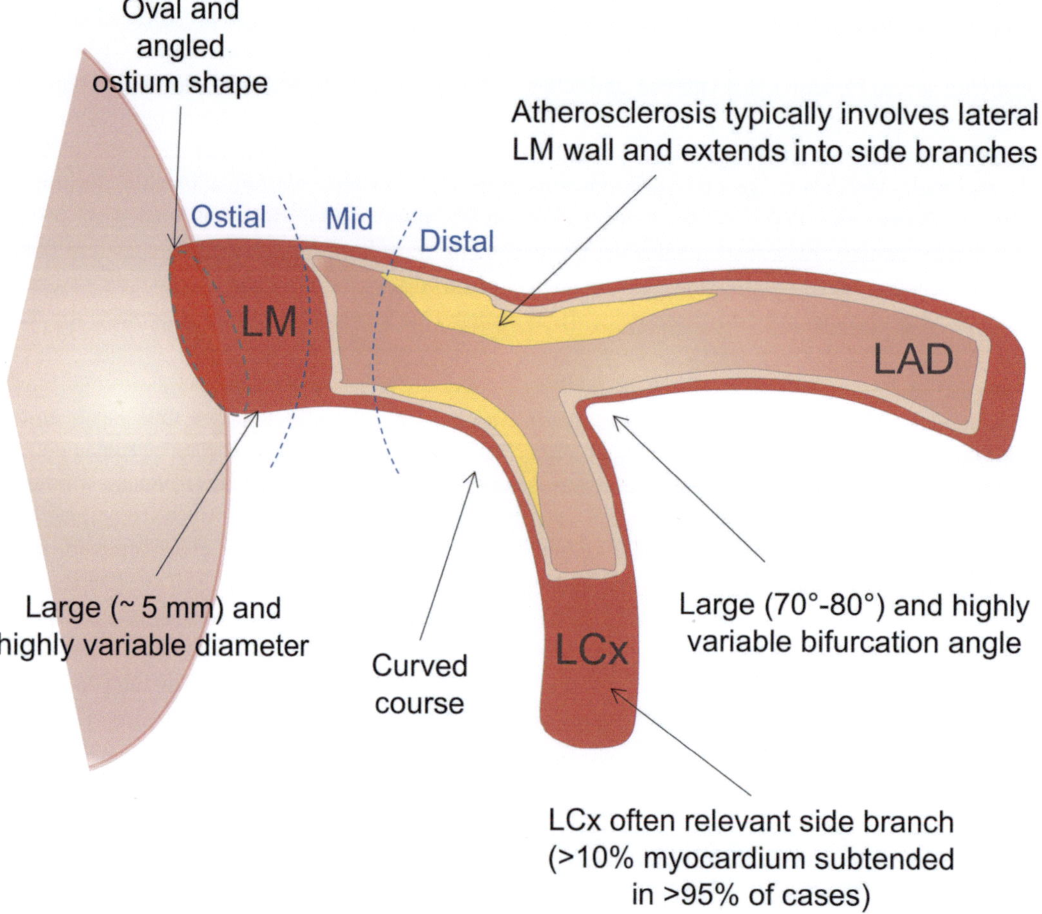

Fig. 12.1 Schematic representation of major LM anatomical features. LM, left main; LCx, left circumflex

approximately 4%, and isolated LM disease is detected in only 5% to 10% of these patients [17]. In addition to native disease, iatrogenic LM disease (i.e., dissection or ostial stenosis after catheterization or aortic valve surgery) is a rare but well-documented procedural complication [18]. LM atherosclerotic disease is usually diffuse, with frequent involvement of the bifurcation. Distal disease that involves the bifurcation with LAD and LCx is more common than ostial or mid-shaft disease. When atheroma develops within the LM course (i.e., mid-shaft or distal segments), it is often characterized by positive remodeling, which may preserve lumen dimensions. In contrast, LM ostial stenoses may be the consequence of localized negative vessel remodeling [15]. Shorter anatomic LM stems tend to develop ostial stenoses while longer anatomic LM stems usually develop distal bifurcation lesions [19]. When the LM bifurcation is diseased, atherosclerotic plaques are commonly more prevalent at the lateral walls and extend into the divisional branches. Previous intracoronary imaging studies showed that LM atherosclerotic disease extends into proximal LAD in 90% of cases, proximal LCx in 66% of cases, and both branches in 62% of cases [15, 20].

12.3   Practical Tips and Tricks for Correct Assessment of Left Main by OCT

OCT is a light-based imaging modality operating in the near-infrared spectrum to generate high-resolution images of the coronary vessel wall and lumen [21]. In contrast to IVUS, which utilized ultrasound and can be performed with the catheter disengaged from the artery, OCT requires the selection and positioning of a guiding catheter precisely at the ostium to allow an adequate flush of the lumen during pullback [22, 23]. A blood-free field in fact is required for image acquisition, which is usually achieved by injection of contrast die or saline during an automated pullback of the OCT catheter. This renders adequate assessment of ostial/proximal LM disease technically difficult by OCT [23]. In contrast, OCT enables high-resolution imaging of the LM lumen and vessel wall in the mid and distal LM segments [11]. Compared with IVUS, OCT provides higher spatial resolution (10–15 μm vs. 100 μm), in spite of a lower tissue penetration (2.0 mm vs. 10 mm) [24]. In order to allow an accurate imaging of the LM using OCT and to obtain good image quality, some practical tips and tricks regarding the acquisition technique are pivotal (Fig. 12.2a–b):

1. Aim at the best alignment of the guiding catheter (and check with a test injection before acquisition), which needs to be fully engaged, but not deeply intubated, and coaxial with the LM stem centerline (Fig. 12.2a);
2. Consider using one guidewire only (systematically feasible for baseline LM scanning and often feasible for post-PCI check); this reduces the total arc of the cross-sectional image obscured by the wire artifact, and limits the artifacts related to the straightening of the side-branch (usually LCx) curvature and to the reduction of the bifurcation angle (Fig. 12.2a).
3. Use enhanced contrast injection protocol (6 ml/s) in the case of large-sized LM (Fig. 12.2a).

Adopting these technical tips, a retrospective analysis from our group showed that OCT can be effectively used to assess non-ostial LM segments. Artifacts hindering a reliable LM lumen analysis by OCT, in fact, are substantially confined to the more proximal segments (artifact rates, 43.3%), whereas they are less frequent in the mid-shaft segment (11.4%) and infrequent in other segments of LM bifurcation (i.e., distal LM: 2.1%; ostial LAD: 1.9%; ostial LCx: 0%) [11] (Fig. 12.3). Of note, LM length as imaged by OCT was about 3 mm shorter compared with that measured by quantitative coronary angiography analysis (8.4 ± 5.1 mm vs. 11.6 ± 5.1 mm, $p = 0.001$) due to the systematic missing of the ostium [11]. Another recent study by Roule et al. confirmed very low rates of artifacts during OCT imaging of left main bifurcation (mid LM: 5.8%; distal LM 3.6%, ostial LAD 2.6%, and ostial LCX 0%) [25]. Taken together, these data support the feasibility of OCT assessment of

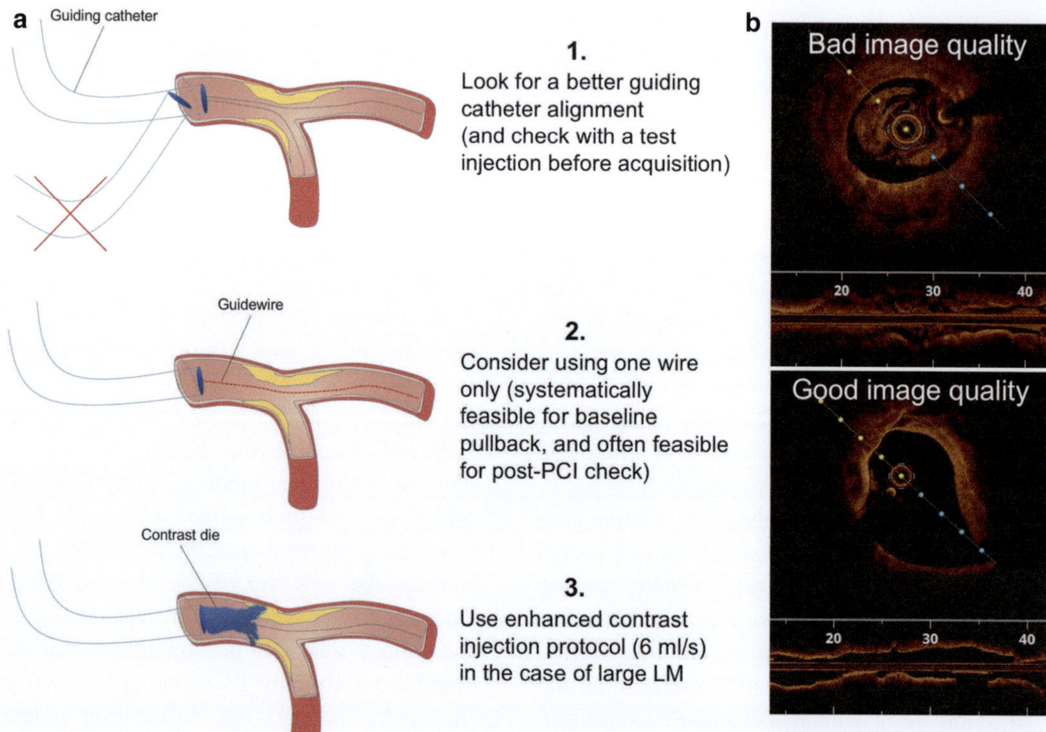

Fig. 12.2 Practical aspects to be considered when performing OCT imaging of LM bifurcation to improve image quality. Checking for a perfect guiding catheter alignment, using a single guidewire (whenever possible) to limit the area obscured by wire artifact, and using an enhanced contrast injection (i.e., 6 ml/s) usually allow to obtain good image quality during an OCT pullback of the left main (**a**). An example of bad OCT image quality of left main due to insufficient clearance of blood, improved after adopting these technical considerations (**b**). PCI, percutaneous coronary intervention; LM, left main

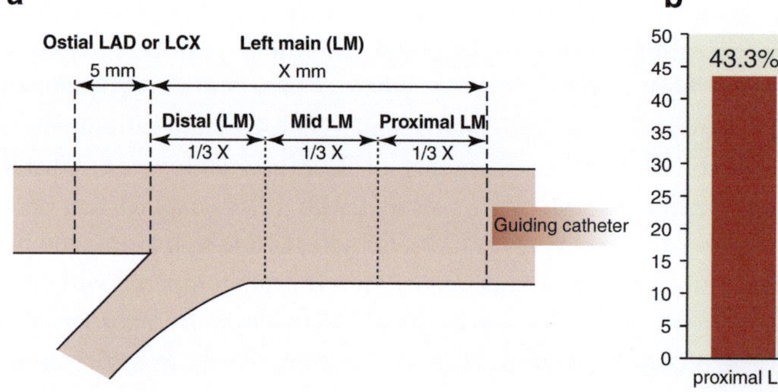

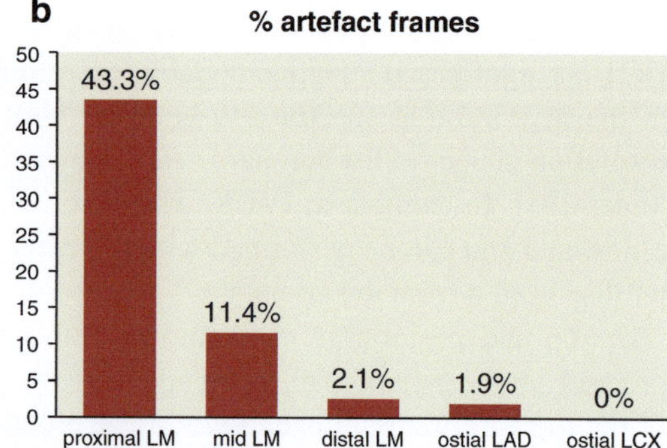

Fig. 12.3 Segments of LM bifurcation (**a**). Frequency of OCT artifacts according to different LM segments (**b**). Artifacts hindering a reliable LM lumen analysis by OCT are typically confined to the more proximal segment, whereas they are less frequent in the mid-shaft, and infrequent in other segments of LM bifurcation. LM, left main; LAD, left anterior descending; LCx, left circumflex. Adapted from Burzotta et al. [11], with permission from the Publisher

mid-distal LM (where artifacts are rare). In contrast, the assessment of the ostial/proximal LM segment by OCT is limited because of systematic missing of the LM ostium and the increased rate of artifact occurrence, so that its evaluation should be reserved to IVUS.

12.4 Use of OCT for the Definition of LM Disease and for the Assessment of Plaque Morphology

While several IVUS studies have assessed LM disease severity using different parameters, limited data on the use of OCT to define the significance of LM stenosis are available [8]. The traditional MLA cut-off value of 6 mm^2 was prospectively validated in the LITRO study confirming the feasibility of treatment deferral in patients with angiographically intermediate LM stenosis and MLA >6 mm^2 [9]. Consequently, the use of IVUS to assess the severity of LM lesions has a Class IIa recommendation in the most recent ESC guidelines on myocardial revascularization [26]. Nevertheless, a number of studies evaluating the relation between IVUS-derived MLA and FFR provided inconsistent results [8]. This might be due, at least in part, to the differences in the study population ethnicity, as significantly smaller MLA cut-off values have been described in Asian compared with non-Asian populations [8, 27, 28]. In particular, a study by Park et al. detected an IVUS-defined MLA of 4.5 mm^2 as the best cut-of value correlating with an abnormal FFR [27]. Consequently, as suggested by a recent Consensus Document on the clinical use of intracoronary imaging, it seems reasonable to defer LM treatment when MLA > 6 mm^2, to treat LM if the MLA < 4.5 mm^2, and to consider further evaluation (such as functional assessment with FFR) if the MLA is between 4.5 and 6 mm^2 [29]. Due to the different image-generation processes, IVUS thresholds cannot be applied to OCT in clinical practice [7]. Data from a head-to-head comparison between IVUS and OCT in LM showed that MLA measured by OCT is 10 to 15% smaller than that derived by IVUS [30]. In a study from our group, including 122 patients undergoing OCT evaluation of angiographically intermediate distal LM stenosis, an MLA cut-off of >4.0 mm^2 helped to identify patients in whom revascularization could be deferred [10]. In the above-mentioned study, the OCT LM criteria for percutaneous or surgical revascularization were: (1) LM area stenosis (AS) $\geq$75%; (2) LM AS >50% but <75% with MLA <4 mm^2 or the presence of plaque ulceration; (3) A critical OCT ostial stenosis on LAD and/or LCx is defined as AS $\geq$75%, or MLA $\leq$2.5 mm^2 in the presence of AS between 50% and 75%. Importantly, clinical outcome after a mean follow-up time of 18 months was not different between patients who had undergone coronary revascularization and those who had been deferred based on OCT assessment [10].

OCT allows a more detailed characterization of coronary plaque morphology compared with IVUS, even in large coronary segments like LM. OCT is able to accurately define plaque type (i.e., fibrous vs. lipid), and to assess fibrous cap thickness, thereby allowing identification of thin-cap fibroatheroma (TCFA) which is known to be the precursor of plaque rupture [31, 32]. Data from our group showed that distal LM segment has usually thinner fibrous cap as compared to other segments, and that plaque ulcerations also tend to cluster in this segment [32]. Previous studies and several case reports suggest that all main plaque morphologies, including plaque rupture, erosion, thrombus, and TCFA, are more frequently detected by OCT compared with IVUS [30, 33, 34]. This can be particularly relevant in patients with acute coronary syndrome, in whom identifying a complicated plaque or thrombus in the LM can make the difference in selecting an appropriate and timely treatment strategy [29].

When OCT is used to assess LM bifurcation disease, it would be advisable to perform, whenever possible, two pullbacks in order to assess both LAD and LCx disease as well. This approach allows to readily determine the atherosclerotic disease distribution at the bifurcation, the side branch involvement, and the length of the disease, thus favoring a thorough procedural planning [29].

12.5 Use of OCT for the Guidance and Optimization of Left Main Bifurcation PCI

OCT is an important tool for the interventional cardiologist during a LM PCI, both for planning and optimization of the procedure [10, 12, 13] (Fig. 12.4), as it allows to assess the following:

1. *Risk of side branch compromise*: the evaluation of ostial side branch disease and/or the presence of atherosclerotic disease in the proximal or distal segments of the main vessel can be useful to prevent (or at least try to avoid) side branch compromise after stent implantation in the main vessel due to plaque or carina "shift". The evidence of a "vulnerable" carina or the presence of significant main vessel disease (in particular, high calcific burden) are predictors of plaque/carina shift toward the side branch after main vessel stenting [35].

2. *Stent length*: OCT allows identifying the best proximal and distal "landing zones" for the stent, which are represented, whenever possible, by coronary segments free from atherosclerotic disease and with a circular shape. A normal reference coronary segment is identified by OCT as an area with a tree-layered structure of the vessel wall (i.e., intima, media, and adventitia) [36]. This approach enables a precise definition of the ideal stent length, thus minimizing the risk to have a "geographical miss" and to leave diseased coronary segments untreated. When the stent is implanted, OCT assessment of edge segments may show if the intended landing zones were covered and if residual stenosis or dissections are present.

3. *Stent sizing*: after defining the atherosclerotic plaque distribution and identifying the "healthy" reference segments, OCT can be used for stent sizing. Due to the large size of LM and to the mismatch usually observed

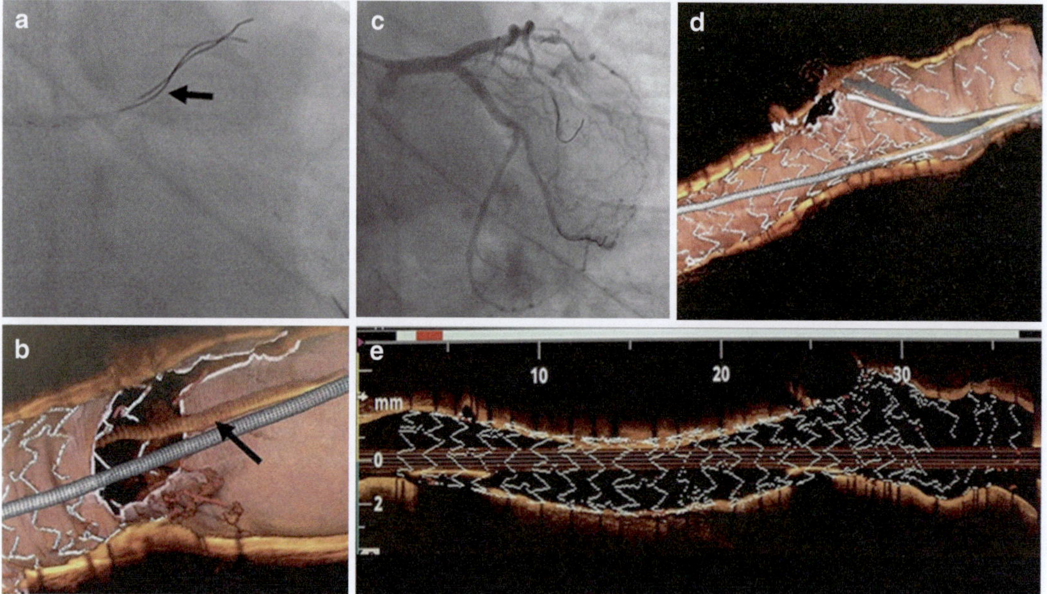

Fig. 12.4 Examples of OCT use for the guidance and optimization of a complex LM bifurcation PCI. Panels (**a**) and (**b**) show a distal rewiring (black arrow) on coronary angiography and 3D OCT reconstruction, respectively, during a LM PCI performed using the culotte technique. The final angiographic result is shown in (**c**). Post-PCI OCT imaging shows an optimal result as assessed by 3D image reconstructions, with good side branch orifice opening (**d**) and optimal stent expansion and apposition (**e**). From Burzotta et al. [14], with permission from the Publisher

compared to the LAD and LCx, the selection of the best stent diameter can be challenging using bi-dimensional angiograms only. The high resolution of OCT along with blood clearance provides sharp vessel lumen definition and allows automated measurements of lumen dimensions, which are more reproducible than with IVUS. However, unlike IVUS, the limited penetration depth of OCT light signal at the atherosclerotic lesion site may result in the loss of external elastic lamina (EEL) visibility in case of a large plaque burden [12, 36]. For these reasons, whenever possible, a "normal" landing zone should be selected, and EEL-based sizing should be attempted in order to select the appropriate stent sizing and to guarantee a good coverage of LM by stent struts, and appropriate scaffolding towards the side branch ostium.

4. *Selection of the "proximal optimization technique" (POT) balloon*: the "POT" allows tapering the proximal main vessel, achieving good stent apposition, and opening the side branch ostium to facilitate rewiring. OCT sizing of length and diameter of the proximal main vessel, as well as assessment of plaque morphology and bifurcation "geometry", are of particular importance for the selection of an appropriate balloon for the "POT", including length, diameter, and type (e.g., semi-compliant, non-compliant). This may help avoiding to jeopardize the side branch ostium, as well as the proximal stent edge when the lesion is not fully covered proximally, and the POT balloon may extend into the plaque [12, 36].

5. *Check of side branch rewiring*: experimental studies by Foin et al. [37] and clinical investigations by Alegría-Barrero et al. [38] showed that side branch rewiring critically affects scaffolding of the side branch ostium and the extent of stent malapposition at the bifurcation. Guidewire position can be evaluated and optimized by OCT. For this purpose, using the longitudinal OCT view and automated three-dimensional reconstruction may help to identify the optimal wire position in distal stent cell recrossing (i.e., near the carina), and to exclude accidental abluminal rewiring, in particular in the presence of complex anatomies and when two-stent techniques are used (Fig. 12.4) [39].

6. *Identification of the mechanisms responsible for side branch "compromise"* after main vessel stenting: OCT imaging can be useful to understand whether a side branch stenting can be avoided or not ("provisional" approach), and to guide, in some cases, the selection of the most appropriate two-stent strategy. For example, in case of evidence of "carina shift" after main vessel stenting without significant side branch disease, a kissing balloon inflation may re-establish the normal bifurcation geometry without the need of a second stent. In contrast, evidence of significant plaque shift and/or ostial side branch dissection after main vessel stenting may prompt the decision to convert a single stent to a dual stent strategy [35].

7. *PCI optimization*: suboptimal PCI results are frequent after angiographically guided stent implantation. Stent underexpansion is associated with higher risk of in-stent restenosis and target vessel failure, and currently available OCT systems provide dedicated tools that efficiently identify areas of underexpansion [36]. The occurrence and entity of stent underexpansion can be reduced by appropriately sized postdilation, but modifying fibrocalcified plaques before stent implantation (i.e., lesion preparation) can be as important [36]. An IVUS study by Kang et al. found minimal stent area (MSA) cut-off values that should be reached to prevent angiographic in-stent restenosis on a segmental basis: >8 mm^2 for LM, >6 mm^2 for ostial LAD, >5 mm^2 for ostial LCx and > 7 mm^2 for the polygon of confluence [40]. Although these IVUS cut-offs cannot be directly applied to OCT, they can serve as a reference, keeping in mind the systematic 10–15% underestimation of lumen dimension by OCT as compared to IVUS. Malapposition is another frequent finding after stenting, particularly in bifurcation PCI, and OCT is the best available intravascular imaging technique to assess it. Despite the

lack of robust evidence linking stent malapposition to adverse clinical and procedural outcomes [41], it is still advisable to aim for a good stent apposition for a number of reasons: (1) stent strut coverage is delayed on malapposed struts, and uncovered struts have been associated with a higher risk of stent thrombosis; (2) malapposed struts may directly increase the risk of ST, and overlapping segments of malapposed struts might amplify this risk; (3) major malapposition may favor accidental abluminal rewiring [38, 42].

The ROCK I study, a multicenter, retrospective observational study including 122 patients undergoing LM PCI, evaluated the acute and midterm angiographic outcome of OCT-guided PCI, as compared with standard angiographic guidance with or without IVUS [13]. OCT guidance detected four cases of stent underexpansion (7.2%) and six cases of acute malapposition (10.9%). After a median follow-up of 207 days, late lumen loss of LM tended to be lower in the OCT group (0.12 ± 0.41 vs. 0.26 ± 0.52 mm, $p = 0.10$), and was significantly reduced in the distal portion of the main vessel (0.03 ± 0.45 vs. 0.24 ± 0.53 mm, $p = 0.025$). Adverse event rates were similar in the two groups [13]. More recently, a prospective, multicenter trial, the LEMON study, investigated whether patients might benefit from OCT-guided PCI for mid/distal LM according to a pre-specified protocol [12]. Successful stent expansion was defined as MSA/reference MLA >80% in both proximal and distal stent sections. Primary endpoint was the procedural success, defined as TIMI 3 flow in all vessels + residual stenosis <50% by QCA + adequate stent expansion according to LEMON criteria. The primary endpoint was achieved in 86% of patients. Adequate stent expansion was observed in 86% of cases, while significant edge dissection was detected in 30% and residual significant struts malapposition in 24% of cases. The operator's strategy was modified by OCT guidance in 24% of cases. MACE-free survival was 98.6% at 1-year follow-up [12]. Although these results are very encouraging, the impact of an OCT-guided strategy on clinical outcome after LM PCI, as compared with angiography-guided or IVUS-guided LM PCI, needs to be further investigated in future larger randomized trials [43, 44]. The European trial on Optical Coherence Tomography Optimized Bifurcation Event Reduction (OCTOBER), a prospective, randomized, controlled, superiority, multicenter trial, assessing the 2-year clinical outcomes after OCT-guided vs. standard guided (i.e., angiography ± IVUS) revascularization of patients requiring complex bifurcation treatment, will include a substantial group of patients with significant LM bifurcation disease and will hopefully provide a response to this question [43].

12.6 Conclusions

Accurate assessment of LM stem is critical in defining treatment strategies and selecting revascularization options in order to improve patient prognosis. We have witnessed a continuous evolution in invasive intracoronary techniques enabling a detailed assessment of both function and anatomy of LM disease. While IVUS is still considered the invasive imaging modality of choice for the evaluation of ostial LM stenosis, OCT imaging, thanks to its unprecedented spatial resolution, is emerging as a valid alternative to IVUS, in particular for the assessment of midshaft and distal LM stenosis. OCT imaging has the potential to improve the assessment of LM disease severity, aid the choice of the revascularization strategy, guide LM PCI, and optimize its result. Although a growing body of data is already available on the use of OCT imaging for LM disease assessment and treatment, ongoing large prospective randomized trials will provide us with a more definitive evidence in this regard. These advances may substantially influence patient outcomes in what is a rapidly evolving field of coronary intervention.

References

1. El-Menyar AA, Al Suwaidi J, Holmes DR Jr. Left main coronary artery stenosis: state-of-the-art. Curr Probl Cardiol. 2007;32:103–93.
2. Cheezum MK, Liberthson RR, Shah NR, Villines TC, O'Gara PT, Landzberg MJ, Blankstein R. Anomalous

aortic origin of a coronary artery from the inappropriate sinus of Valsalva. J Am Coll Cardiol. 2017;69:1592–608.

3. Naganuma T, Chieffo A, Meliga E, Capodanno D, Park SJ, Onuma Y, Valgimigli M, Jegere S, Makkar RR, Palacios IF, Costopoulos C, Kim YH, Buszman PP, Chakravarty T, Sheiban I, Mehran R, Naber C, Margey R, Agnihotri A, Marra S, Capranzano P, Leon MB, Moses JW, Fajadet J, Lefevre T, Morice MC, Erglis A, Tamburino C, Alfieri O, Serruys PW, Colombo A. Long-term clinical outcomes after percutaneous coronary intervention versus coronary artery bypass grafting for ostial/midshaft lesions in unprotected left main coronary artery from the DELTA registry: a multicenter registry evaluating percutaneous coronary intervention versus coronary artery bypass grafting for left main treatment. JACC Cardiovasc Interv. 2014;7:354–61.

4. Chieffo A, Tanaka A, Giustino G, Briede I, Sawaya FJ, Daemen J, Kawamoto H, Meliga E, D'Ascenzo F, Cerrato E, Stefanini GG, Capodanno D, Mangiameli A, Templin C, Erglis A, Morice MC, Mehran R, Van Mieghem NM, Nakamura S, De Benedictis M, Pavani M, Varbella F, Pisaniello M, Sharma SK, Tamburino C, Tchetche D, Colombo A, Investigators D. The DELTA 2 registry: a multicenter registry evaluating percutaneous coronary intervention with new-generation drug-eluting stents in patients with obstructive left main coronary artery disease. JACC Cardiovasc Interv. 2017;10:2401–10.

5. Isner JM, Kishel J, Kent KM, Ronan JA Jr, Ross AM, Roberts WC. Accuracy of angiographic determination of left main coronary arterial narrowing. Angiographic--histologic correlative analysis in 28 patients. Circulation. 1981;63:1056–64.

6. Neumann FJ, Sousa-Uva M, Ahlsson A, Alfonso F, Banning AP, Benedetto U, Byrne RA, Collet JP, Falk V, Head SJ, Juni P, Kastrati A, Koller A, Kristensen SD, Niebauer J, Richter DJ, Seferovic PM, Sibbing D, Stefanini GG, Windecker S, Yadav R, Zembala MO. 2018 ESC/EACTS guidelines on myocardial revascularization. Kardiol Pol. 2018;76:1585–664.

7. Bing R, Yong AS, Lowe HC. Percutaneous transcatheter assessment of the left main coronary artery: current status and future directions. JACC Cardiovasc Interv. 2015;8:1529–39.

8. Mintz GS, Lefevre T, Lassen JF, Testa L, Pan M, Singh J, Stankovic G, Banning AP. Intravascular ultrasound in the evaluation and treatment of left main coronary artery disease: a consensus statement from the European Bifurcation Club. EuroIntervention. 2018;14:e467–74.

9. de la Torre Hernandez JM, Hernandez Hernandez F, Alfonso F, Rumoroso JR, Lopez-Palop R, Sadaba M, Carrillo P, Rondan J, Lozano I, Ruiz Nodar JM, Baz JA, Fernandez Nofrerias E, Pajin F, Garcia Camarero T, Gutierrez H, Group LS. Prospective application of pre-defined intravascular ultrasound criteria for assessment of intermediate left main coronary artery lesions results from the multicenter LITRO study. J Am Coll Cardiol. 2011;58:351–8.

10. Dato I, Burzotta F, Trani C, Romano A, Paraggio L, Aurigemma C, Porto I, Leone AM, Niccoli G, Crea F. Optical coherence tomography guidance for the management of angiographically intermediate left main bifurcation lesions: early clinical experience. Int J Cardiol. 2017;248:108–13.

11. Burzotta F, Dato I, Trani C, Pirozzolo G, De Maria GL, Porto I, Niccoli G, Leone AM, Schiavoni G, Crea F. Frequency domain optical coherence tomography to assess non-ostial left main coronary artery. EuroIntervention. 2015;10:e1–8.

12. Amabile N, Range G, Souteyrand G, Godin M, Boussaada MM, Meneveau N, Cayla G, Casassus F, Lefevre T, Hakim R, Bagdadi I, Motreff P, Caussin C. Optical coherence tomography to guide percutaneous coronary intervention of the left main coronary artery: the LEMON study. EuroIntervention. 2020.

13. Cortese B, Burzotta F, Alfonso F, Pellegrini D, Trani C, Aurigemma C, Rivero F, Antuna P, Orrego PS, Prati F. Role of optical coherence tomography for distal left main stem angioplasty. Catheter Cardiovasc Interv. 2020;96:755–61.

14. Burzotta F, Lassen JF, Banning AP, Lefevre T, Hildick-Smith D, Chieffo A, Darremont O, Pan M, Chatzizisis YS, Albiero R, Louvard Y, Stankovic G. Percutaneous coronary intervention in left main coronary artery disease: the 13th consensus document from the European bifurcation Club. EuroIntervention. 2018; 14:112–20.

15. Oviedo C, Maehara A, Mintz GS, Araki H, Choi SY, Tsujita K, Kubo T, Doi H, Templin B, Lansky AJ, Dangas G, Leon MB, Mehran R, Tahk SJ, Stone GW, Ochiai M, Moses JW. Intravascular ultrasound classification of plaque distribution in left main coronary artery bifurcations: where is the plaque really located? Circ Cardiovasc Interv. 2010;3:105–12.

16. Medrano-Gracia P, Ormiston J, Webster M, Beier S, Young A, Ellis C, Wang C, Smedby O, Cowan B. A computational atlas of normal coronary artery anatomy. EuroIntervention. 2016;12.845–54.

17. Giannoglou GD, Antoniadis AP, Chatzizisis YS, Damvopoulou E, Parcharidis GE, Louridas GE. Prevalence of narrowing >or=50% of the left main coronary artery among 17,300 patients having coronary angiography. Am J Cardiol. 2006;98:1202–5.

18. Eshtehardi P, Adorjan P, Togni M, Tevaearai H, Vogel R, Seiler C, Meier B, Windecker S, Carrel T, Wenaweser P, Cook S. Iatrogenic left main coronary artery dissection: incidence, classification, management, and long-term follow-up. Am Heart J. 2010;159:1147–53.

19. Maehara A, Mintz GS, Castagna MT, Pichard AD, Satler LF, Waksman R, Laird JR Jr, Suddath WO, Kent KM, Weissman NJ. Intravascular ultrasound assessment of the stenoses location and morphology in the left main coronary artery in relation to anatomic left main length. Am J Cardiol. 2001;88:1–4.

20. Arbab-Zadeh A, DeMaria AN, Penny WF, Russo RJ, Kimura BJ, Bhargava V. Axial movement of the intravascular ultrasound probe during the cardiac cycle: implications for three-dimensional reconstruction and

measurements of coronary dimensions. Am Heart J. 1999;138:865–72.

21. Jang IK, Tearney GJ, MacNeill B, Takano M, Moselewski F, Iftima N, Shishkov M, Houser S, Aretz HT, Halpern EF, Bouma BE. In vivo characterization of coronary atherosclerotic plaque by use of optical coherence tomography. Circulation. 2005;111:1551–5.

22. Johnson PM, Patel J, Yeung M, Kaul P. Intra-coronary imaging modalities. Curr Treat Options Cardiovasc Med. 2014;16:304.

23. Johnson TW, Raber L, Di Mario C, Bourantas CV, Jia H, Mattesini A, Gonzalo N, de la Torre Hernandez JM, Prati F, Koskinas KC, Joner M, Radu MD, Erlinge D, Regar E, Kunadian V, Maehara A, Byrne RA, Capodanno D, Akasaka T, Wijns W, Mintz GS, Guagliumi G. Clinical use of intracoronary imaging. Part2: acute coronary syndromes, ambiguous coronary angiography findings, and guiding interventional decision-making: an expert consensus document of the European Association of Percutaneous Cardiovascular Interventions. EuroIntervention. 2019;15:434–51.

24. Jang IK. Optical coherence tomography or intravascular ultrasound? JACC Cardiovasc Interv. 2011;4:492–4.

25. Roule V, Rebouh I, Lemaitre A, Bignon M, Ardouin P, Sabatier R, Labombarda F, Blanchart K, Beygui F. Evaluation of left main coronary artery using optical frequency domain imaging and its pitfalls. J Interv Cardiol. 2020;2020:4817239.

26. Neumann FJ, Sousa-Uva M, Ahlsson A, Alfonso F, Banning AP, Benedetto U, Byrne RA, Collet JP, Falk V, Head SJ, Juni P, Kastrati A, Koller A, Kristensen SD, Niebauer J, Richter DJ, Seferovic PM, Sibbing D, Stefanini GG, Windecker S, Yadav R, Zembala MO, Group ESCSD. 2018 ESC/EACTS Guidelines on myocardial revascularization. Eur Heart J. 2019;40:87–165.

27. Park SJ, Ahn JM, Kang SJ, Yoon SH, Koo BK, Lee JY, Kim WJ, Park DW, Lee SW, Kim YH, Lee CW, Park SW. Intravascular ultrasound-derived minimal lumen area criteria for functionally significant left main coronary artery stenosis. JACC Cardiovasc Interv. 2014;7:868–74.

28. Kang SJ, Lee JY, Ahn JM, Song HG, Kim WJ, Park DW, Yun SC, Lee SW, Kim YH, Mintz GS, Lee CW, Park SW, Park SJ. Intravascular ultrasound-derived predictors for fractional flow reserve in intermediate left main disease. JACC Cardiovasc Interv. 2011;4:1168–74.

29. Johnson TW, Raber L, di Mario C, Bourantas C, Jia H, Mattesini A, Gonzalo N, de la Torre Hernandez JM, Prati F, Koskinas K, Joner M, Radu MD, Erlinge D, Regar E, Kunadian V, Maehara A, Byrne RA, Capodanno D, Akasaka T, Wijns W, Mintz GS, Guagliumi G. Clinical use of intracoronary imaging. Part 2: acute coronary syndromes, ambiguous coronary angiography findings, and guiding interventional decision-making: an expert consensus document of the

30. Fujino Y, Bezerra HG, Attizzani GF, Wang W, Yamamoto H, Chamie D, Kanaya T, Mehanna E, Tahara S, Nakamura S, Costa MA. Frequency-domain optical coherence tomography assessment of unprotected left main coronary artery disease-a comparison with intravascular ultrasound. Catheter Cardiovasc Interv. 2013;82:E173–83.

31. Vergallo R, Uemura S, Soeda T, Minami Y, Cho JM, Ong DS, Aguirre AD, Gao L, Biasucci LM, Crea F, Yu B, Lee H, Kim CJ, Jang IK. Prevalence and predictors of multiple coronary plaque ruptures: in vivo 3-vessel optical coherence tomography imaging study. Arterioscler Thromb Vasc Biol. 2016;36: 2229–38.

32. Dato I, Burzotta F, Trani C, Romano A, Porto I, Aurigemma C, Niccoli G, Leone AM, Crea F. Angiographically intermediate left main bifurcation disease assessment by frequency domain optical coherence tomography (FD-OCT). Int J Cardiol. 2016;220:726–8.

33. Bezerra HG, Attizzani GF, Sirbu V, Musumeci G, Lortkipanidze N, Fujino Y, Wang W, Nakamura S, Erglis A, Guagliumi G, Costa MA. Optical coherence tomography versus intravascular ultrasound to evaluate coronary artery disease and percutaneous coronary intervention. JACC Cardiovasc Interv. 2013;6:228–36.

34. Chandrasekar B, Alanbaei M. Intracoronary imaging identifies plaque rupture underlying left main thrombosis in acute myocardial infarction without angiographically evident atherosclerosis. Eur Heart J. 2020;41:4448.

35. Watanabe M, Uemura S, Sugawara Y, Ueda T, Soeda T, Takeda Y, Kawata H, Kawakami R, Saito Y. Side branch complication after a single-stent crossover technique: prediction with frequency domain optical coherence tomography. Coron Artery Dis. 2014;25:321–9.

36. Raber L, Mintz GS, Koskinas KC, Johnson TW, Holm NR, Onuma Y, Radu MD, Joner M, Yu B, Jia H, Meneveau N, de la Torre Hernandez JM, Escaned J, Hill J, Prati F, Colombo A, di Mario C, Regar E, Capodanno D, Wijns W, Byrne RA, Guagliumi G, Group ESCSD. Clinical use of intracoronary imaging. Part 1: guidance and optimization of coronary interventions. An expert consensus document of the European Association of Percutaneous Cardiovascular Interventions. Eur Heart J. 2018;39:3281–300.

37. Foin N, Torii R, Alegria E, Sen S, Petraco R, Nijjer S, Ghione M, Davies JE, Di Mario C. Location of side branch access critically affects results in bifurcation stenting: insights from bench modeling and computational flow simulation. Int J Cardiol. 2013;168:3623–8.

38. Alegria-Barrero E, Foin N, Chan PH, Syrseloudis D, Lindsay AC, Dimopolous K, Alonso-Gonzalez R, Viceconte N, De Silva R, Di Mario C. Optical coherence tomography for guidance of distal cell recrossing

in bifurcation stenting: choosing the right cell matters. EuroIntervention. 2012;8:205–13.

39. Okamura T, Onuma Y, Yamada J, Iqbal J, Tateishi H, Nao T, Oda T, Maeda T, Nakamura T, Miura T, Yano M, Serruys PW. 3D optical coherence tomography: new insights into the process of optimal rewiring of side branches during bifurcational stenting. EuroIntervention. 2014;10:907–15.

40. Kang SJ, Ahn JM, Song H, Kim WJ, Lee JY, Park DW, Yun SC, Lee SW, Kim YH, Lee CW, Mintz GS, Park SW, Park SJ. Comprehensive intravascular ultrasound assessment of stent area and its impact on restenosis and adverse cardiac events in 403 patients with unprotected left main disease. Circ Cardiovasc Interv. 2011;4:562–9.

41. Prati F, Romagnoli E, La Manna A, Burzotta F, Gatto L, Marco V, Fineschi M, Fabbiocchi F, Versaci F, Trani C, Tamburino C, Alfonso F, Mintz GS. Long-term consequences of optical coherence tomography findings during percutaneous coronary intervention: the Centro Per La Lotta Contro L'infarto - Optimization Of Percutaneous Coronary Intervention (CLI-OPCI) LATE study. EuroIntervention. 2018;14:e443–51.

42. Souteyrand G, Amabile N, Mangin L, Chabin X, Meneveau N, Cayla G, Vanzetto G, Barnay P, Trouillet C, Rioufol G, Range G, Teiger E, Delaunay R, Dubreuil O, Lhermusier T, Mulliez A, Levesque S, Belle L, Caussin C, Motreff P, Investigators P. Mechanisms of stent thrombosis analysed by optical coherence tomography: insights from the national PESTO French registry. Eur Heart J. 2016;37:1208–16.

43. Holm NR, Andreasen LN, Walsh S, Kajander OA, Witt N, Eek C, Knaapen P, Koltowski L, Gutierrez-Chico JL, Burzotta F, Kockman J, Ormiston J, Santos-Pardo I, Laanmets P, Mylotte D, Madsen M, Hjort J, Kumsars I, Ramunddal T, Christiansen EH. Rational and design of the European randomized optical coherence tomography optimized bifurcation event reduction trial (OCTOBER). Am Heart J. 2018;205:97–109.

44. Miyazaki Y, Muramatsu T, Asano T, Katagiri Y, Sotomi Y, Nakatani S, Takahashi K, Kogame N, Higuchi Y, Ishikawa M, Kyono H, Yano M, Ozaki Y, Serruys PW, Okamura T, Onuma Y. Online three-dimensional OFDI-guided versus angiography-guided PCI in bifurcation lesions: design and rationale of the randomised OPTIMUM trial. EuroIntervention. 2021;16:1333–41.

A Clinical Appraisal of Optical Coherence Tomography for Left Main Stem Intervention

13

Erick Sanchez-Jimenez and Bernardo Cortese

13.1 Introduction

Recent advances in patients with left main steam (LM) coronary lesions, specifically with low and intermediate *Synergy between PCI with Taxus and Cardiac Surgery* (SYNTAX) Score or those otherwise not eligible for coronary artery bypass grafting (CABG), have made percutaneous coronary intervention (PCI) a viable option for treatment. The 2018 European Society of Cardiology (ESC) myocardial revascularization guidelines set PCI as class I, level of evidence A for low SYNTAX score (0–22) and class IIa, level of evidence A for intermediate SYNTAX score [1–3].

Although LM PCI remains a technically challenging and complex procedure, the improved results in recent clinical studies with short- and long-term outcomes have refined the safety, technique, and use of imaging to guide the procedure. The imaging guidance to optimize stent implantation, patient selection, use of newer stents, and safely achieving optimal procedural results is paramount to improve outcomes [4, 5].

Indeed, the clinical outcome of the studies is not only related to the intra-procedural and immediate post-procedural factors (as discussed in the previous chapter) such as lesion preparation, stent sizing, stent selection, stent implantation, edge disease, edge dissection, tissue protrusion, stent malapposition, stent underexpansion, and minimum stent area characteristics, but also depend on pre-procedural factors such as patient selection in the case of intermediate lesions, the presence of bifurcation lesion with the choice of one- vs. two-stent strategy and the technique used for PCI [6, 7]. Moreover, center experience and minimum operator volume of 25 patients per year play a critical role in order to have a sustained clinical benefit for the patient [3].

In addition, suboptimal PCI results in the LM setting tends to affect the clinical outcomes and survival rate of patients more than PCI in any other coronary territory.

13.2 Role of Intravascular Imaging to Improve Clinical Outcomes in Left Main Intervention

Intravascular imaging (technical details provided in the previous chapter) is now strongly associated with improved PCI outcomes in non-LM lesion with both randomized trials and meta-analyses accounting for the utility of either intravascular ultrasound (IVUS) or optical coherence tomography (OCT) [8–10].

E. Sanchez-Jimenez · B. Cortese (✉)
Fondazione Ricerca e Innovazione Cardiovascolare, Milano, Italy

In the case of LM lesions, the 2018 ESC revascularization guidelines advocated, as class IIa recommendation, the use of imaging to guide PCI in this setting. Nevertheless, the specific indication for intravascular imaging to improve PCI in the setting of unprotected LM lesions was advocated only for IVUS and not yet for OCT [3].

Despite the high-quality evidence of imaging with IVUS to guide PCI specifically in the LM to decrease the risk of cardiovascular death and major adverse cardiovascular events (MACE), its widespread use is still not standardized [11, 12]. This under-utilization can be attributed to the time-consuming procedure. For OCT more factors can be added for a suboptimal penetration, including the use of iodinated contrast (especially in the more vulnerable patients) which is associated with an increased risk of acute kidney injury. Interestingly, in a study coordinated by our group, we showed that OCT use for LM PCI was not associated with an increase in contrast use or procedural time after a run-in period aimed at achieving a sufficient expertise [13]. Finally, depending on the healthcare system, there may be a financial disincentive to perform imaging when considering the intravascular imaging incremental expense. Yet, in some countries such as Japan, this incremental expense is fully reimbursed and consequently, the penetration of intravascular imaging is much higher than in other geographical areas [14].

Kinnaird et al. performed a study using the British Cardiovascular Intervention Society database aiming to explore the temporal change in the use of intravascular imaging for unprotected LM PCI between 2007 and 2014. Out of the included 11,264 patients, after propensity matching a pool of 5056 pairs of subjects was created, with or without imaging use. At first glance it is evident the increase in intravascular imaging use over time, from 30.2% in 2007 to 50.2% in 2014; also the OCT use did increase over the last 3 years of the study (Fig. 13.1). The frequent use of imaging was associated with some clinical presentations as stable angina, bifurcation LM disease, and previous PCI, yet some other clinical factors favoring the use of imaging were trainee first operator and left ventricular ejection fraction (EF) less than 30%. The study concluded that the implementation of intravascular imaging was associated with a lower rate of coronary complications, in-hospital death, major cardiovascular adverse events, and in-hospital major bleedings. A reduction of 46% and 34% in 30-day and 12-month mortality, respectively, was also demonstrated (Table 13.1) [15].

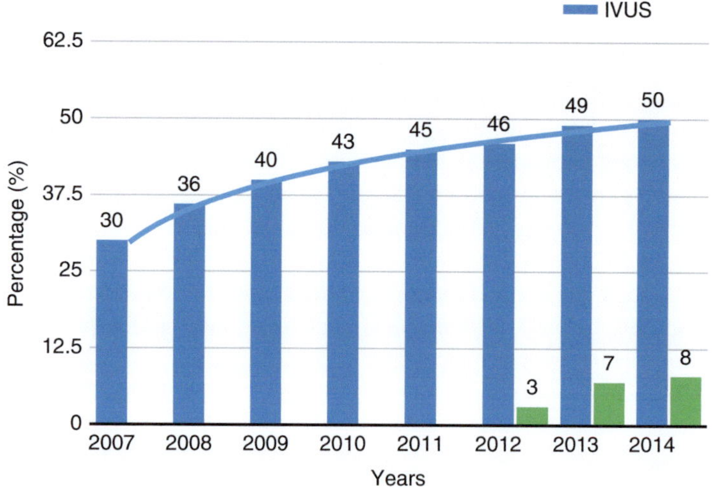

Fig. 13.1 Temporal changes in the use of imaging for left main stem percutaneous coronary intervention in the British Cardiovascular Society database

Table 13.1 Procedural and clinical outcomes by imaging status for unprotected left main stem percutaneous coronary intervention in the British Cardiovascular Society database

	No imaging $n = 6.208$ (%)	Imaging $n = 5.056$ (%)	p value
Procedural outcomes			
Left main PCI success	5.530 (97.2)	4.530 (98.0)	0.017
Coronary complications	493 (8.7)	330 (7.0)	0.003
Clinical outcomes			
Emergency CABG	20 (0.3)	4 (0.08)	0.009
In-hospital major bleed	85 (1.4)	44 (0.9)	0.014
In-hospital death	280 (4.6)	72 (1.5)	<0.001
In-hospital MACE	340 (6.6)	112 (2.3)	<0.001
Mortality at 30 days	366 (6.6)	122 (2.9)	<0.001
Mortality at 12 months	790 (15.5)	335 (0.9)	<0.001

PCI, percutaneous coronary intervention; CABG, coronary artery bypass grafting; MACE, major adverse cardiovascular events

13.3 Assessment of Intermediate Lesions in the Left Main Stem

The most important reason to treat an intermediate lesion is the final clinical outcome: with any treatment option you want to be sure to have an outcome which is better than the one expected if the lesion is left untreated. This assumption is particularly important if the coronary lesion is attributable to the LM, because in most cases a recurrence in this segment is associated with bad outcome, including impaired survival rate. The Spanish multicenter prospective trial LITRO proved that it was safe to delay the revascularization of intermediate LM lesions with minimal luminal area (MLA) > 6 mm^2 obtained by imaging, with favorable clinical results after 2 years [16].

LM atherosclerosis is often underestimated by coronary angiography. Several studies demonstrated that a very high percentage of patients with angiographically normal LM have atherosclerotic disease by imaging evaluation. Conversely, 50% of angiographically ambiguous lesions had a significant stenosis. Those coronary lesions with a 30–70% plaque burden, specifically in the context of multi-vessel disease, can be underestimated [17].

There are some reasons for such discrepancy between angiography and imaging associated with mistakes when evaluating a LM lesion. Diffuse atherosclerotic disease in any coronary artery may lead to a false normal reference segment, but short LM makes it difficult to identify a normal reference segment, and the presence of arterial remodeling can aggravate this issue. Therefore, the only way to obviate at this is to have a careful evaluation of the three vessel layers, which is possible only by means of intravascular imaging. Correlation between angiography and necropsy or imaging appears to be better in non-LM lesions possibly because of similar geometric issues in the LM. Finally, significant inter- and intra-observer variability in the angiographic assessment of LM disease seems higher in this segment (Fig. 13.2) [18, 19].

These topics are very important from the clinical point of view since LM disease can change the whole treatment approach for patients with low SYNTAX scores. A patient with one or two vessel disease would be managed by PCI but the implication of the LM can change the management radically to coronary artery bypass grafting (CABG).

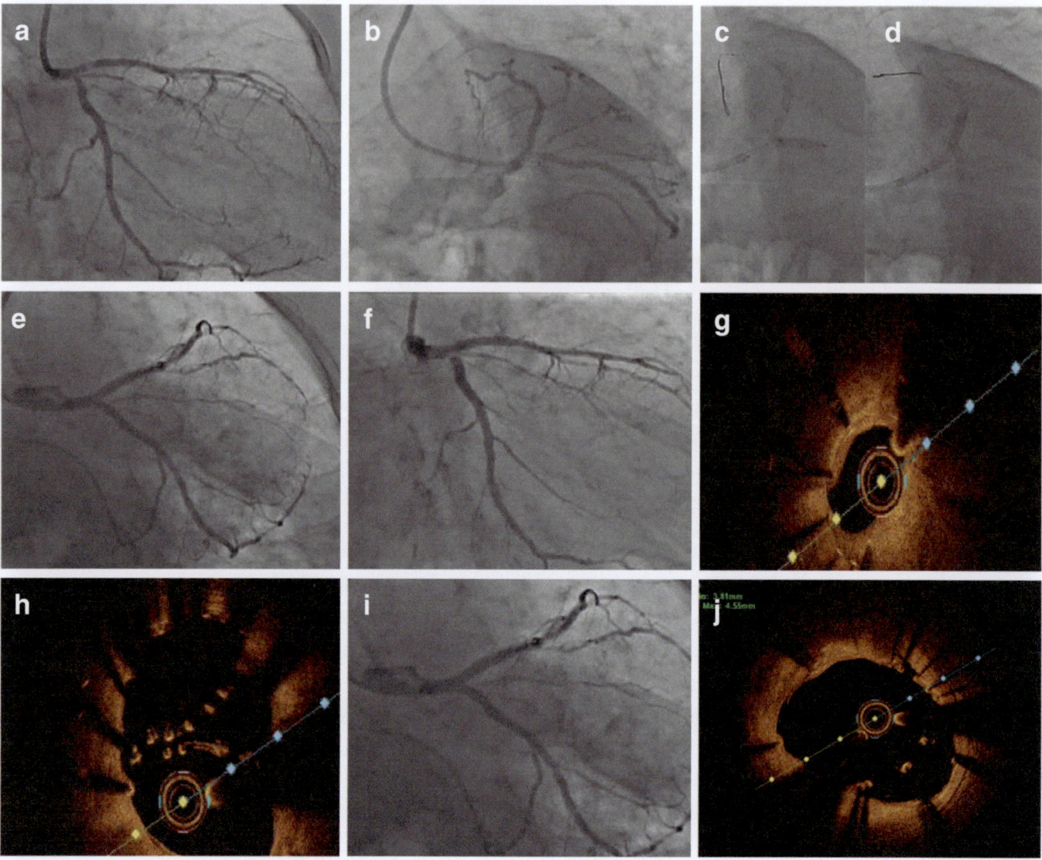

Fig. 13.2 Case of a 65-year-old lady with hypertension and diabetes who presents with unstable angina. Diagnostic angiogram right caudal (**a**) and spider (**b**) views were showing left main stem (LM) bifurcation lesion, Medina 1.1.1 (positive FFR in the left anterior descending-LAD). The case was managed with T-stenting technique. After lesion preparation, percutaneous transluminal coronary angioplasty (PTCA) in the ostium of the circumflex coronary artery (CX) with drug-eluting stent (DES) Xience 3.0 × 12 mm (**c**) was done, followed by DES Stentys 3–3.5 × 22 mm implantation to the LM-LAD (**d**), then kissing balloon inflation (KBI) and finalized with proximal optimization technique. Final optimal angiographic result is shown (**e**). During the index procedure the patient did not undergo intravascular imaging assessment. Patient returned with stable angina 6 months later, an angiography performed showed probable in-stent restenosis (ISR) of the LAD and CX (**f**). OCT demonstrated ISR and stent underexpansion of the ostial LAD (**g**) and double stent line in the LMS lumen (**h**). Stent underexpansion could have been avoided using OCT at the end of the first procedure to evaluate for optimal minimal luminal area (MLA). The double stent into the LMS probably was caused by displacement of the CX stent during the delivery of the self-expanding Stentys due to the splittable sheath. To overcome this complication we decided to do pre-dilatation with KBI using two non-compliant (NC) balloons, 3 × 20 mm on LMS-LDA and 3 × 15 mm on LMS-CX, then PTCA on LM with NC balloon 4.5 × 12 mm in order to crush protruded struts of CX stent and finally KBI with drug-coated balloon 3.5 × 20 mm on LM-LAD and 3 × 20 on CX. Final angiographic result (**i**) and OCT run (**j**) show an improved result.

13.4 Clinical Data Supporting the Use of OCT Over IVUS

As previously discussed, advantages of OCT over IVUS in terms of detailed imaging resolution of vessel layers, stent struts apposition, stent expansion, final minimal luminal area, discovery of tissue protrusion, new thrombus, and edge dissections after stenting have been already established in other coronary territories different than LM [20, 21].

One study about the pathophysiology of culprit lesion in acute myocardial infarction indicated that OCT was superior to IVUS and coronary angiography, in: (a) detecting plaque rupture, OCT (73%) compared to IVUS (40%) and angiography alone (47%), $p = 0.021$; (b) detecting plaque erosion (23%, 0%, and 3%, respectively; $p = 0.003$), and (c) assessing the presence of thrombus (100%, 33%, and 100%; $p < 0.001$). The incidence of thin cap fibroatheroma was 83%, which was only detectable by OCT [22].

There is an assumption that OCT can lose some imaging quality while performing the procedure at the LM but some studies are demonstrating the opposite. Cortese et al. conducted a retrospective study (ROCK I) with 112 patients undergoing LM PCI. One group of 55 patients with OCT guidance and one group of 57 patients with standard guidance (10 with IVUS) were compared in terms of late lumen loss (LLL) ether in the LM or the distal segment (LAD/CX) as a primary endpoint and MACE as a secondary endpoint, after 6 months. LLL was defined as the difference in minimal lumen diameter (MLD) between the immediate post-PCI result and the angiographic follow-up; MLD distribution in the two groups can be analyzed in Fig. 13.3. The OCT assistance helped to obtain optimal stent deployment and improved angiographic outcomes in terms of late lumen loss and percent diameter stenosis after 6 months. The beneficial impact of OCT guidance was more relevant in the distal segment of the LM (Table 13.2) [13].

In addition, a prospective trial (LEMON) was completed recently proving the performance of OCT when treating mid- and distal part of the LM using three OCT runs from the main branch to the main vessel, first for pre-PCI analysis, second after proximal optimization technique (POT) and side branch rewiring, and third post-PCI after procedure optimization. Although the primary endpoint was procedural success which was obtained in 86% of patients, there were no complications during procedure nor MACE at 30 days, and 1-year survival from MACE was 98.6% (Table 13.3) [23].

Is OCT not inferior to IVUS in the management of LM lesions treated with PCI? As mentioned previously, while the accurate diagnosis and the stent results are important, the clinical outcome is the most important goal when comparing tools to improve PCI as indicated by another study named ROCK II, a retrospective multicenter study which involved 15 LM PCI-expert centers. ROCK II enrolled 730 patients undergoing distal LM PCI divided into three groups according to the use of intravascular imaging or not to assist the intervention: OCT, IVUS, or angiography alone (Fig. 13.4). In the study, the median follow-up was 33 months using latest generation DES and the population was considerably large including diabetic patients with a clinical presentation ranging from stable patients to ST-elevation myocardial infarction. One important value for this study, which confirmed the previous ROCK I findings, was the equal amount of contrast volume used between groups and a new finding including procedural time without significant differences between the groups. After propensity matching, we obtained three groups of 100 patients each which did not show significant baseline and procedural differences between the populations. Despite the use of similar amount of contrast media, the risk of acute kidney injury was lower in the intravascular imaging groups. Moreover, the two-stent strategy had the lowest percentage (15%) in the OCT group, showing a possible way to reduce the total amount of metal implanted in such complex lesions (Table 13.4) [24].

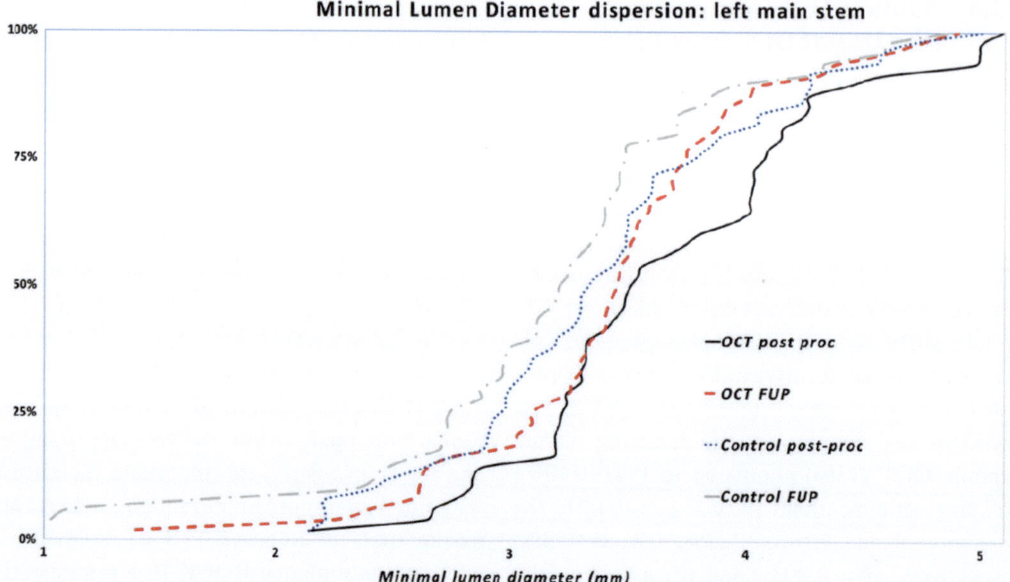

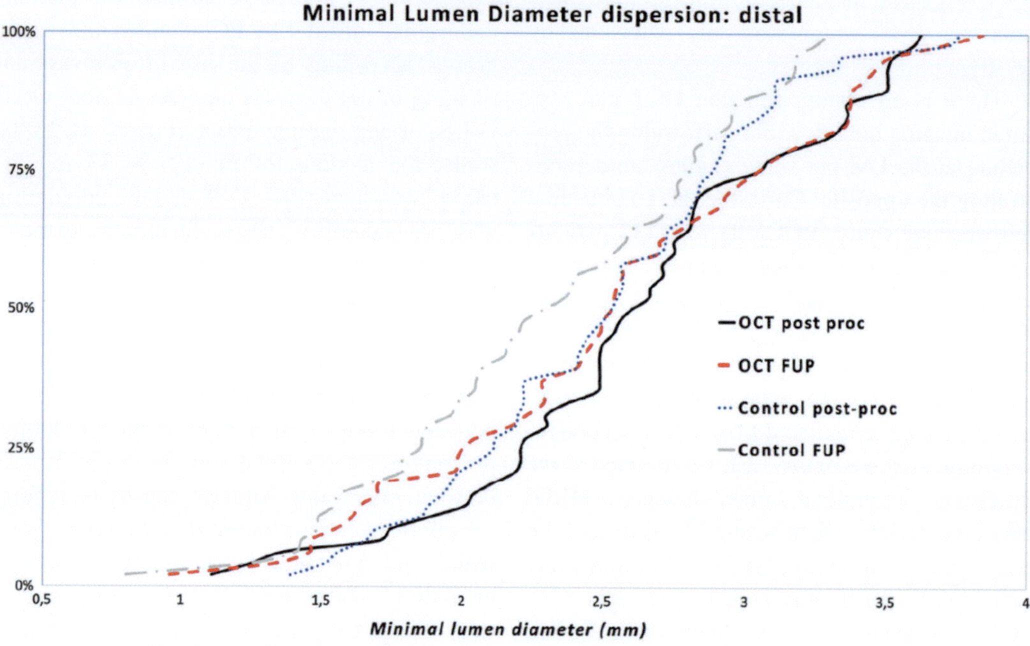

Fig. 13.3 Example of coregistered angio-optical coherence tomography (OCT) display in the cathlab. (**a**) Angiogram. The small white line in the left main (LM) indicates the position of the OCT imaging probe and the parallel red lines indicate the stent malapposition in the LM. The parallel large white lines in the left anterior descending artery (LAD) indicates the stent. (**b**) Cross-sectional OCT image corresponding to the location of the white marker in the angiogram, LM. Red dotted line tracing showing the stent in the LM and malapposition from 1 o'clock to10 o'clock, leaving a gap between the stent and the coronary intima. (**c**) Longitudinal view of the OCT pullback from distal (LAD-left) to proximal (LM-right). Between 25 and 45 mm it can be appreciated LAD stent well apposed, as shown by the automatic white color stained. On the right along with the cursor the LM stent, red color stained showing the malapposition and the white color stained in the middle showing well apposed stent

Table 13.2 ROCK I study final results summary and comparison between groups

	OCT group $n = 55$	Standard group $n = 57$	p value
Primary outcome			
LLL in LM, mm	0.12	0.26	0.10
LLL in distal portion, mm	0.03	0.24	0.025
Secondary outcome			
MACE, *n (%)*	4 (7.2)	5 (8.7)	0.82
Cardiac death, *n (%)*	0 (0)	2 (03.5)	0.49
Myocardial infarction, *n (%)*	1 (1.8)	1 (1.7)	0.88

LLL, late lumen loss; LM, left main; MACE, major adverse cardiovascular events; OCT, optical coherence tomography

Table 13.3 LEMON prospective trial for OCT guidance in the left main stem PCI clinical outcomes

Description	Results (%) after final OCT run
Primary endpoint (procedural success)[a]	86
Adequate stent expansion	86
Edge dissection	30
Strut malapposition	24
OCT modified operator strategy	26
1 year survival free from MACE	98.6

MACE, Major adverse cardiovascular events; AKI, acute kidney injury
[a] Procedural success definition: residual angiographic stenosis <50% + TIMI (Thrombolysis In Myocardial Infarction) flow grade 3 in all branches + adequate stent expansion by OCT analysis (LEMON criteria)

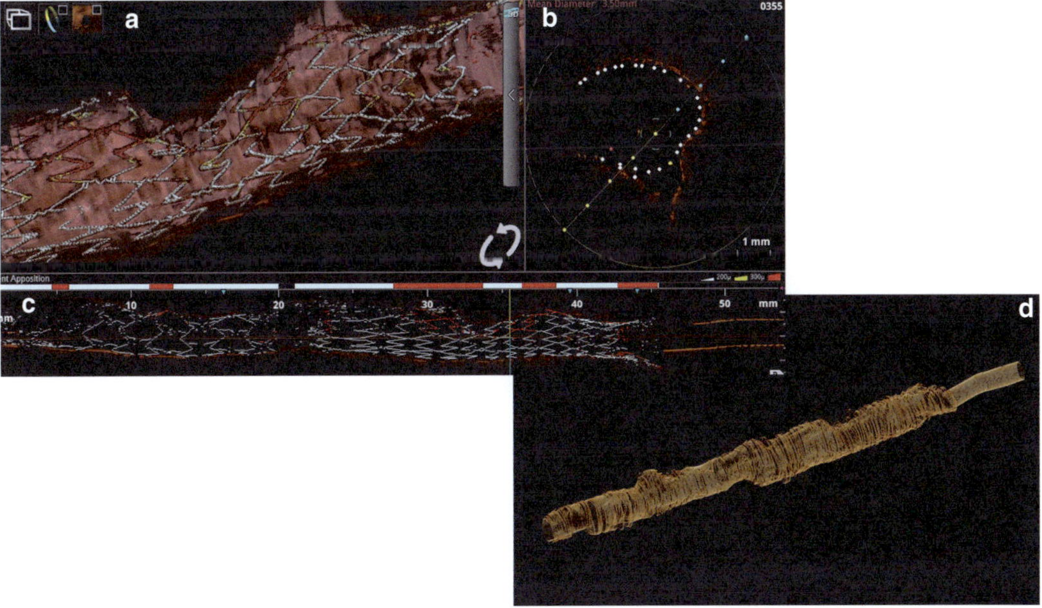

Fig. 13.4 ROCK II study design flow chart

Table 13.4 Baseline clinical and procedural characteristics of the overall population in the ROCK II study

	Angiography	Intravascular imaging	p Value	OCT	IVUS	p Value
Number of patients	353	377	–	162	215	–
Male, n (%)	272 (76.7)	286 (76)	0.92	120 (74.3)	166 (77.1)	0.73
Age, years, (mean ± SD)	71 (10)	67 (10)	0.76	69 (10)	69.5 (11)	0.77
Hypertension, n (%)	258 (73.4)	290 (77)	0.40	134 (83.1)	187 (73.7)	0.20
Diabetes, n (%)	120 (34.3)	94 (24.9)	0.03	26 (16.7)	65 (29.9)	0.06
Previous CABG, n (%)	64 (19)	34 (9.1)	0.003	13 (8.1)	19 (9.4)	0.42
Previous PCI, n (%)	141 (40.2)	151 (40.2)	0.99	52 (32.4)	95 (44.7)	0.10
LVEF, (mean ± SD)	51 (9)	53 (9)	0.11	55 (10)	52 (10)	0.34
Stable angina, n (%)	134 (38)	147 (39.4)	0.46	74 (45.3)	75 (34.6)	0.17
Unstable angina, n (%)	99 (27.7)	90 (24)	0.36	49 (30.8)	43 (20)	0.12
NSTEMI, n (%)	85 (24.3)	83 (22.1)	0.57	44 (27.4)	39 (18.5)	0.21
STEMI, n (%)	42 (12.3)	41 (11.5)	0.33	16 (9.6)	26 (12.4)	0.81
SYNTAX score	26.5 (7.5)	19.9 (7.6)	0.01	19.9 (8.7)	19.9 (7.3)	0.95
Three-vessel disease, n (%)	115 (39.8)	49 (25.9)	0.03	30 (21.9)	33 (28.4)	0.84
Total contrast use (mean ± SD)	220 (100)	220 (105)	0.67	225 (131)	220 (100)	0.46
Total procedural time in minutes (mean ± SD)	84 (40)	90 (41)	0.22	92 (45)	88 (50)	0.51
Two-stent technique, n (%)	64 (18.5)	53 (21.7)	0.42	20 (15.5)	33 (25.7)	0.07

IVUS, intravascular ultrasound; OCT, optical coherence tomography; CABG, coronary artery bypass grafting; PCI, percutaneous coronary intervention; LVEF, left ventricular ejection fraction; NSTEMI, non-ST elevation myocardial infarction; STEMI, ST elevation myocardial infarction

Table 13.5 ROCK II study final results and comparison between techniques

	OCT (%)	IVUS (%)	Angiography (%)	p Value
TFL at 12 months (Primary endpoint)	12.7		21.2	$p = 0.039$
	11.7	13.5	–	$p = 0.26$
Total deaths rate (Secondary endpoint)	4.4		13.9	$p = 0.02$
	2.6	5.0	–	$p = 0.02$
Procedural success	98.7		94.7	$p = 0.04$
	99.3	99.0	–	$p = 1.0$

OCT, optical coherence tomography; IVUS, intravascular ultrasound; TLF, target lesion failure (composite of cardiac death, target vessel myocardial infarction, and target lesion revascularization)

ROCK II most important results are summarized in Tables 13.4 and 13.5. Intravascular imaging was found superior to angiography, and OCT was found similar to IVUS in terms of primary endpoint target lesion failure (TLF), a composite of cardiac death, target vessel MI and target lesion revascularization, but with an improved survival rate (secondary endpoint). These results were confirmed also by propensity matching analysis, with the TLF significantly reduced in the intravascular imaging vs. angiographic guid-ance and with no difference between OCT and IVUS. After matching score groups were done, the OCT group had 0% peri-procedural MI complication, contrary to IVUS with 1% and angiography alone with 6% (Fig. 13.5) Catheter Cardiovasc Interv. 2022 Feb;99(3):664-673.

Miura et al. also compared OCT to IVUS in terms of composite of cardiac death, myocardial infarction, and target lesion revascularization but in the setting of LM bifurcation PCI with single stent crossover across the side branch and kissing

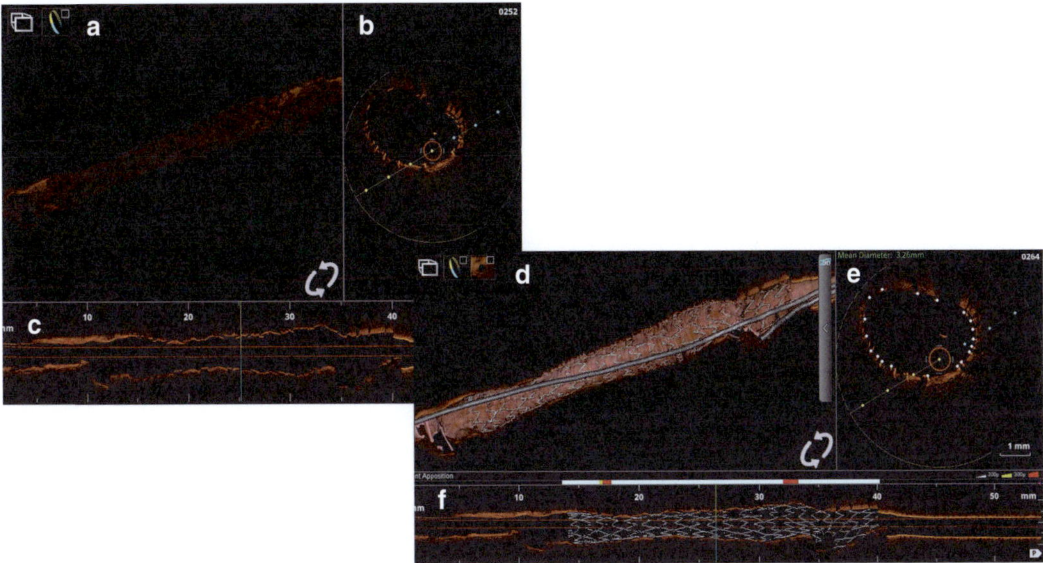

Fig. 13.5 Rock II study Kaplan-Meier curves for primary endpoint target lesion failure in the three groups. IVUS, intravascular ultrasound; OCT, optical coherence tomography

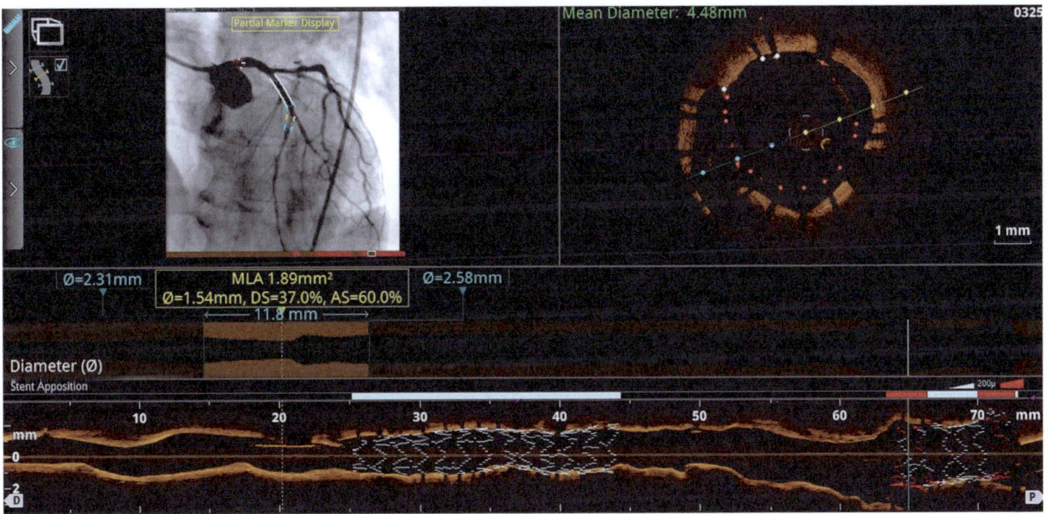

Fig. 13.6 OCT assessment after LM stenting, showing stent malapposition

balloon inflation. One issue within the study is that only 58 (17.5%) of patients underwent OCT-guided procedure among the 331 patients enrolled. After 12 months of follow-up, the rate of the cumulative primary endpoint was not significantly different between the two groups, both before and after propensity score adjustments. An interesting phenomenon in this study is that the balloon for POT was smaller in the OCT group, probably due to the limited visibility in the proximal portion of the LM, although the restenosis rate was similar between the groups [25] (Fig. 13.6).

13.5 Ongoing Clinical Studies for LM PCI with OCT Guidance

Although data to present has been promising for the use of OCT in the management of LM lesions, the majority of studies have been retrospective. *The need of prospective trials to validate the most important findings in the previous studies has to encourage the scientific community to design new trials* (Table 13.6).

Studies dedicated to LM will provide more support for the use of OCT to guide a PCI in terms of feasibility, safety, and clinical outcomes. There is a prospective ongoing study named SOLEMN, evaluating the stent strut coverage with follow-up to 12 months, an important factor implicated in the pathogenesis of stent thrombosis (ST) which in turn is one of the most important causes of mortality after stent implantation. As a secondary outcome, the study will evaluate major cardiovascular events [26–28].

Alongside, the OPTICO-LM and VIP-LM studies, comparing prospectively OCT to physiologic testing (FFR and FFR/iFR respectively) would help to determine the optimal MLA in intermediate lesions at the LM. In addition, OPTICO-LM will evaluate the clinical outcome accounting for MACE at 1 year of follow-up [29, 30].

Finally, the OCT safety will be tested in a French study comparing the management of exclusively non-ostial LM lesions during PCI in a randomized fashion with a group of OCT-guided patients to a group of angiography alone-guided patients, both assessed by physiologic measures, and will include either stable coronary artery disease and acute coronary syndrome (ACS) patients. The aim of this study is to analyze the hypothesized superiority of OCT over angiography and will give a pathway to develop more trials focused on OCT to strengthen this imaging tool [31] (Fig. 13.7).

13.6 Optimizing the Use of OCT in the LM with a Non-stent-Based Approach

Drug-coated balloons (DCB) have been used initially for the management of in-stent restenosis (ISR) with excellent results and recently became a very important tool also for the treatment of de novo coronary lesions (including small coronary artery disease), with strong and growing evidence supported by studies like BASKET-SMALL 2 and PICCOLETO 2 [32, 33].

In the setting of general bifurcation lesions, the use of DCB has been particularly attractive as those lesions are associated with an increased incidence of complications such as ST, ISR, incomplete coverage of the bifurcation area, scaffolding of the side branch ostium, and others. A few studies showed that DCB, as adjuvant therapy on top of DES (and also aiming at reducing the total stent length), is safe and effective to treat selected bifurcation lesions, offering similar angiographic results compared to a full-DES strategy, with few complications and the potential advantage of shortening DAPT in case of solo-DCB PCI, specifically in patients with multiple co-morbidities and at high bleeding risk [34, 35].

Recently, on top of paclitaxel, also sirolimus has been used as a drug of choice for DCBs. Preliminary data from the EASTBOURNE registry (interim analysis in 642 patients with 1 year follow-up) showed a very low TLR (2.5%), myocardial infarction (2.3%), total death (1%), and MACE rates (5.8%), showing good immediate performance and an adequate and encouraging safety profile. Some patients treated with DCB for ISR in the LM have been included, and these data will be analyzed in an ad hoc study [36].

Recently the randomized study EBC MAIN for LM bifurcation management showed how a stepwise layered provisional strategy was associated with lower MACE compared to systematic

Table 13.6 Ongoing studies for left main stem intervention outcomes with OCT

Study name	Type	N	Patient	Comparators	Follow up	Primary Outcome	Secondary Outcome	Country
SOLEMN [26]	Single group	75	SCAD. LMS lesion >50%	OCT to OCT follow-up	3 m, 6 m and 12 m	Stent strut coverage	MACE	USA
OPTICO-LM [29]	Single group	104	ACS and SCAD. LMS lesion <50%	OCT to FFR	1 year	Validation of MLA with OCT on intermediate LMS lesions	MACE and clinical at 1 year	Germany, Switzerland, and Japan
VIP-LMS [30]	Single group	53	SCAD and NSTEMI LMS 40–70% stenosis	OCT and IVUS to iFR and FFR	No	Accuracy of OCT and IVUS in predicting functionally significant LMS stenosis	OCT MLD and MLA	Brazil
DOCTORS-LM [31]	Randomized control group	188	ACS and SCAD non-ostial LMS disease	OCT group vs. control (fluoroscopy group)	No	OCT-guided PCI is superior to LMS PCI guided by fluoroscopy, assessed by FFR	OCT safety	France

OCT, optical coherence tomography; SCAD, stable coronary artery disease; LMS, left main stem; m, moths; MACE, major adverse cardiovascular effects; U.S.A., United States of America; ACS, acute coronary syndrome; FFR, flow fractional reserve; MLA, minimal luminal area; NSTEMI, non-ST elevation myocardial infarction; IVUS, intravascular ultrasound; iFR, instantaneous wave-free ratio; MLD, minimal luminal diameter; PCI, percutaneous coronary intervention

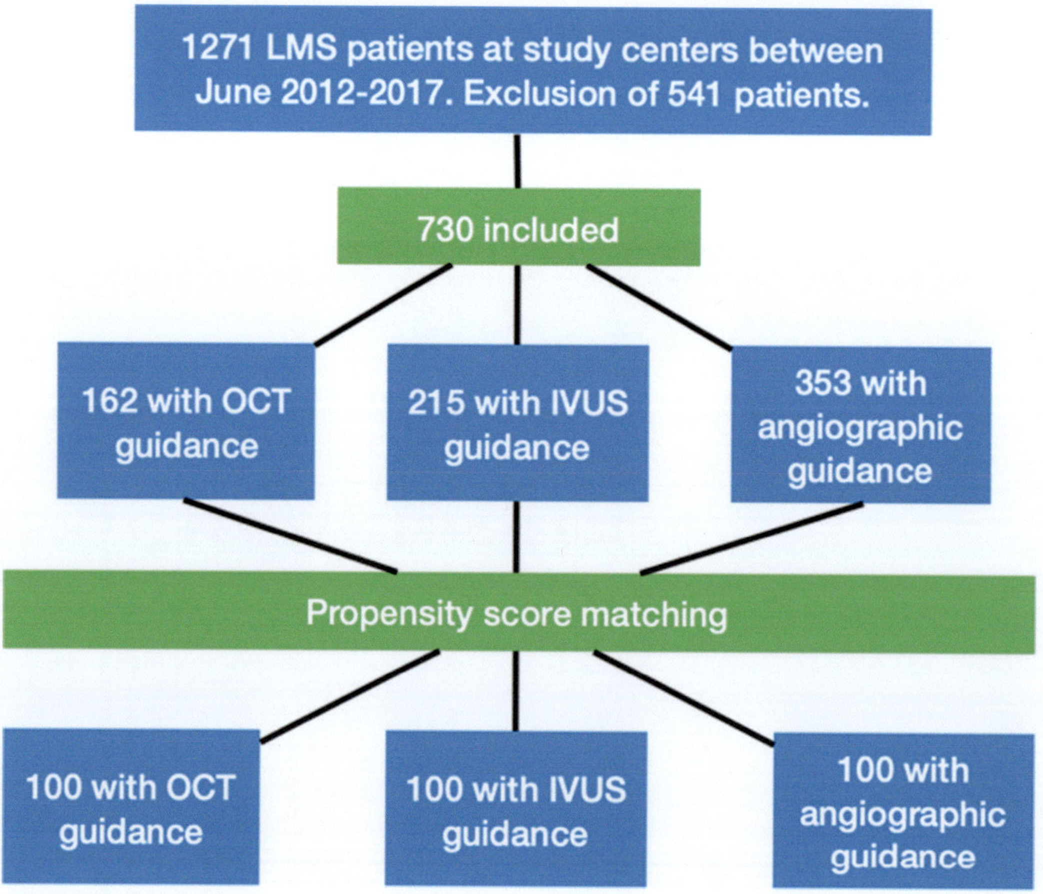

Fig. 13.7 Optical coherence tomography (OCT) images with stent under-expansion of a patient treated with a direct stent from the left main (LM) to the left anterior descending (LAD) artery. (**a**) 3D navigation view with stent display, asterisk in the notch showing the site of stent underexpansion. (**b**) Cross-sectional OCT image corresponding to the location of interest, white dotted line fol-lowing stent struts well apposed but under-expanded. (**c**) Longitudinal view of the OCT pullback from distal (LAD-left) to proximal (ostial LM-right). Between 30 and 40 mm it can be observed LM stent under-expansion as marked by the red color stained. (**d**) 3D navigation view of the LM-LAD with the stent. The asterisk shows the site of under-expansion

dual stent implantation (14.7% vs. 17.7%, respectively, $p = 0.34$), although the difference was not statistically significant [7, 37].

The utilization of a DCB to LM PCI in the side branch could be an option, but more studies are needed before suggesting this as one of the default strategies for complex LM bifurcation lesions. Based on these considerations, the use of OCT would help to better analyze the LM lesion and decide the best possible management, taking into consideration the premise of utilization as least metal as possible to have good angiographic results and less long-term complications (Fig. 13.8).

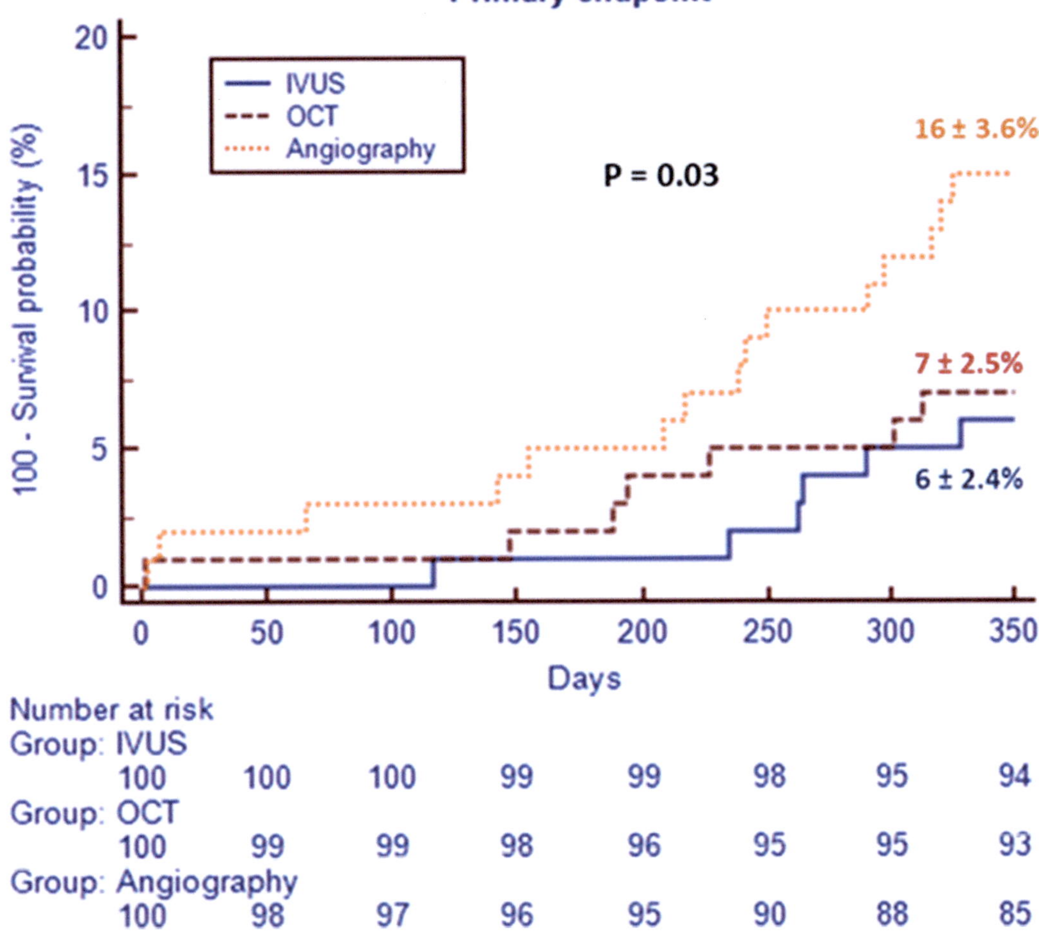

Fig. 13.8 OCT images of percutaneous coronary intervention of a patient treated with a provisional side-branch stenting technique at the left main (LM) bifurcation lesion, Medina 1.1.0. (**a**) 3D imaging of the stent in the artery (LAD to LM, left to right) after kissing balloon inflation and proximal optimization technique, showing a spot of open-cell at the bifurcation of the circumflex (Cx) (asterisk). (**b**) Cross-sectional OCT image of the LAD with well stent apposition. (**c**) Longitudinal view of the OCT pullback from distal (LAD-left) to proximal (LM-right). (**d**) 3D navigation view with stent display, a guidewire from the LM (right) to the LAD (left) and a guidewire appreciated from the LM to the Cx (right-down). (**e**) Cross-sectional OCT image corresponding to the LAD, white dotted line following stent struts well apposed to the wall. (**f**) Longitudinal view of the OCT pullback from distal (LAD-left) to proximal (LM-right). From 14 to 40 mm the stent implanted can be appreciated. At the level of 35 mm in the bifurcation, the well form carina (white arrow), the Cx roof (yellow arrow) well apposed and the cell opening can be seen

13.7 Future Perspective

Clinical studies have demonstrated that the use of intravascular imaging improves the outcome in the setting of LM PCI, compared to angiography alone. Such benefits of intravascular imaging guidance may be greatest in high-risk patients and complex lesions.

Even though IVUS has more clinical studies supporting the superiority over angiography, recently OCT was tested in some first-line pivotal studies and even larger ones. This imaging technique was found non-inferior to IVUS in terms of clinical endpoints on the long term, and has been demonstrated to lead to improved assessment of the immediate performance of PCI, due to the inherently higher spatial resolution and the ability to detect potential suboptimal stent implantation.

References

1. Holm NR, Mäkikallio T, Lindsay MM, Spence MS, Erglis A, Menown IBA, et al. Percutaneous coronary angioplasty versus coronary artery bypass grafting in the treatment of unprotected left main stenosis: updated 5-year outcomes from the randomised, non-inferiority NOBLE trial. Lancet. 2020;395(10219):191–9.
2. Stone GW, Kappetein AP, Sabik JF, Pocock SJ, Morice M-C, Puskas J, et al. Five-year outcomes after PCI or CABG for left main coronary disease. N Engl J Med. 2019;381(19):1820–30.
3. Neumann F-J, Sousa-Uva M, Ahlsson A, Alfonso F, Banning AP, Benedetto U, et al. 2018 ESC/EACTS Guidelines on myocardial revascularization. Eur Heart J. 2019;40(2)
4. Alfonso F, Kastrati A. Ten-year follow-up of left main coronary artery revascularization: still equipoise between percutaneous interventions and surgery? Circulation. 2020;141:1447–51.
5. Buccheri S, Franchina G, Romano S, Puglisi S, Venuti G, D'Arrigo P, et al. Clinical outcomes following intravascular imaging-guided versus coronary angiography-guided percutaneous coronary intervention with stent implantation: a systematic review and Bayesian network meta-analysis of 31 studies and 17,882 patients. JACC Cardiovasc Interv. 2017;10(24)
6. Nashef SAM, Roques F, Sharples LD, Nilsson J, Smith C, Goldstone AR, et al. EuroSCORE II. Eur J Cardiothorac Surg. 2012;41(4).
7. Hildick-Smith D, Egred M, Banning A, Brunel P, Ferenc M, Hovasse T, et al. The European bifurcation club left main coronary stent study: a randomized comparison of stepwise provisional vs. systematic dual stenting strategies (EBC MAIN). Eur Heart J. 2021;ehab283:1–11.
8. Bavishi C, Sardar P, Chatterjee S, Khan AR, Shah A, Ather S, et al. Intravascular ultrasound–guided vs angiography-guided drug-eluting stent implantation in complex coronary lesions: meta-analysis of randomized trials. Am Heart J. 2017;185:26–34.
9. Steinvil A, Zhang Y-J, Lee SY, Pang S, Waksman R, Chen S-L, et al. Intravascular ultrasound-guided drug-eluting stent implantation: an updated meta-analysis of randomized control trials and observational studies. Int J Cardiol. 2016;216:133–9.
10. Meneveau N, Souteyrand G, Motreff P, Caussin C, Amabile N, Ohlmann P, et al. Optical coherence tomography to optimize results of percutaneous coronary intervention in patients with Non-ST-elevation acute coronary syndrome: results of the multicenter, randomized DOCTORS (Does Optical Coherence Tomography Optimize Results of Stenting) study. Circulation. 2016;134(13):906–17.
11. de la Torre Hernandez JM, Baz Alonso JA, Gómez Hospital JA, Alfonso Manterola F, Garcia Camarero T, Gimeno de Carlos F, et al. Clinical impact of intravascular ultrasound guidance in drug-eluting stent implantation for unprotected left main coronary disease: pooled analysis at the patient-level of 4 registries. JACC Cardiovasc Interv. 2014;7(3)
12. Park SJ, Kim YH, Park DW, Lee SW, Kim WJ, Suh J, et al. Impact of intravascular ultrasound guidance on long-term mortality in stenting for unprotected left main coronary artery stenosis. Circ Cardiovasc Interv. 2009;2(3):167–77.
13. Cortese B, Burzotta F, Alfonso F, Pellegrini D, Trani C, Aurigemma C, et al. Role of optical coherence tomography for distal left main stem angioplasty. Catheter Cardiovasc Interv. 2020;96(4):755–61.
14. Koskinas KC, Nakamura M, Räber L, Colleran R, Kadota K, Capodanno D, et al. Current use of intracoronary imaging in interventional practice – results of a European Association of Percutaneous Cardiovascular Interventions (EAPCI) and Japanese Association of Cardiovascular Interventions and Therapeutics (CVIT) Clinical Practice Survey. EuroIntervention. 2018;14(4):475–84.
15. Kinnaird T, Johnson T, Anderson R, Gallagher S, Sirker A, Ludman P, et al. Intravascular imaging and 12-month mortality after unprotected left main stem PCI: an analysis from the British cardiovascular intervention society database. JACC Cardiovasc Interv. 2020;13(3):346–57.
16. de la Torre Hernandez JM, Hernández Hernandez F, Alfonso F, Rumoroso JR, Lopez-Palop R, Sadaba M, et al. Prospective application of pre-defined intravascular ultrasound criteria for assessment of intermediate left main coronary artery lesions: results from the multicenter LITRO study. J Am Coll Cardiol. 2011;58(4):351–8.
17. Jasti V, Ivan E, Yalamanchili V, Wongpraparut N, Leesar MA. Correlations between fractional flow reserve and intravascular ultrasound in patients with an ambiguous left main coronary artery stenosis. Circulation. 2004;110(18):2831–6.
18. Chieffo A, Latib A, Caussin C, Presbitero P, Galli S, Menozzi A, et al. A prospective, randomized trial of intravascular-ultrasound guided compared to angiography guided stent implantation in complex coronary lesions: the AVIO trial. Am Heart J. 2013;165(1):65–72.
19. Kang S-J, Cho Y-R, Park G-M, Ahn J-M, Kim W-J, Lee J-Y, et al. Intravascular ultrasound predictors for edge restenosis after newer generation drug-eluting stent implantation. Am J Cardiol. 2013;111(10):1408–14.
20. Ali ZA, Maehara A, Généreux P, Shlofmitz RA, Fabbiocchi F, Nazif TM, et al. Optical coherence tomography compared with intravascular ultrasound and with angiography to guide coronary stent implantation (ILUMIEN III: OPTIMIZE PCI): a randomised controlled trial. Lancet. 2016;388(10060):2618–28.

21. Soeda T, Uemura S, Park SJ, Jang Y, Lee S, Cho JM, et al. Incidence and clinical significance of poststent optical coherence tomography findings: one-year follow-up study from a multicenter registry. Circulation. 2015;132(11):1020–9.

22. Kubo T, Imanishi T, Takarada S, Kuroi A, Ueno S, Yamano T, et al. Assessment of culprit lesion morphology in acute myocardial infarction. ability of optical coherence tomography compared with intravascular ultrasound and coronary angioscopy. J Am Coll Cardiol. 2007;50(10):933–9.

23. Amabile N, Rangé G, Souteyrand G, Godin M, Boussaada MM, Meneveau N, et al. Optical coherence tomography to guide percutaneous coronary intervention of the left main coronary artery: the LEMON study. EuroIntervention. 2021;17(2):124–31.

24. Cortese B, de la Torre Hernandez JM, Lanocha M, Ielasi A, Giannini F, Campo G, D'Ascenzo F, Latini RA, Krestianinov O, Alfonso F, Trani C, Prati F, Linares JA, Sardella G, Wlodarczak A, Viganò E, Camarero TG, Stella P, Sozykin A, Fineschi M, Burzotta F. Optical coherence tomography, intravascular ultrasound or angiography guidance for distal left main coronary stenting. The ROCK cohort II study. Catheter Cardiovasc Interv. 2022;99(3):664–73. https://doi.org/10.1002/ccd.29959. Epub 2021 Sep 28.

25. Miura K, Tada T, Shimada T, Ohya M, Murai R, Kubo S, et al. Three-dimensional optical coherence tomography versus intravascular ultrasound in percutaneous coronary intervention for the left main coronary artery. Heart Vessels. 2021;36(5):630–7.

26. Vidovich M. Synergy optical coherence tomography in left main PCI (SOLEMN). Clinicaltrials.gov Identifier NCT03474432. 2019.

27. Takano M, Yamamoto M, Xie Y, Murakami D, Inami S, Okamatsu K, et al. Serial long-term evaluation of neointimal stent coverage and thrombus after sirolimus-eluting stent implantation by use of coronary angioscopy. Heart. 2007;93(11).

28. Finn A, Joner M, Nakazawa G, Kolodgie F, Newell J, John MC, et al. Pathological correlates of late drug-eluting stent thrombosis: strut coverage as a marker of endothelialization. Circulation. 2007;115(18).

29. Raeber L. Comparison of optical coherence tomography-derived minimal lumen area, invasive fractional flow reserve and FFRCT (OPTICO-LM). Clinicaltrials.gov Identifier NCTO3820492. 2019.

30. Chamie D. Imaging and physiology for intermediate left main stem stenosis (VIP-LMS). Clinicaltrials.org NCT04531007. 2020.

31. Meneveau N. Does OCT optimise results of stenting on the left main stem (DOCTORS-LM). Clinicaltrials.gov Identifier: NCT04391413. 2020.

32. Jeger R, Farah A, Ohlow M-A, Mangner N, Möbius-Winkler S, Leibundgut G, et al. Drug-coated balloons for small coronary artery disease (BASKET-SMALL 2): an open-label randomised non-inferiority trial. Lancet. 2018;392(10150):849–56.

33. Cortese B, di Palma G, Guimaraes MG, Piraino D, Orrego PS, Buccheri D, et al. Drug-coated balloon versus drug-eluting stent for small coronary vessel disease: PICCOLETO II randomized clinical trial. JACC Cardiovasc Interv. 2020;13(24):2840–9.

34. Rathore S, Tehrani S, Prvulovic D, Araya M, Lefèvre T, Banning AP, et al. Drug coated balloons and their role in bifurcation coronary angioplasty: appraisal of the current evidence and future directions. Expert Rev Med Devices. 2020;17(10).

35. Berland J, Lefèvre T, Brenot P, Fajadet J, Motreff P, Guerin P, et al. DANUBIO - a new drug-eluting balloon for the treatment of side branches in bifurcation lesions: six-month angiographic follow-up results of the DEBSIDE trial. EuroIntervention. 2015;11(8):868–76.

36. Cortese B, Testa L, di Palma G, Heang TM, Bossi I, Nuruddin AA, et al. Clinical performance of a novel sirolimus-coated balloon in coronary artery disease: EASTBOURNE registry. J Cardiovasc Med. 2021;22(2):94–100.

37. Chen S-L, Zhang J-J, Han Y, Kan J, Chen L, Qiu C, et al. Double kissing crush versus provisional stenting for left main distal bifurcation lesions. J Am Coll Cardiol. 2017;70(21):2605–17.

The Role of Intravascular Imaging for Post-procedural and Long-Term Evaluation of the Revascularized Left Main

Akiko Maehara, Gary S. Mintz, and Martin B. Leon

Post-procedural left main stent expansion to predict long-term outcomes In non-left main (LM) coronary artery lesions, numerous studies using intravascular ultrasound (IVUS) or optical coherence tomography (OCT) have shown the absolute minimum stent area (MSA) to be the most powerful predictor for future major adverse cardiac events (MACE) after percutaneous coronary intervention (PCI), including stent thrombosis and restenosis [1–6].

In 403 unprotected LM lesions treated with first generation drug-eluting stents (DES) (in this study the sirolimus-eluting Cypher [Cordis, Miami, FL, USA] stent), Kang et al. [7] reported that the MSA cut-offs that best differentiated 9-month angiographic binary restenosis were 8.2 mm^2 for the LM trunk, 7.2 mm^2 for the polygon of confluence at the bifurcation, 6.3 mm^2 for the ostial left anterior descending (LAD), and 5.0 mm^2 for the ostial left circumflex (LCX) (if stented). Patients with stent underexpansion at any one of these four locations had increased rates of MACE at 2 years, mainly due to a reste-

notic ostial LCX. An IVUS substudy from the EXCEL trial (randomized DES versus coronary artery bypass grafting [CABG] in patients with LM disease) showed larger MSA cut-offs that best differentiated 3-year lesion-specific outcomes (either definite/probable stent thrombosis or ischemia-driven target lesion revascularization [TLR]): 9.8 mm^2 for the LM, 7.3 mm^2 for the ostial LAD, and 5.7 mm^2 for the ostial LCX (if stented). In particular, the LM MSA was independently associated with LM-related MACE [8]. The approximately 1.0 mm^2 larger cut-offs in EXCEL compared with the Korean study by Kang et al. can be explained by the two very different patient populations. Compared with Asians, Caucasians have larger bodies, greater left ventricular mass, and larger LM coronary arteries [9]. A substudy of the NOBLE trial (randomized DES versus CABG in patients with LM disease) also reported that a larger final LM MSA was associated with fewer LM-related revascularizations, although post-PCI IVUS was available in only 224 (~one-third) of the PCI cohort [10]. Finally, de la Torre Hernández et al. [11] compared 124 patients treated using a pre-specified PCI protocol (target LM MSA >80–90% of reference lumen area and LAD or LCX MSA >90% of reference lumen area without edge dissection or stent deformation and with stent edge plaque burden <40%) versus 124 propensity-score matched patients with IVUS-guided LM stenting but without a pre-specified

A. Maehara · M. B. Leon (✉)
Columbia University, New York, NY, USA

Cardiovascular Research Foundation,
New York, NY, USA
e-mail: mleon@crf.org

G. S. Mintz
Cardiovascular Research Foundation,
New York, NY, USA

© Springer Nature Switzerland AG 2022
B. Cortese (ed.), *Left Main Coronary Revascularization*,
https://doi.org/10.1007/978-3-031-05265-1_14

Table 14.1 Post-procedure minimum stent areas of each segment of LM, ostial LAD, or LCX reported in IVUS studies

Cohort	Study type	# of lesions (% distal bifurcation)	Minimum stent area (mm^2)		
			LM	Ostial LAD	Ostial LCX
Kang et al. [7]	Retrospective observational	403 (83%)	10.2 ± 2.4 in 403 lesions	8.1 ± 1.8 in 336 lesions	5.6 ± 1.4 in 104 lesions
NOBLE [10]	Substudy in randomized trial	224 (91%)	12.5 ± 3.0	NA	NA
EXCEL [8]	Substudy in randomized trial	505 (80%)	9.9 ± 2.3 in 505 lesions	7.5 ± 2.3 in 337 lesions	6.3 ± 2.0 in 85 lesions
Spanish registry [11]	IVUS with guidance	124 (65%)	11.8 (10.2, 12.6)	8.5 (7.4, 9.2)	7.0 (6.3, 7.6)
Spanish registry [11]	IVUS without guidance	124 (62%)	10.0 (8.1, 11.2)	7.4 (6.6, 8.2)	6.1 (5.4, 6.5)

Vales are shown mean ± standard deviation or median (first quartile, third quartile). IVUS = intravascular ultrasound; LAD = left anterior descending artery; LCX = left circumflex; LM = left main; NA = not available

PCI protocol. Patients treated with the pre-specified IVUS-guidance PCI protocol achieved stent expansion optimization in 88% versus 65% after IVUS guidance without a protocol; the LM median MSA measured 11.8 mm^2 (10.2–12.6) versus 10.0 mm^2 (8.1–11.2), respectively, substantially different.

Table 14.1 summarizes the mean LM, ostial LAD, and ostial LCX MSA measurements from each of these four studies. Compared with the data from Kang et al., from EXCEL, and from patients in the Spanish registry treated without the pre-specified PCI protocol, the cohort from NOBLE and the Spanish registry patients treated with pre-specified PCI guidance protocol showed substantially larger LM MSAs.

When treating a distal LM bifurcation lesion, the location of re-wiring in the LCX is important to optimize stent expansion and coverage at the carina [12]. Among 127 LM lesions in the EXCEL IVUS substudy treated with a two-stent technique (62 T-stents, 25 crush, 35 culotte, and 5 simultaneous kissing stents) with final IVUS evaluation, a stent gap at the carina was found in 11% (14/127), and incomplete crush (>0.5 mm crushed stent thickness) was found in 28% (36/127) [13]. The importance of wire position and re-positioning the wire, if necessary, may be answered in the ongoing OCTOBER trial in true bifurcation (including LM) lesions in which a pre-specified OCT-guided protocol requires repositioning the side branch guidewire if the crossing point is suboptimal [12]. Figure 14.1 illustrates a patient with failed CABG and a distal LM lesion treated with culotte stenting who suffered stent thrombosis 2 months after DES implantation possibly due to an underexpanded stent at the ostial LCX along with a small gap and uncovered dissection at the carina.

LM Stent Vessel Wall Malapposition Based on the fractal nature of epicardial coronary artery geometry, the appropriate balloon diameter when performing PCI in the LM is typically ≥1 mm larger compared with the proximal LAD; thus, after stenting from the LAD to the LM using a stent sized to the distal stent edge landing zone in the LAD, the proximal edge of the stent in the LM is almost always significantly malapposed [14]. If the balloon used for the proximal optimization technique (POT) is not appropriately sized or positioned (just proximal to the carina and reaching up to the proximal edge of main vessel stent), proximal stent edge struts may float in the LM [15]. Figure 14.2 illustrates such a case leading to aberrant re-wiring of the stent. It is recommended to choose an appropriately sized POT balloon based on pre-IVUS evaluation of LM and adjusted based on post-stent IVUS evaluation, if necessary. Conversely, acute malapposition of LM stents is not associated with stent failure (stent thrombosis or restenosis) unless there is stent underexpansion [7, 16].

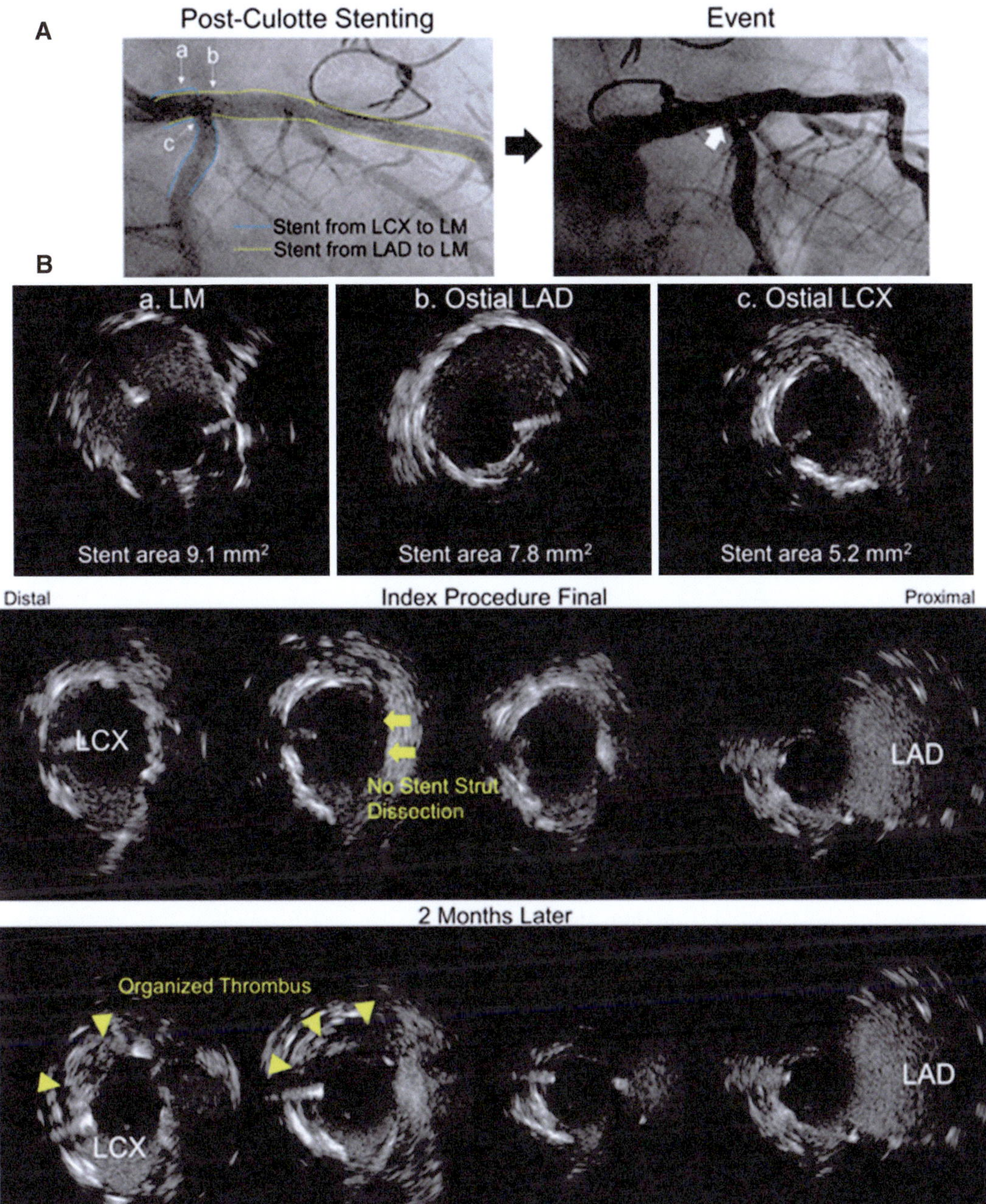

Fig. 14.1 Late stent thrombosis due to underexpanded circumflex ostial stent with gap and residual dissection. Because of bypass graft occlusion, an unprotected distal left main (LM) lesion was treated with culotte stenting. Top panel: (**a**) Coronary angiogram post-culotte stenting (yellow and blue dotted lines) and 2 months later during a stent thrombosis event (severe stenosis, white arrow) at the ostial left circumflex (LCX). (**b**) Post-procedure intravascular ultrasound (IVUS) findings at index: Stent area measured 9.1 mm² at distal LM, 7.8 mm² at ostial left anterior descending artery (LAD), and 5.2 mm² at ostial LCX. Bottom panel: Matched post-procedural and 2-month intravascular ultrasound (IVUS) images. Post-procedural IVUS showed a small medial dissection without stent struts at the carina side of the ostial LCX (yellow arrows), and 2-month IVUS showed organized thrombus at the ostial LCX. It can be speculated that during the index procedure, the distal pathway of re-wiring the LCX resulted in a gap at the carina along with a small medial dissection and a relatively underexpanded stent at the ostial LCX. All of these may have contributed to the late stent thrombosis

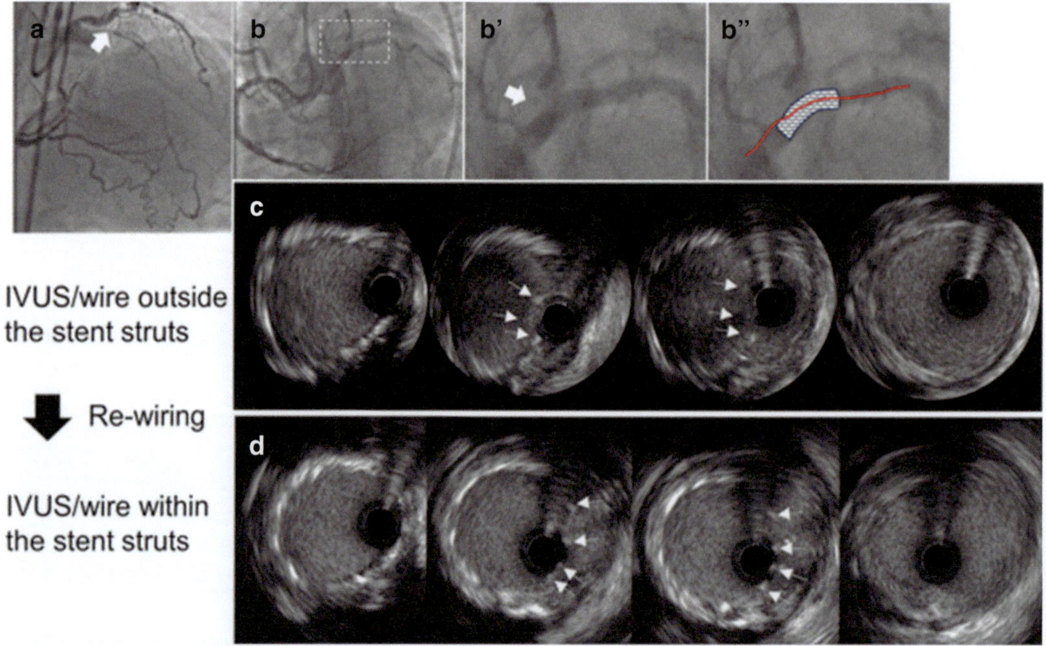

Fig. 14.2 Aberrant rewiring of an ostial left main stent due to prior proximal edge malapposed struts. (**a**) and (**b**) show a coronary angiogram. (**b'**) and (**b"**) (**b'** with annotation) are the magnified images of the dotted rectangle in (**b**). Four months prior, the patient suffered a myocardial infarction, and the culprit lesion (proximal left circumflex [LCX] to distal left main [LM]) was stented. The left anterior descending artery (LAD) lesion was an ostial chronic total occlusion (CTO) (white arrows in **a** and **b'**); staged percutaneous coronary intervention (PCI) to the LAD was planned. To identify the proximal cap of the LAD CTO, a guidewire was introduced from the LM to the LCX, and intravascular ultrasound was performed. At the proximal edge of the prior stent, the wire was outside of the stent struts (**b"** and **c**). After re-wiring, the guidewire was confirmed to be within the stent (**d**). To avoid aberrant rewiring, proximal optimization during the index procedure is recommended, with confirmation by IVUS

Covering the Aorto-ostial Junction and LM Stent Deformation Kang et al. [16] evaluated 493 lesions (half in the LM) in which the proximal end of a stent was positioned at or near the coronary ostium. The coverage of ostium by stent and the amount of protrusion of the stent into the aorta were not related to ostial restenosis if there was no significant residual plaque burden. In the EXCEL IVUS substudy, the prevalence of strut protrusion into the aorta was 54.7%, and the protrusion length measured 2.9 ± 1.7 mm [17].

Longitudinal stent deformation has been reported with second-generation DES [18]. Among 1489 consecutive lesions treated with second-generation DES, acute longitudinal stent deformation was found in 1.1% (17/1489) of lesions. The most common site of deformation was the proximal edge of the stent, especially at the LM ostium location (8.3% of LM lesions). In the EXCEL IVUS substudy, the prevalence of LM stent deformation was 6.5% (33/506 lesions with analyzable IVUS), and 82% were at the ostial LM [17]. LM lesions with stent deformation had worse 3-year MACE compared with LM lesions without stent deformation (28.0% vs. 13.4%, $p = 0.02$) even after adjusting for LM MSA or other clinical factors.

Stent Edge Residual Disease or Dissection Because the average length of the LM segment is approximately 10 mm and the LM is frequently diffusely diseased [19], in most LM PCIs, the LM segment is fully covered by the stent such that stent edge issues (residual disease or edge dissection) are mostly related to the distal stent edge in either the LAD or the LCX. Both IVUS and OCT studies show that a stent edge landing zone with a greater amount of disease (plaque burden, calcium, lipidic plaque) is associated with an edge dissection [20, 21] that, in turn, may be associated with late events [5, 20]. In particular, a large dissection (dissection length > 3 mm, dissection angle >60°, dissection flap ≥200 µm) along with a smaller lumen area (<5.0 mm^2 by IVUS or <4.5 mm^2 by OCT) is associated with worse outcomes and, thus, should be covered by an additional stent. Similarly, a stent edge with a plaque burden >50% by IVUS or lipid-rich plaque >180° by OCT is also associated with edge restenosis and should be covered [22, 23].

LCX Ostium as the Most Frequent Location of Restenosis Table 14.2 summarizes restenosis location after treatment of unprotected LM lesions irrespective of the technique [24–26] in which the average IVUS usage was 48%. Restenosis was most frequent at the LCX ostium: 45% of TLR and 67% of angiographic binary restenosis after provisional stenting and 84% of

Table 14.2 Location of target lesion revascularization or angiographic binary restenosis after unprotected left main bifurcation lesions were treated with percutaneous coronary intervention

Study name	Population	IVUS use	Restenosis measures	Rate of restenosis or TLR stratified by stent type and stenting technique			
				Provisional stenting		Two-stent techniques	
				First-generation DES	Second-generation DES	First-generation DES	Second-generation DES
PRECOMBAT-2 [19]	334 ULM lesions treated with EES and 327 ULM lesions treated with SES	90%	8~10-month binary restenosis	3.6%	5.1%	16.9%	15.2%
			% of LCX ostium location	36%	70%	75%	100%
Pooled bifurcation studies [20]	689 ULM lesions treated with first-generation DES and 214 ULM lesions treated with second-generation DES	39%	3-year TLR	5.5%	6.7%	17.8%	3,8%
			% of LCX ostium location	32%	78%	85%	67%
DKCRUSH-V [21]	482 true bifurcation ULM lesions with second-generation DES; DK crush versus provisional stentings	42%	1-year binary restenosis	–	14.6%	–	7,1%
			% of LCX ostium location	–	83%	–	73%
Weighted average	A total of 531 ULM lesions treated with provisional stenting and 372 ULM lesions treated with two-stent techniques	48%	% of LCX ostium location in 8-month ~1-year binary restenosis	67%		79%	
			% of LCX ostium location in 3-year TLR	45%		84%	

DES = drug-eluting stents; DK = double kissing; EES = everolimus-eluting stents; IVUS = intravascular ultrasound; LCX = left circumflex; SES = sirolimus-eluting stents; TLR = target lesion revascularization; ULM = unprotected left main

TLR and 79% of angiographic binary restenosis after two-stent techniques. Thus, optimization of the LCX ostium is most important during IVUS-guided PCI. This requires IVUS pullback from both the LCX as well as the LAD because we have shown that the side branch evaluation from main vessel pullback (i.e., oblique view of the LCX when imaging from the LAD to the LM) has modest sensitivity and poor specificity to diagnose disease in the side branch [27].

Evidence that Using IVUS Guidance During LM Revascularization Improves Outcomes There are two small randomized trials, multiple registries, and four meta-analyses that have compared outcomes between IVUS-guided versus angiography-guided PCI for the treatment of unprotected LM lesions (Fig. 14.3) [28–32]. Compared with randomized trials or registries that did not include LM lesions [33–35], the impact of IVUS guidance when treating LM lesions was more prominent for reducing mortality than for reducing repeat revascularization. The most important British Cardiovascular Intervention Society (BCIS) registry report compared 5056 lesions with IVUS guidance versus 6208 lesions without IVUS guidance using 1-year mortality as the primary endpoint [32]. Very strikingly, the main separation of mortality was observed within 30 days (mortality between IVUS vs. angiography guidance; 2.9% vs. 6.6%, adjusted hazard ratio [HR] 0.54 [0.43–0.68] at 30 days; 9.0% vs. 15.5%, adjusted HR 0.66 [0.57–0.77] at 1 year); similar patterns have been observed in prior studies [31, 34, 35]. IVUS can identify suboptimal stent results (stent underexpansion or residual edge disease or dissection), and these suboptimal findings are the strongest predictors for subacute stent thrombosis, although subacute stent thrombosis is rare. In the BCIS analysis, the greatest benefit of IVUS guidance was in the hands of interventional cardiologists with the greatest PCI experience [32], indicating that the most experienced interventionalists were also the ones most knowledgeable of how to use intravascular imaging to optimize their procedures.

Mechanism of Stent Failure Intravascular imaging can delineate three major mechanisms of in-stent restenosis (ISR) including (1) stent underexpansion or other mechanical complications (stent fracture, deformation, or chronic stent recoil), (2) excessive neointimal hyperplasia (NIH), and (3) neoatherosclerosis (defined as new in-stent atherosclerosis such as lipidic or calcified plaque evolving from NIH). The rate of these three causes depends on the stent type and the duration from stent implantation. In our OCT report including 171 non-LM ISR lesions within second-generation DES, the prevalence of stent underexpansion was 56% within 1 year from DES implantation and 48% beyond 1 year from DES implantation [36]. Among 114 ISR lesions beyond 1 year (3.3 ± 1.9 years) from DES implantation, the prevalence of neoatherosclerosis was 29%. Stent fracture or deformation was found in 10.5% (6/57) within 1 year and 11.4% (13/114) beyond 1 year. Although there are no such studies exclusively for LM lesions, the mechanism is likely to be the same. Examples are shown in Figs. 14.4 and 14.5. Coronary angiography is unable to differentiate among these mechanisms. It is very important to evaluate the mechanism of every stent failure using intravascular imaging to choose the appropriate treatment strategy.

Acceleration of Calcium in Left Main Post-CABG In long-term serial angiographic studies after CABG, there is progressive narrowing in the native coronary arteries proximal to the distal graft anastomosis [37, 38]. Using IVUS, we compared 41 patients with patent grafts to the left coronary artery (mean duration from CABG of 8.2 ± 6.1 years) versus 45 patients without prior CABG and showed that LM disease proximal to the patent graft had greater calcium with negative remodeling compared with LM disease in non-CABG patients [39]. In a second study using OCT, we compared LM disease in 76 CABG patients with a patent graft to the left coronary artery versus LM disease in 146 propensity-matched non-CABG patients [40]. CABG patients had greater amounts of calcium (thicker calcium, larger calcium angle, and longer calcium length) compared with non-CABG patients as well as a greater prevalence of a calcified nodule

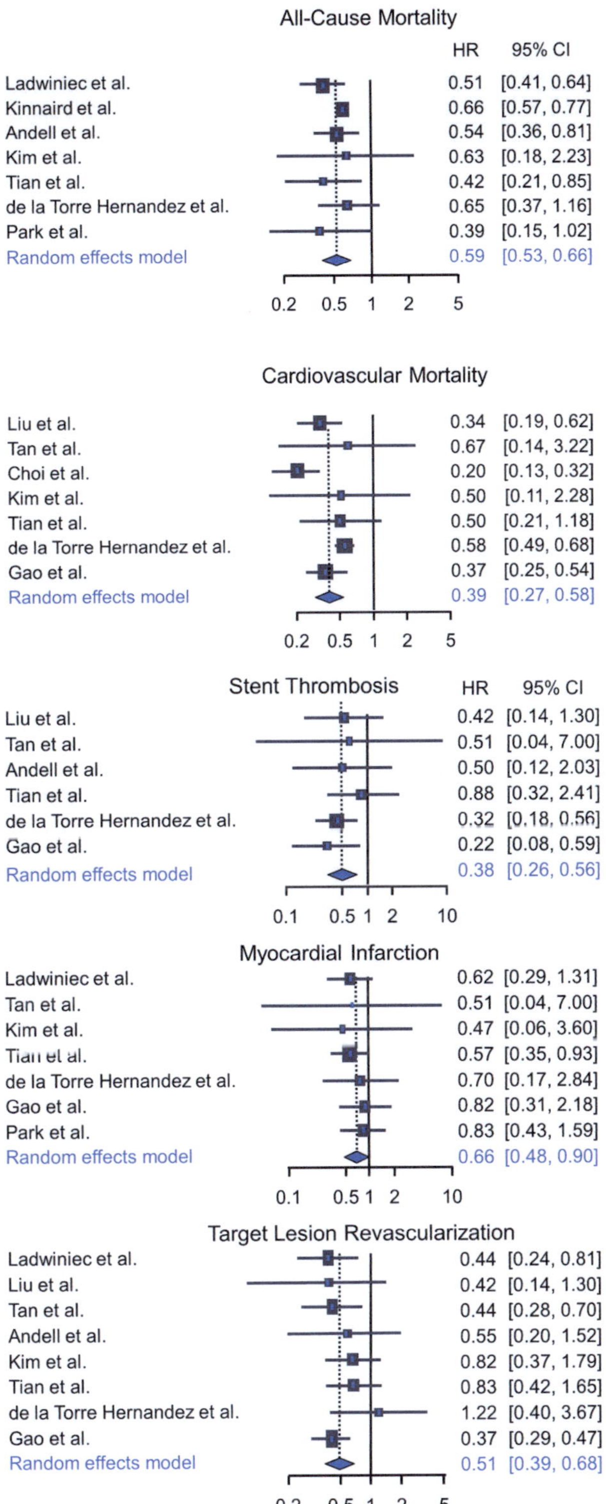

Fig. 14.3 Summary plot for the outcomes from meta-analysis of 11 studies of left main coronary artery disease treated with drug-eluting stents. CI = confidence interval; HR = hazard ratio; TLR = target lesion revascularization. Reprinted from Am J Cardiol 128; Elgendy, IY, et al. 92, Copyright (2020), with permission from Elsevier Inc

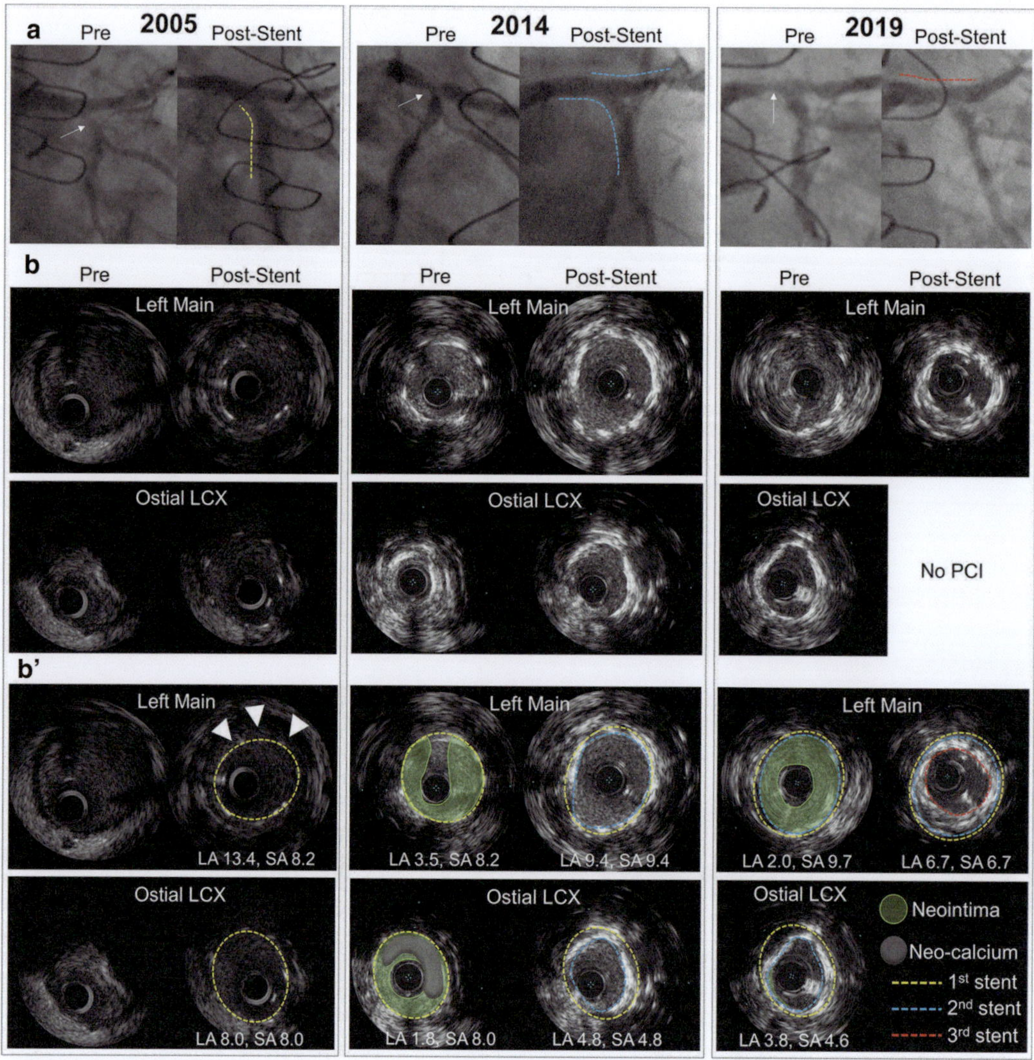

Fig. 14.4 Distal left main lesion stent failure due to neo-intimal hyperplasia and neoatherosclerosis. (**a**) shows coronary angiograms; (**b** and **b'**) (same image of **b** with annotation) show intravascular ultrasound (IVUS) images of the distal left main coronary artery (LM) and the ostial left circumflex (LCX). This patient had prior bypass grafting. Angiography in 2005 showed an occluded saphenous vein graft to the LCX and a patent internal mammary artery anastomosed to the left anterior descending artery (LAD). A severe ostial LCX lesion was treated with a drug-eluting stent (DES, yellow dotted lines in **a**) that slightly protruded into the distal LM and appeared to be malapposed (white triangles in **b'**). In 2014, coronary angiography showed severe stenosis at the distal LM and ostial LCX and LAD; IVUS showed calcification within the stent (neoatherosclerosis, gray area in **b'**) within the ostial LCX stent, whereas the distal LM had significant neointimal hyperplasia (NIH, green area in **b'**). The LM to LCX and LAD lesion was treated using two stents (crush technique, blue dotted lines). Post-procedure IVUS showed good stent expansion of the distal LM (stent area measured 9.4 mm^2), although stent expansion of ostial LCX was modest (minimum stent area [MSA] 4.8 mm^2) due to calcification inside the stent. In 2019, severe distal LM stenosis was found, and IVUS showed excessive NIH (green area) in the LM stent and a patent LCX stent with minimal NIH. A new stent (red dotted line) was implanted in the LM with a final MSA of only 6.7 mm^2 due to three layers of stents. IVUS delineated the mechanism of in-stent restenosis (NIH and neoatherosclerosis) and confirmed the most achievable revascularization result each time. LA = lumen area; SA = stent area

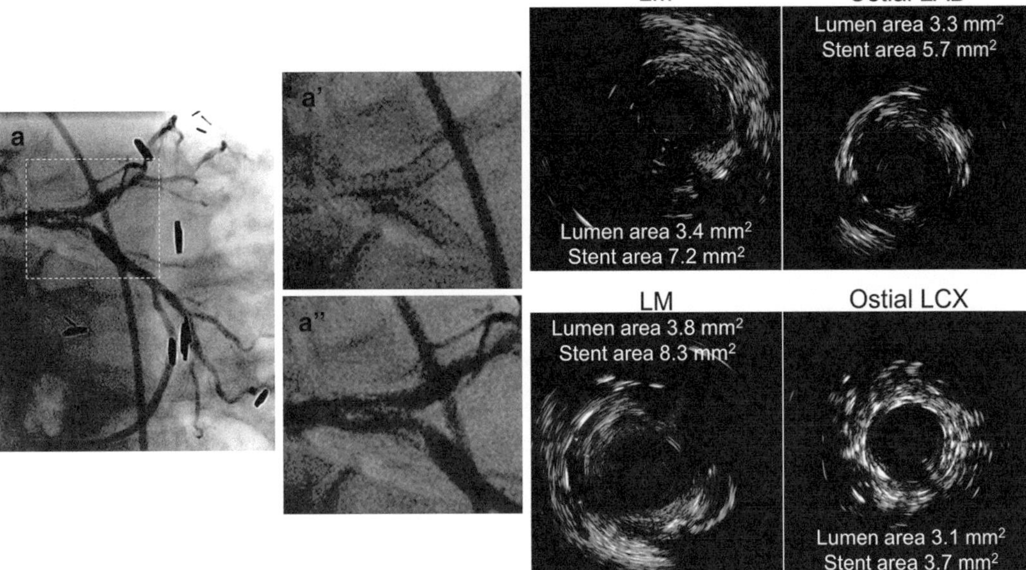

Fig. 14.5 In-stent restenosis in the simultaneous kissing stent due to stent underexpansion and neointimal hyperplasia. (**a**, **a′**, and **a″**) (same image as **a′**, but with contrast) are angiograms showing distal left main (LM) to ostial left circumflex (LCX) restenosis in a patient with LM disease previously treated with simultaneous kissing stents. Intravascular ultrasound (IVUS) shows adequate stent expansion of the distal LM and ostial left anterior descending (LAD) with modest amounts of neointimal hyperplasia (NIH); however, the ostial LCX stent was severely underexpanded with only modest NIH accumulation

(37% vs. 14%), more calcium at the carina that is spared from plaque or calcium accumulation in the atherosclerosis without CABG (30% vs. 14%), and more thin calcium (26% vs. 17%, similar to what was seen in dialysis patients). These findings suggested that reduced flow within the LM in the setting of a patent graft likely leads to vessel shrinkage and non-atherosclerotic calcium progression.

References

1. Fujii K, Carlier SG, Mintz GS, Yang YM, Moussa I, Weisz G, et al. Stent underexpansion and residual reference segment stenosis are related to stent thrombosis after sirolimus-eluting stent implantation: an intravascular ultrasound study. J Am Coll Cardiol. 2005;45:995–8. https://doi.org/10.1016/j.jacc.2004.12.066.
2. Lee SY, Shin DH, Kim JS, Kim BK, Ko YG, Choi D, et al. Intravascular ultrasound predictors of major adverse cardiovascular events after implantation of everolimus-eluting stents for long coronary lesions. Rev Esp Cardiol (Engl Ed). 2017;70:88–95. https://doi.org/10.1002/ccd.24560.
3. Song HG, Kang SJ, Ahn JM, Kim WJ, Lee JY, Park DW, et al. Intravascular ultrasound assessment of optimal stent area to prevent in-stent restenosis after zotarolimus-, everolimus-, and sirolimus-eluting stent implantation. Catheter Cardiovasc Interv. 2014;83:873–8. https://doi.org/10.1002/ccd.24560.
4. Soeda T, Uemura S, Park SJ, Jang Y, Lee S, Cho J, et al. Incidence and clinical significance of post-stent optical coherence tomography findings: one-year follow-up study from a multicenter registry. Circulation. 2015;132:1020–9. https://doi.org/10.1161/CIRCULATIONAHA.114.014704.
5. Prati F, Romagnoli E, La Manna A, Burzotta F, Gatto L, Marco V, et al. Long-term consequences of optical coherence tomography findings during percutaneous coronary intervention: the Centro Per La Lotta Contro L'infarto - Optimization Of Percutaneous Coronary Intervention (CLI-OPCI) LATE study. EuroIntervention. 2018;14:e443–51. https://doi.org/10.4244/EIJ-D-17-01111.
6. Katagiri Y, De Maria GL, Kogame N, Chichareon P, Takahashi K, Chang CC, et al. Impact of post-procedural minimal stent area on 2-year clinical outcomes in the SYNTAX II trial. Catheter Cardiovasc Interv. 2019;93:E225–34. https://doi.org/10.1002/ccd.28105.

7. Kang SJ, Ahn JM, Song H, Kim WJ, Lee JY, Park DW, et al. Comprehensive intravascular ultrasound assessment of stent area and its impact on restenosis and adverse cardiac events in 403 patients with unprotected left main disease. Circ Cardiovasc Interv. 2011;4:562–9. https://doi.org/10.1161/CIRCINTERVENTIONS.111.964643.

8. Maehara A, Mintz G, Serruys P, Kappetein A, Kandzari D, Schampaert E, et al. Impact of final minimum stent area by IVUS on the 3-year outcome after PCI of left main coronary disease: the EXCEL trial. J Am Coll Cardiol. 2017;69(11 suppl):963.

9. Skowronski J, Cho I, Mintz GS, Wolny R, Opolski MP, Cha MJ, et al. Inter-ethnic differences in normal coronary anatomy between Caucasian (Polish) and Asian (Korean) populations. Eur J Radiol. 2020;130:109185. https://doi.org/10.1016/j.ejrad.2020.109185.

10. Ladwiniec A, Walsh SJ, Holm NR, Hanratty CG, Makikallio T, Kellerth T, et al. Intravascular ultrasound to guide left main stem intervention: a sub-study of the NOBLE trial. EuroIntervention. 2020;16:201–9. https://doi.org/10.4244/EIJ-D-19-01003.

11. de la Torre Hernández JM, Camarero TG, Alonso JAB, Hospital JAG, Fernandez GV, Hwang DHL, et al. The application of predefined optimization criteria for intravascular ultrasound guidance of left main stenting improves outcomes. EuroIntervention. 2020;16:210–7. https://doi.org/10.4244/EIJ-D-19-01057.

12. Holm NR, Andreasen LN, Walsh S, Kajander OA, Witt N, Eek C, et al. Rational and design of the European randomized Optical Coherence Tomography Optimized Bifurcation Event Reduction Trial (OCTOBER). Am Heart J. 2018;205:97–109. https://doi.org/10.1016/j.ahj.2018.08.003.

13. Fujimura T, Maehara A, Matsumura M, Banning A, Ungi I, et al. TCT-382 technical issues in 2-stent distal left main bifurcation treatment: an EXCEL trial intravascular ultrasound substudy. J Am Coll Cardiol. 2019;74(13 suppl):B379.

14. Finet G, Gilard M, Perrenot B, Rioufol G, Motreff P, Gavit L, et al. Fractal geometry of arterial coronary bifurcations: a quantitative coronary angiography and intravascular ultrasound analysis. EuroIntervention. 2008;3:490–8. https://doi.org/10.4244/eijv3i4a87.

15. Burzotta F, Lassen JF, Lefèvre T, Banning AP, Chatzizisis YS, Johnson TW, et al. Percutaneous coronary intervention for bifurcation coronary lesions: the 15th consensus document from the European Bifurcation Club. EuroIntervention. 2021;16:1307–17. https://doi.org/10.4244/EIJ-D-20-00169.

16. Kang SJ, Ahn JM, Kim WJ, Lee JY, Park DW, Lee SW, et al. Intravascular ultrasound assessment of drug-eluting stent coverage of the coronary ostium and effect on outcomes. Am J Cardiol. 2013;111:1401–7. https://doi.org/10.1016/j.amjcard.2013.01.291.

17. Kim SY, Maehara A, Banning A, Merkely B, Ungi I, van Boven AJ, et al. Frequency and impact of acute stent deformation after PCI of left main coronary artery disease: an EXCEL trial intravascular ultrasound substudy. 2017. https://www.tctmd.com/slide/tct-44-frequency-and-impact-acute-stent-deformation-after-pci-left-main-coronary-artery. Accessed 26 Apr 2021.

18. Inaba S, Weisz G, Kobayashi N, Saito S, Dohi T, Dong L, et al. Prevalence and anatomical features of acute longitudinal stent deformation: an intravascular ultrasound study. Catheter Cardiovasc Interv. 2014;84:388–96. https://doi.org/10.1002/ccd.25411.

19. Motreff P, Rioufol G, Gilard M, Caussin C, Ouchchane L, Souteyrand G, et al. Diffuse atherosclerotic left main coronary artery disease unmasked by fractal geometric law applied to quantitative coronary angiography: an angiographic and intravascular ultrasound study. EuroIntervention. 2010;5:709–15. https://doi.org/10.4244/eijv5i6a117.

20. Kobayashi N, Mintz GS, Witzenbichler B, Metzger DC, Rinaldi MJ, Duffy PL, et al. Prevalence, features, and prognostic importance of edge dissection after drug-eluting stent implantation: An ADAPT-DES intravascular ultrasound substudy. Circ Cardiovasc Interv. 2016;9:e003553. https://doi.org/10.1161/CIRCINTERVENTIONS.115.003553.

21. Chamié D, Bezerra HG, Attizzani GF, Yamamoto H, Kanaya T, Stefano GT, et al. Incidence, predictors, morphological characteristics, and clinical outcomes of stent edge dissections detected by optical coherence tomography. JACC Cardiovasc Interv. 2013;6:800–13. https://doi.org/10.1016/j.jcin.2013.03.019.

22. Kang SJ, Cho YR, Park GM, Ahn JM, Kim WJ, Lee JY, et al. Intravascular ultrasound predictors for edge restenosis after newer generation drug-eluting stent implantation. Am J Cardiol. 2013;111:1408–14. https://doi.org/10.1016/j.amjcard.2013.01.288.

23. Ino Y, Kubo T, Matsuo Y, Yamaguchi T, Shiono Y, Shimamura K, et al. Optical coherence tomography predictors for edge restenosis after everolimus-eluting stent implantation. Circ Cardiovasc Interv. 2016;9:e004231. https://doi.org/10.1161/CIRCINTERVENTIONS.116.004231.

24. Kim YH, Park DW, Ahn JM, Yun SC, Song HG, Lee JY, et al. Everolimus-eluting stent implantation for unprotected left main coronary artery stenosis. The PRECOMBAT-2 (Premier of Randomized Comparison of Bypass Surgery versus Angioplasty Using Sirolimus-Eluting Stent in Patients with Left Main Coronary Artery Disease) study. JACC Cardiovasc Interv. 2012;5:708–17. https://doi.org/10.1016/j.jcin.2012.05.002.

25. Lee JM, Hahn JY, Kang J, Park KW, Chun WJ, Rha SW, et al. Differential prognostic effect between first- and second-generation drug-eluting stents in coronary bifurcation lesions: patient-level analysis of the Korean bifurcation pooled cohorts. JACC Cardiovasc Interv. 2015;8:1318–31. https://doi.org/10.1016/j.jcin.2015.05.014.

26. Chen SL, Zhang JJ, Han Y, Kan J, Chen L, Qiu C, et al. Double kissing crush versus provisional stenting for left main distal bifurcation lesions: DKCRUSH-V

randomized trial. J Am Coll Cardiol. 2017;70:2605–17. https://doi.org/10.1016/j.jacc.2017.09.1066.

27. Oviedo C, Maehara A, Mintz GS, Tsujita K, Kubo T, Doi H, et al. Is accurate intravascular ultrasound evaluation of the left circumflex ostium from a left anterior descending to left main pullback possible? Am J Cardiol. 2010;105:948–54. https://doi.org/10.1016/j.amjcard.2009.11.029.

28. Elgendy IY, Gad M, Mintz GS. Meta-analysis of intravascular ultrasound-guided drug-eluting stent implantation for left main coronary disease. Am J Cardiol. 2020;128:92–3. https://doi.org/10.1016/j.amjcard.2020.05.013.

29. Liu XM, Yang ZM, Liu XK, Zhang Q, Liu CQ, Han QL, et al. Intravascular ultrasound-guided drug-eluting stent implantation for patients with unprotected left main coronary artery lesions: a single-center randomized trial. Anatol J Cardiol. 2019;21:83–90. https://doi.org/10.14744/AnatolJCardiol.2018.21447.

30. de la Torre Hernandez JM, Baz Alonso JA, Gómez Hospital JA, Alfonso Manterola F, Garcia Camarero T, Gimeno de Carlos F, et al. Clinical impact of intravascular ultrasound guidance in drug-eluting stent implantation for unprotected left main coronary disease: pooled analysis at the patient-level of 4 registries. JACC Cardiovasc Interv. 2014;7:244–54. https://doi.org/10.1016/j.jcin.2013.09.014.

31. Andell P, Karlsson S, Mohammad MA, Götberg M, James S, Jensen J, et al. Intravascular ultrasound guidance is associated with better outcome in patients undergoing unprotected left main coronary artery stenting compared with angiography guidance alone. Circ Cardiovasc Interv. 2017;10:e004813. https://doi.org/10.1161/CIRCINTERVENTIONS.116.004813.

32. Kinnaird T, Johnson T, Anderson R, Gallagher S, Sirker A, Ludman P, et al. Intravascular imaging and 12-month mortality after unprotected left main stem PCI: an analysis from the British Cardiovascular Intervention Society database. JACC Cardiovasc Interv. 2020;13:346–57. https://doi.org/10.1016/j.jcin.2019.10.007.

33. Hong SJ, Kim BK, Shin DH, Nam CM, Kim JS, Ko YG, et al. Effect of intravascular ultrasound-guided vs angiography-guided everolimus-eluting stent implantation: the IVUS-XPL randomized clinical trial. JAMA. 2015;314:2155–63. https://doi.org/10.1001/jama.2015.15454.

34. Zhang J, Gao X, Kan J, Ge Z, Han L, Lu S, et al. Intravascular ultrasound versus angiography-guided drug-eluting stent implantation: the ULTIMATE trial. J Am Coll Cardiol. 2018;72:3126–37. https://doi.org/10.1016/j.jacc.2018.09.013.

35. Maehara A, Mintz GS, Witzenbichler B, Weisz G, Neumann FJ, Rinaldi MJ, et al. Relationship between intravascular ultrasound guidance and clinical outcomes after drug-eluting stents. Circ Cardiovasc Interv. 2018;11:e006243. https://doi.org/10.1161/CIRCINTERVENTIONS.117.006243.

36. Song L, Mintz GS, Yin D, Yamamoto MH, Chin CY, Matsumura M, et al. Characteristics of early versus late in-stent restenosis in second-generation drug-eluting stents: an optical coherence tomography study. EuroIntervention. 2017;13:294–302. https://doi.org/10.4244/EIJ-D-16-00787.

37. Guthaner DF, Robert EW, Alderman EL, Wexler L. Long-term serial angiographic studies after coronary artery bypass surgery. Circulation. 1979;60:250–9. https://doi.org/10.1161/01.cir.60.2.250.

38. Bourassa MG, Campeau L, Lespérance J, Grondin CM. Changes in grafts and coronary arteries after saphenous vein aortocoronary bypass surgery: results at repeat angiography. Circulation. 1982;65:90–7. https://doi.org/10.1161/01.cir.65.7.90.

39. Shang Y, Mintz GS, Pu J, Guo J, Kobayashi N, Franklin-Bond T, et al. Bypass to the left coronary artery system may accelerate left main coronary artery negative remodeling and calcification. Clin Res Cardiol. 2013;102:831–5. https://doi.org/10.1007/s00392-013-0598-6.

40. Wolny R, Mintz GS, Matsumura M, Kim SY, Ishida M, Fujino A, et al. Left coronary artery calcification patterns after coronary bypass graft surgery: an in-vivo optical coherence tomography study. Catheter Cardiovasc Interv. 2020; https://doi.org/10.1002/ccd.29220.

Follow-up of Left Main Patients Treated with PCI or CABG

15

Ahmad Alkhalil, Miguel Alvarez Villela, Y. Kobayashi, and Azeem Latib

15.1 Background

Percutaneous coronary intervention (PCI) for the treatment of left main coronary artery (LMCA) disease has been extensively studied as an alternative to coronary artery bypass surgery (CABG). Although a definitive uniform answer remains elusive, PCI seems to be an acceptable alternative for certain patients with favorable anatomy. The details regarding patient selection and optimal technique for PCI have been comprehensively addressed in this book. In this chapter, we will summarize current evidence on the angiographic and clinical follow-up after the revascularization of LMCA disease.

Whether CABG or PCI is the preferred method for revascularization, the ideal follow-up strategy for these patients remains a topic of debate. Given the large amount of myocardium supplied by the LMCA and its branches, adverse events resulting from lesion failure after PCI can lead to catastrophic outcomes. Hence, careful attention is required when deciding on several aspects of care after left main revascularization.

For clinicians, important considerations when providing care for these patients are: (1) What is the incidence and time course of adverse events after LMCA PCI and CABG, (2) How can dual-antiplatelet therapy impact this risk, and (3) Can invasive coronary angiography detect early lesion failure and reduce adverse outcomes. We review each of these issues separately.

15.2 Incidence and Time Course of Adverse Events After LMCA Revascularization

Patients revascularized with PCI or CABG have different short-term risk profiles for adverse events. While CABG carries a higher up-front risk of MI, stroke, and bleeding surrounding the surgery, PCI has lower periprocedural risk with a higher risk of target lesion failure (TLF) due to stent thrombosis (ST) and restenosis in the months following revascularization. On the other hand, long-term risk follows a similar pattern after either procedure, accumulating steadily over time [1–3].

The risk of ischemic events after LMCA PCI is dictated by an interplay of different patient characteristics and procedural factors. The overall burden and complexity of coronary disease, an initial presentation with acute coronary syndrome (ACS), and the presence of non-cardiac

A. Alkhalil
Stony Brook University Hospital, Stony Brook, NY, USA

M. Alvarez Villela
Montefiore Medical Center, Bronx, NY, USA

Department of Cardiology, Lenox Hill Hospital - Northwell Health, New York, USA

Y. Kobayashi · A. Latib (✉)
Montefiore Medical Center, Bronx, NY, USA

© Springer Nature Switzerland AG 2022
B. Cortese (ed.), *Left Main Coronary Revascularization*,
https://doi.org/10.1007/978-3-031-05265-1_15

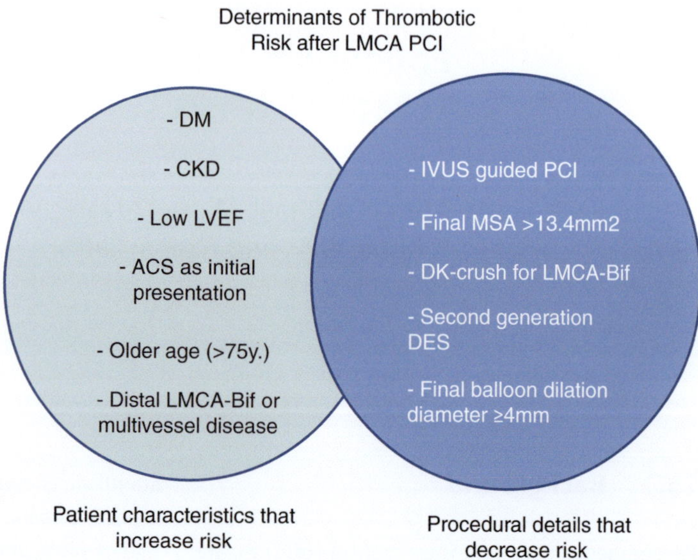

Fig. 15.1 Determinants of thrombotic event risk after LMCA PCI

comorbidities result in higher risk. Meanwhile, procedural and device-related factors such as the number and type of stents placed, stenting technique applied, and the use of intravascular imaging to guide the procedure influence the risk of downstream events (Fig. 15.1).

Registry data indicate that the risk of ST and target lesion revascularization (TLR) follows a bimodal distribution, clustering in the first 50 days after PCI and rising again 150 days after the procedure, while the risk of MACE is accumulated at a steadier rate over time. This is likely explained by the different drivers for each risk. Procedural factors and the pattern of stent drug elution could explain the time course of ST and TLR, while comorbid conditions would explain the pattern of incidence of MACE such as non-target lesion-related MI, stroke, and non-cardiac death [4].

This pattern is reflected in other registries, where the greatest risk of cardiac death and myocardial infarction after LMCA PCI is accumulated within the first 6 months, at a rate of 19.1 in the first 30 days and 2.7 and 2.3 per 10,000 patient-days in the subsequent 30–90-day and 90–180-day periods (Fig. 15.2) [5].

Data from the two most recent clinical trials of PCI vs. CABG using second-generation DES, >70% IVUS-guided PCI, and high prevalence of LMCA-Bifurcation lesions show ST rates of 1.3–1.8% at 5 years. Non-fatal MI rates in the

PCI arm vary between 6.9%–10.7% and overall MACE is 22–28% at this same time point. In the EXCEL trial, nearly 50% of all ST cases reported in the first 3 years occurred within 30 days. A similar pattern was seen in NOBLE, where 66% of the ST cases in the first year occurred within the first 30 days of follow-up [6, 7].

The relevance of procedural technique is illustrated in the DK-Crush III and V trials where LMCA bifurcation (LMCA-Bif) stenting with the DK-Crush technique resulted in lower ST rates compared to the Culotte technique (0% vs. 1%, $p = 0.25$) or provisional side-branch stenting strategy (0.4% vs. 3.3%, $p = 0.22$) at 1 year, in patients with otherwise similar clinical characteristics [8, 9].

The use of IVUS is an independent predictor of reduced adverse events among patients with LMCA-Bif disease but not in those with ostial or mid-shaft lesions according to data from one national registry. Overall, IVUS can lead to a 10% absolute reduction in the risk of a composite of cardiac death, TLR, and MI at 3 years (HR = 0.54, 95% CI: 0.34–0.90, $p = 0.02$). The use of IVUS also results in lower rates of ST (0.6% vs. 2.2%, $p = 0.04$) [10]. Its benefit upon long-term mortality has been confirmed by other observational studies [11].

Moreover, in a recent ad-hoc analysis from the NOBLE trial [12], post-PCI IVUS assessment and adequate stent expansion were associated

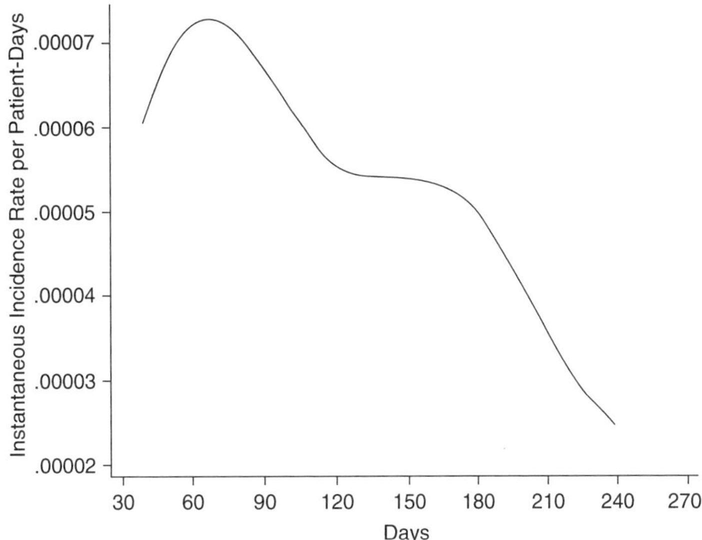

Fig. 15.2 Adjusted instantaneous incidence rate/patient-days of cardiac mortality and MI during the first year of follow-up in patients taking dual antiplatelet therapy. Adapted from Palmerini T et al. Journal of the American College of Cardiology. 2009 Apr 7;53(14):1176–81

with reduced left main stent target lesion revascularization (LMS TLR) but not overall MACCE (death, stroke, myocardial infarction, or ischemia-driven revascularization). A minimal stent area (MSA) of more than 13.4 mm² (upper tertile) was associated with less overall revascularization and LMS TLR. Indeed, none of the 77 patients who had MSA more than 13.4 mm² required LMS TLR at 5 years follow-up and only four patients (5.2%) required repeat revascularization.

Among patient characteristics, the factors most consistently associated with high risk of ST, TLF, and MACE after PCI in observational and randomized studies is an initial presentation with ACS, CKD, older age, peripheral arterial disease, low LVEF, and DM [5, 13].

The risk of adverse events after CABG is dictated by similar factors. Determinants of adverse events after CABG are chronic obstructive pulmonary disease (COPD), diabetes mellitus (DM), higher EuroSCORE, and the need for emergent revascularization and previous PCI [13, 14]. Although outcomes in patients with a higher complexity of disease (SYNTAX score) and multivessel disease favor CABG [3, 13], the use of arterial conduits clearly influences outcomes after surgery [15].

The risk profile of CABG as compared to PCI is best appraised by the six randomized controlled trials (RCT) comparing these two therapies in patients with LMCA disease. Mostly,

these studies included patients with a low prevalence of diabetes (15–30%), preserved LVEF, and low prevalence of CKD. LMCA-Bif lesions had a high prevalence and patients randomized to PCI were mostly treated with provisional side-branch stenting per protocol [2, 3, 13, 16–18]. The primary outcome was a composite of MACE (death, stroke, and MI) that has variably included target vessel revascularization (TVR) in the PCI arm. Graft occlusion in the CABG arm is also reported. Excluding differences in outcome definitions, the importance of newer DES use in PCI and LIMA use in CABG is illustrated when comparing results between these studies. The LE MANS trial, with high usage of BMS and low rate of LIMA use, has the highest rate of adverse outcomes in the PCI arm [16]. The SYNTAX trial, with the highest overall complexity of disease, low usage of IVUS, and use of the Taxus stent, follows in adverse event rates [13].

Although ST and graft occlusion are presented together as leading to unplanned revascularization and show similar rates in these trials, these two outcomes are not comparable in terms of the associated risk. Occlusion of arterial grafts is a rare event, and while occlusion of venous grafts could result in MI, it is less likely to result in acute mortality [19]. By contrast, ST carries a 50–70% risk of MI or cardiac death [20].

Table 15.1 provides an overview of the incidence of adverse outcomes in these trials along

Table 15.1 Summary of randomized controlled trials comparing PCI vs. CABG in patients with LMCA

PCI

Study name (year)	Age (years)	ACS (%)	Distal LMCA-Bif (%)	IVUS guided PCI (%)	Stent (DES generation)	ST 1 → 5 years	MI 1 → 5 years	MACE 1→ 5 years
EXCEL (2019)	66.0 ± 9.6	39	79%	77%	EES (2nd)	1.3%[a] → 1.8%	5.6%[a] → 10.7%	15.4%[a] → 22%
NOBLE (2016)	66.2 ± 9.9	18	87%	74%	BES (2nd)	0.3% → 1.3%	1.9% → 6.9%	7.1% → 28%
Le MANS (2015)	60.6 ± 10.5	NR	48%	Yes (%NR)	Mostly BMS, rare DES (1st)	0% → 0%[b]	1.9% → 8.7%[b]	38% → 52%[b]
PRECOMBAT (2010)	61.8 ± 10.0	50	64%	91%	SES (1st)	0% → 0.3%	1.3% → 2.0%	8.7% → 17.5%
SYNTAX (2011)	65.4 ± 9.8	29	61%	Rare	PES (1st)	NR →5.1%	4.3% → 8.2%	15.8% → 36.9%
Boudriot (2011)	66 (62–73)	Excluded	74%	Yes (%NR)	SES (1st)	0% → N/A[c]	3% → N/A[c]	19% → N/A[c]

CABG

Study name (year)	EuroScore	LIMA use (%)	DM prevalence (%)	Stroke 1 → 5 yrs. (%)	Graft occlusion 1 → 5 yrs. (%)	MI 1 → 5 years	MACE 1→ 5 years
EXCEL (2019)	NR	99%	28%	2.5%[a] →4.3%	3.6%[a] → 6%	7.4[a] → 9.8	14.7%[a] → 19%
NOBLE (2016)	2 (IQR:2;4)	96%	15.2%	1% → 1.7%	1.2% → 4.1%	1.4% → 1.9%	7.1% → 18%
Le MANS (2015)	3.5 ± 2.3	72%	17%	3.8% → 6.3%[b]	NR	5.6% → 10.4[b]	25% → 62%[b]
PRECOMBAT (2010)	2.8 ± 1.9	94%	30%	0.3% → 0.7%	1%	1.0% → 1.7%	6.7% → 14.3%
SYNTAX (2011)	3.9 ± 2.9	NR	25.6%	NR → 4.3%	4% → NR	4.1% → 4.8%	13.6% → 31%
Boudriot (2011)	2.4 (IQR:1,5; 3.7)	99%	33%	2%	NR	3% → N/A[c]	13.9% → N/A[c]

ACS: Acute coronary syndrome, LMCA: Left main coronary artery, Bif: Bifurcation, IVUS: Intravascular ultrasound, ST: Stent thrombosis, MI: Myocardial infarction, MACE: Major adverse cardiovascular events. BMS: Bare metal stent, EES: Everolimus-eluting stent, BES: Biolimus-eluting stent, SES: Sirolimus-eluting stent, PES: Placlitaxel-eluting stent

NR = not reported

[a]Signals 3-year outcome

[b]Signals 10-year outcome

[c]Not applicable, only 1-year follow-up was performed

LIMA: Left-internal mammary artery, MI: Myocardial infarction, MACE: Major adverse cardiovascular events

with an outline of the relevant patient and procedural characteristics.

15.3 Dual Antiplatelet Therapy Duration

Among patients undergoing PCI, the use of more potent P2Y12 inhibitors and longer regimens of dual-antiplatelet therapy (DAPT) protect against thrombotic events. However, they also increase the risk of life-threatening bleeding. Patients with the highest complexity of coronary disease resulting in higher thrombotic risk also generally carry the highest burden of comorbidities, portending the highest risk of bleeding.

This paradigm is clearly exemplified in patients with LMCA disease. Compared to the general population of patients undergoing PCI, this group carries a very high risk of MACE, TLR, and ST [4] as well as a marked risk for bleeding after hospital discharge [21].

There is growing attention to the need for refining DAPT to balance ischemic and bleeding risks after PCI. Several contemporary RCTs have studied shortened DAPT duration as an option to decrease the risk of bleeding events. However, these studies are generally underpowered for the

detection of ST and the population of patients with LMCA disease is grossly underrepresented within them [1, 22–24]. Hence, extrapolation of these findings to patients with LMCA PCI should be done with caution. DAPT duration should be decided with attention to specific procedural details and patient risk factors as described above (Fig. 15.1).

There are currently no data from dedicated randomized studies addressing the question of ideal DAPT duration for this patient population. RCTs comparing PCI to CABG have almost uniformly used 12 months as the protocolized DAPT duration for all PCI patients. Contemporary registry data indicate that 12 months is the duration of DAPT prescribed in 75–86% of patients undergoing LMCA PCI in real-world scenarios. Clopidogrel is the most widely investigated P2Y12 inhibitor in this patient population, but Ticagrelor is used in close to one-third of cases in current registries. Prasugrel use is rare [25, 26].

DAPT clearly influences the risk of adverse events after LMCA PCI. In one registry, a fourfold increase in the risk of cardiac death and MI was seen in the first 30 days after DAPT discontinuation, this risk was higher in patients receiving less than a total 6 months of DAPT (Fig. 15.3) [5]. A duration of <3 months resulted in a 1-year

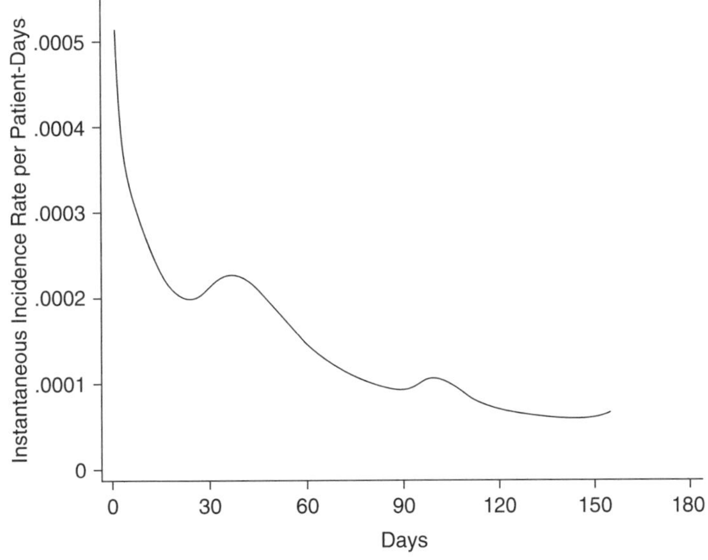

Fig. 15.3 Adjusted instantaneous incidence rate/patient-days of cardiac mortality and MI after clopidogrel discontinuation. Adapted from Palmerini T et al. Journal of the American College of Cardiology. 2009 Apr 7;53 (14):1176–81

ST rate of 4.3% compared to 1.8% in those receiving 12 months in another contemporary registry report [25].

Stenting technique should be an important consideration for deciding on DAPT duration. A patient-level pooled analysis of five nationwide multicenter registries showed an increase in TLF with early DAPT discontinuation (<1 year) in patients with LMCA-Bif treated with non-DK-Crush two-stent strategies (HR: 3.3 (95% CI: 1.5–7.3) despite a high IVUS usage rate (80%) [26]. In the DK-Crush III and V studies, the duration of DAPT was also at least 12 months with a resulting 3-year ST rate of 1% (vs. 3.7% with Culotte) and 0.4% (vs. 4.3% with provisional stenting) as discussed above [8, 9].

These data indicate that DAPT cessation can unmask procedural shortcomings such as stent mal-apposition and under-expansion, triggering the occurrence of stent failure and MACE. Hence extensive consideration of anatomical complexity and procedural technique is needed when deciding on DAPT duration.

Importantly, DAPT also reduces the risk of non-lesion-related events. MACE in general, including ischemic stroke, increase in incidence after cessation of DAPT following LMCA PCI [3]. Moreover, patients with angiographic LMCA disease benefit from prolonged DAPT whether these lesions were treated with PCI or not [27].

Current AHA/ACC guidelines provide no specific recommendations on DAPT for patients with LMCA PCI. DAPT recommendations are based on clinical presentation: 12 months (Class I) for ACS versus 6 months (Class I) for stable ischemic heart disease. Formal assessment of patient bleeding risk is recommended with use of the "DAPT" score, to help weigh the benefit of prolonging DAPT beyond the minimal recommendation (Class IIb) [28]. This score integrates different patient and procedural characteristics, not including LMCA disease, to position the patient on a scale of −2 to 9 reflecting greater bleeding to greater thrombotic risk. A score of ≤2 favors DAPT discontinuation and a score ≥2 favors uninterrupted DAPT [29].

European guidelines give similar recommendations suggesting the use of two different risk estimation tools to determine ideal DAPT duration in the general PCI population: "PRECISE-DAPT" at the time of PCI and the "DAPT" score after 12 months of uneventful DAPT therapy [1]. The "PRECISE-DAPT" score estimates the 1-year risk of bleeding while on DAPT after PCI, a score of 25 is used as a cut-off to decide on DAPT duration of 3–6 months or 12–24 months [30].

A post-hoc analysis from the EXCEL study suggests that there is no benefit of extending DAPT beyond 1 year on outcomes like death, MI, and stroke, or all-cause mortality [31]. However, given that there are no dedicated studies comparing DAPT duration in LMCA PCI population to date, the duration of DAPT in this setting may need an individualized approach, especially if a distal LMCA bifurcation lesion was treated with a two-stent technique.

DAPT after CABG can reduce the rate of vein graft occlusion. It is recommended for at least 12 months after surgery by American (Class IIb) [28] and European guidelines (Class IC) [1] in patients who present with ACS, unless there is high bleeding risk. DAPT was used in this manner in RCTs of PCI vs. CABG in patients with LMCA disease; therefore 12 months of DAPT after CABG is recommended in the absence of increased bleeding risk or prior bleeding events.

The ideal regimen for patients who require concomitant anticoagulation or "triple therapy" after LMCA PCI is unknown. Recent trials addressing this issue have not included or have not reported on the number of patients with LMCA PCI in their studies [24, 32]. Early interruption of ASA may be considered in patients with high bleeding risk (PRECISE-DAPT score ≥25), especially if low-risk procedural and patient features are present (Fig. 15.1).

15.4 Role of Non-invasive and Invasive Ischemia Testing After LMCA PCI

Finally, we discuss the role of non-invasive and invasive testing after LMCA PCI including myocardial perfusion imaging, exercise stress testing, stress echocardiography, coronary computed tomography angiography, and invasive coronary angiography.

15.4.1 Myocardial Perfusion Imaging

The value of myocardial perfusion imaging (MPI) with single-photon emission computerized tomography (SPECT) is limited in the evaluation of LMCA disease. Despite its high sensitivity in identifying large myocardial ischemia, this modality cannot specifically identify patients with isolated LMCA lesions. Efforts to improve its accuracy by implementing different techniques such as attenuation-corrected SPECT and identifying non-perfusion abnormalities such as transient ischemic dilatation, the clinical utility of SPECT in LM disease remains inadequate [33]. Hence, this imaging modality is generally not advisable as a method of follow-up after LMCA revascularization.

15.4.2 Exercise Stress Testing

The utility of exercise stress testing is limited in identifying LMCA disease. While some studies have suggested marked and prolonged duration of ECG changes, as well as exertional hypotension as predictors of LMCA disease, these seem to be mostly present in patients with other concomitant coronary diseases [34]. One large registry-based study showed how none of the variables obtained during supine cycle exercise stress test can accurately identify patients with isolated LMCA disease [35].

15.4.3 Stress Echocardiography

The addition of echocardiography substantially increases the sensitivity of ECG stress testing. Exercise stress echocardiography (SE) can identify signs of severe myocardial ischemia beyond ECG changes in patients with LMCA disease, such as exercise-induced decrease in ejection fraction, wall motion abnormalities (WMA), and increased left ventricular cavity size [36].

There are few data regarding the utility of Dobutamine stress echocardiography (DSE) in this patient group. DSE does not elicit the classic signs of severe ischemia seen with exercise, such as severe and prolonged ECG changes, drop in ejection fraction, and LV dilation, but prevalence of stress-induced WMA is comparable to that seen with exercise SE and can serve to identify up to 98% of patients with LMCA disease. WMA, however, don't easily discriminate between these patients and those with multivessel coronary disease [36].

Important physiologic and technical factors can limit the accuracy of DSE, such as failure to elicit ischemic response due to concomitant beta-blockade, critical LMCA stenosis limiting blood flow at rest, or poor acoustic windows limiting visualization of all LV segments [37]. Despite a higher incidence of ventricular arrhythmias during DSE in patients with LMCA disease compared with other patient groups, serious adverse events seem rare [36].

Generally, SE or DSE are considered more sensitive and accurate than MPI for identifying LMCA disease [38].

15.4.4 Coronary Computed Tomography Angiography

Coronary computed tomography angiography (CCTA) is a promising technique for non-invasive follow-up after LMCA stenting. Although the assessment of coronary stents by CCTA is challenging due to artifacts produced by stent struts, the accuracy of CCTA to assess in-stent restenosis is reasonable in relatively large size stents (>3 mm of nominal diameter) [39]. Roura et al. reported that elective 6-month CCTA follow-up after LMCA PCI was associated with lower all-cause mortality compared to clinical follow-up (2.6% vs. 8.4%, $p = 0.05$) [40]. This was a small observational single-center study with a historical control arm. Hence, results should be interpreted with caution.

Currently, non-invasive CT-based fractional flow reserve (CT-FFR) is available. This technology allows the assessment of ischemic burden without

Table 15.2 Comparison of follow-up modality and event rates in PCI arm from PRECOMBAT, EXCEL, and NOBLE trials

Study	PCI no	Follow-up modality	Length of follow-up	Event rates
PRECOMBAT [17] 2015	300 pts	Routine angiography 8–10 months	5 years	Death from any cause, MI, stroke, or ischemia-driven target vessel revascularization 52 (17.5%)
EXCEL [6] 2019	948 pts	Clinical follow-up at 1, 6, and 12 months (routine angiography was not permitted)	5 years	Death, stroke, myocardial infarction, or ischemia-driven revascularization 198/933 (22.4%)
NOBLE [7] 2020	592 pts	Clinical follow-up	5 years	All-cause mortality, non-procedural myocardial infarction, repeat revascularization, or stroke 165/592 (28%)

the need for invasive angiography. However, the available analytic algorithms are not validated for previous stenting within the same vessel [41]. A more sophisticated algorithm to address that issue is being developed and might be of great value in the non-invasive assessment after LMCA stenting.

The PULSE clinical trial [42] is currently underway to assess the role of routine CCTA assessment after LMCA PCI as compared to clinical and ischemia-driven follow-up. It is a prospective, multicenter, open-label, randomized controlled trial. A sample size of 550 patients (275 per group) is required to have an 80% chance of detecting, as significant at the 5% level, a 7.5% relative reduction in the primary combined outcome. Follow-up will be for at least 18 months after randomization.

15.4.5 Invasive Coronary Angiogram

Overall, patients who undergo LMCA PCI represent a high-risk subset with increased likelihood of adverse events. Hence, invasive assessment with coronary angiography (CA) is justified in the US guidelines in the presence of recurrent symptoms or signs of ischemia [43]. Furthermore, according to the European guidelines, a late (3–12 months) surveillance angiography may be considered, irrespective of the symptoms (Class IIb) [44].

There are no randomized studies examining the utility of routine CA after LMCA PCI. One single-center retrospective study (sample size 190 pts) suggests that routine CA can lead to a reduction in cardiac mortality (0% vs. 7%, $p = 0.01$), and an increase in urgent target vessel revascularization (15.4% vs. 5%, $p = 0.01$) [45]. Another observational study reported similar findings with lower all-cause mortality (6% vs. 14%, $p = 0.01$), and cardiac mortality (3% vs. 6%, $P = 0.04$) associated with the routine CA after unprotected left main PCI. But this was at the cost of increased target lesion revascularization (15% vs. 5%, p < 0.001). However, these studies have several limitations including retrospective nature and larger scale randomized controlled trials are needed to address this issue [46].

Contemporary clinical trials comparing LMCA PCI to CABG such as EXCEL or NOBLE did not implement a routine angiography strategy to follow-up patients post-procedurally, which is a typical clinical practice in North America and Europe. On the other hand, patients enrolled in the PRECOMBAT study from Korea underwent routine follow-up angiography. Compared to other LMCA PCI randomized controlled trials, patients in the PRECOMBAT study had lower rates of MI rate in the PCI arm without an increase in the number of revascularization procedures (Tables 15.1 and 15.2).

15.5 Conclusion

Patients who undergo LMCA revascularization should receive close follow-up given the risk of downstream adverse events. Patient characteristics and procedural factors should be considered when estimating the risk of such events. Dual antiplatelet therapy modifies this risk and its duration should be individualized, validated scores in non-LMCA disease may help clinicians balance between the risk of thrombotic and bleeding events in each patient.

Detection of subclinical ischemia could be key in preventing catastrophic clinical events; however, the ideal testing strategy following LMCA revascularization remains controversial and needs further data.

References

1. Valgimigli M, Bueno H, Byrne RA, Collet J-P, Costa F, Jeppsson A, et al. 2017 ESC focused update on dual antiplatelet therapy in coronary artery disease developed in collaboration with EACTS. Eur J Cardiothorac Surg. 2018;53(1):34–78.
2. Stone GW, Kappetein AP, Sabik JF, Pocock SJ, Morice M-C, Puskas J, et al. Five-year outcomes after PCI or CABG for left main coronary disease. N Engl J Med. 2019;381(19):1820–30.
3. Holm NR, Mäkikallio T, Lindsay MM, Spence MS, Erglis A, Menown IB, et al. Percutaneous coronary angioplasty versus coronary artery bypass grafting in the treatment of unprotected left main stenosis: updated 5-year outcomes from the randomised, non-inferiority NOBLE trial. Lancet. 2020;395(10219):191–9.
4. Biolè C, Huczek Z, Nuñez-Gil I, Boccuzzi G, Autelli M, Montefusco A, et al. Daily risk of adverse outcomes in patients undergoing complex lesions revascularization: a subgroup analysis from the RAIN-CARDIOGROUP VII study (veRy thin stents for patients with left mAIn or bifurcatioN in real life). Int J Cardiol. 2019;290:64–9.
5. Palmerini T, Marzocchi A, Tamburino C, Sheiban I, Margheri M, Vecchi G, et al. Temporal pattern of ischemic events in relation to dual antiplatelet therapy in patients with unprotected left main coronary artery stenosis undergoing percutaneous coronary intervention. J Am Coll Cardiol. 2009;53(14):1176–81.
6. Stone GW, Sabik JF, Serruys PW, Simonton CA, Généreux P, Puskas J, et al. Everolimus-eluting stents or bypass surgery for left main coronary artery disease. N Engl J Med. 2016;375(23):2223–35.
7. Mäkikallio T, Holm NR, Lindsay M, Spence MS, Erglis A, Menown IB, et al. Percutaneous coronary angioplasty versus coronary artery bypass grafting in treatment of unprotected left main stenosis (NOBLE): a prospective, randomised, open-label, non-inferiority trial. Lancet. 2016;388(10061):2743–52.
8. Chen S-L, Xu B, Han Y-L, Sheiban I, Zhang J-J, Ye F, et al. Clinical outcome after DK crush versus culotte stenting of distal left main bifurcation lesions: the 3-year follow-up results of the DKCRUSH-III study. JACC Cardiovasc Interv. 2015;8(10):1335–42.
9. Chen X, Li X, Zhang J-J, Han Y, Kan J, Chen L, et al. 3-year outcomes of the DKCRUSH-V trial comparing DK crush with provisional stenting for left main bifurcation lesions. JACC Cardiovasc Interv. 2019;12(19):1927–37.
10. Baz JA, Alfonso FM, Garcia TC, de Carlos Gimeno F, Roura GF, Recalde A, et al. Clinical impact of intravascular ultrasound guidance in drug-eluting stent implantation for unprotected left main coronary disease: pooled analysis at the patient-level of 4 registries. JACC Cardiovasc Interv. 2014;7(3):244–54.
11. Park S-J, Kim Y-H, Park D-W, Lee S-W, Kim W-J, Suh J, et al. Impact of intravascular ultrasound guidance on long-term mortality in stenting for unprotected left main coronary artery stenosis. Circ Cardiovasc Interv. 2009;2(3):167–77.
12. Ladwiniec A, Walsh SJ, Holm NR, Hanratty CG, Makikallio T, Kellerth T, et al. Intravascular ultrasound to guide left main stem intervention: a substudy of the NOBLE trial. EuroIntervention. 2020.
13. Morice M, Serruys P, Kappetein A. Outcomes in patients with de novo left main disease treated with in the synergy between percutaneous coronary intervention with TAXUS and cardiac surgery (SYNTAX) trial. Circulation. 2010;121:2645–53.
14. Min S-Y, Park D-W, Yun S-C, Kim Y-H, Lee J-Y, Kang S-J, et al. Major predictors of long-term clinical outcomes after coronary revascularization in patients with unprotected left main coronary disease: analysis from the MAIN-COMPARE study. Circ Cardiovasc Interv. 2010;3(2):127–33.
15. Galbut DL, Kurlansky PA, Traad EA, Dorman MJ, Zucker M, Ebra G. Bilateral internal thoracic artery grafting improves long-term survival in patients with reduced ejection fraction: a propensity-matched study with 30-year follow-up. J Thorac Cardiovasc Surg. 2012;143(4):844–53.e4.
16. Buszman PE, Buszman PP, Banasiewicz-Szkróbka I, Milewski KP, Żurakowski A, Orlik B, et al. Left Main stenting in comparison with surgical revascularization: 10-year outcomes of the (left main coronary artery stenting) LE MANS trial. JACC Cardiovasc Interv. 2016;9(4):318–27.
17. Ahn J-M, Roh J-H, Kim Y-H, Park D-W, Yun S-C, Lee PH, et al. Randomized trial of stents versus bypass surgery for left main coronary artery disease: 5-year outcomes of the PRECOMBAT study. J Am Coll Cardiol. 2015;65(20):2198–206.
18. Boudriot E, Thiele H, Walther T, Liebetrau C, Boeckstegers P, Pohl T, et al. Randomized comparison of percutaneous coronary intervention with sirolimus-eluting stents versus coronary artery bypass grafting in unprotected left main stem stenosis. J Am Coll Cardiol. 2011;57(5):538–45.

19. Nwasokwa ON. Coronary artery bypass graft disease. Ann Intern Med. 1995;123(7):528–33.
20. Pilgrim T, Vranckx P, Valgimigli M, Stefanini GG, Piccolo R, Rat J, et al. Risk and timing of recurrent ischemic events among patients with stable ischemic heart disease, non–ST-segment elevation acute coronary syndrome, and ST-segment elevation myocardial infarction. Am Heart J. 2016;175:56–65.
21. Généreux P, Giustino G, Witzenbichler B, Weisz G, Stuckey TD, Rinaldi MJ, et al. Incidence, predictors, and impact of post-discharge bleeding after percutaneous coronary intervention. J Am Coll Cardiol. 2015;66(9):1036–45.
22. Vranckx P, Valgimigli M, Jüni P, Hamm C, Steg PG, Heg D, et al. Ticagrelor plus aspirin for 1 month, followed by ticagrelor monotherapy for 23 months vs aspirin plus clopidogrel or ticagrelor for 12 months, followed by aspirin monotherapy for 12 months after implantation of a drug-eluting stent: a multicentre, open-label, randomised superiority trial. Lancet. 2018;392(10151):940–9.
23. Sibbing D, Aradi D, Jacobshagen C, Gross L, Trenk D, Geisler T, et al. Guided de-escalation of antiplatelet treatment in patients with acute coronary syndrome undergoing percutaneous coronary intervention (TROPICAL-ACS): a randomised, open-label, multicentre trial. Lancet. 2017;390(10104):1747–57.
24. Mehran R, Baber U, Sharma SK, Cohen DJ, Angiolillo DJ, Briguori C, et al. Ticagrelor with or without aspirin in high-risk patients after PCI. N Engl J Med. 2019;381(21):2032–42.
25. D'Ascenzo F, Barbero U, Abdirashid M, Trabattoni D, Boccuzzi G, Ryan N, et al. Incidence of adverse events at 3 months versus at 12 months after dual antiplatelet therapy cessation in patients treated with thin stents with unprotected left main or coronary bifurcations. Am J Cardiol. 2020; 125(4):491–9.
26. Rhee T-M, Park KW, Kim C-H, Kang J, Han J-K, Yang H-M, et al. Dual antiplatelet therapy duration determines outcome after 2-but not 1-stent strategy in left main bifurcation percutaneous coronary intervention. JACC Cardiovasc Interv. 2018;11(24):2453–63.
27. Costa F, Adamo M, Ariotti S, Ferrante G, Navarese EP, Leonardi S, et al. Left main or proximal left anterior descending coronary artery disease location identifies high-risk patients deriving potentially greater benefit from prolonged dual antiplatelet therapy duration. EuroIntervention. 2016;11(11):e1222–30.
28. Levine G, Bates E, Bittl J, Brindis R, Fihn S, Fleisher L, et al. Focused update writing group, 2016 ACC/AHA guideline focused update on duration of dual antiplatelet therapy in patients with coronary artery disease. J Am Coll Cardiol. 2016;68(10):1082–115.
29. Yeh RW, Secemsky EA, Kereiakes DJ, Normand S-LT, Gershlick AH, Cohen DJ, et al. Development and validation of a prediction rule for benefit and harm of dual antiplatelet therapy beyond 1 year after percutaneous coronary intervention. JAMA. 2016;315(16):1735–49.
30. Costa F, van Klaveren D, James S, Heg D, Räber L, Feres F, et al. Derivation and validation of the predicting bleeding complications in patients undergoing stent implantation and subsequent dual antiplatelet therapy (PRECISE-DAPT) score: a pooled analysis of individual-patient datasets from clinical trials. Lancet. 2017;389(10073):1025–34.
31. Brener SJ, Serruys PW, Morice MC, Mehran R, Kappetein AP, Sabik JF, et al. Optimal duration of dual antiplatelet therapy after left main coronary stenting. 2018.
32. Vranckx P, Valgimigli M, Windecker S, Steg PG, Hamm C, Jüni P, et al. Long-term ticagrelor monotherapy versus standard dual antiplatelet therapy followed by aspirin monotherapy in patients undergoing biolimus-eluting stent implantation: rationale and design of the GLOBAL LEADERS trial. EuroIntervention. 2016;12(10):1239–45.
33. Rehn T, Griffith LS, Achuff SC, Bailey IK, Bulkley BH, Burow R, et al. Exercise thallium-201 myocardial imaging in left main coronary artery disease: sensitive but not specific. Am J Cardiol. 1981;48(2):217–23.
34. Stone PH, LaFollette L, Cohn K. Patterns of exercise treadmill test performance in patients with left main coronary artery disease: detection dependent on left coronary dominance or coexistent dominant right coronary disease. Am Heart J. 1982;104(1):13–9.
35. Jánosi A, Vertes A. Exercise testing and left main coronary artery stenosis: can patients with left main disease be identified? Chest. 1991;100(1):227–9.
36. Attenhofer CH, Pellikka PA, Oh JK, Roger VL, Sohn D-W, Seward JB. Comparison of ischemic response during exercise and dobutamine echocardiography in patients with left main coronary artery disease. J Am Coll Cardiol. 1996;27(5):1171–7.
37. Thompson C, Bergstrome D, Parlow JL. Limitations of preoperative dobutamine stress echocardiography in identifying severe left main coronary artery stenosis: a report of two cases and a brief review. Can J Anesth. 2003;50(9):933–9.
38. Mahajan N, Polavaram L, Vankayala H, Ference B, Wang Y, Ager J, et al. Diagnostic accuracy of myocardial perfusion imaging and stress echocardiography for the diagnosis of left main and triple vessel coronary artery disease: a comparative meta-analysis. Heart. 2010;96(12):956–66.
39. Ehara M, Kawai M, Surmely JF, Matsubara T, Terashima M, Tsuchikane E, et al. Diagnostic accuracy of coronary in-stent restenosis using 64-slice computed tomography: comparison with invasive coronary angiography. J Am Coll Cardiol. 2007;49(9):951–9.
40. Roura G. Long-term prognostic impact of non-invasive follow-up with computed tomography angiography in patients with left main coronary artery stenting. Minerva Cardioangiol. 2018;66(5):528–35.

41. Modi BN, Sankaran S, Kim HJ, Ellis H, Rogers C, Taylor CA, et al. Predicting the physiological effect of revascularization in serially diseased coronary arteries. Circ Cardiovasc Interv. 2019;12(2):e007577.
42. De Filippo O, Bianco M, Tebaldi M, Iannaccone M, Gaido L, Guiducci V, et al. Angiographic control versus ischaemia-driven management of patients undergoing percutaneous revascularisation of the unprotected left main coronary artery with second-generation drug-eluting stents: rationale and design of the PULSE trial. Open heart. 2020;7(2):e001253.
43. Patel MR, Bailey SR, Bonow RO, Chambers CE, Chan PS, Dehmer GJ, et al. ACCF/SCAI/AATS/AHA/ASE/ASNC/HFSA/HRS/SCCM/SCCT/SCMR/STS 2012 appropriate use criteria for diagnostic catheterization. J Am Coll Cardiol. 2012;59(22):1995–2027.
44. Neumann F-J, Sousa-Uva M, Ahlsson A, Alfonso F, Banning AP, Benedetto U, et al. 2018 ESC/EACTS Guidelines on myocardial revascularization. Eur Heart J. 2019;40(2):87–165.
45. Aurigemma C, Burzotta F, Porto I, Niccoli G, Leone AM, Crea F, et al. Clinical impact of routine angiographic follow-up after percutaneous coronary interventions on unprotected left main. Cardiol J. 2018;25(5):582–8.
46. D'Ascenzo F, Iannaccone M, Pavani M, Kawamoto H, Escaned JP, Varbella F, et al. Planned angiographic control versus clinical follow-up for patients with unprotected left main stem stenosis treated with second generation drug-eluting stents: a propensity score with matching analysis from the FAILS (failure in left main with second generation stents-cardiogroup III study). Catheter Cardiovasc Interv. 2018;92(4):E271–e7.

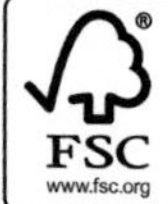

MIX
Papier aus verantwortungsvollen Quellen
Paper from responsible sources
FSC® C105338

If you have any concerns about our products,
you can contact us on
ProductSafety@springernature.com

In case Publisher is established outside the EU,
the EU authorized representative is:
Springer Nature Customer Service Center GmbH
Europaplatz 3, 69115 Heidelberg, Germany

Printed by Libri Plureos GmbH
in Hamburg, Germany